SELF ASSESSMENT
IN
CLINICAL CARDIOLOGY
II

This book is based on a teaching conference

sponsored by

THE UNIVERSITY OF MIAMI SCHOOL OF MEDICINE

and

THE COUNCIL ON CLINICAL CARDIOLOGY

AMERICAN HEART ASSOCIATION

held at Miami, Florida

in cooperation with

HEART ASSOCIATION OF GREATER MIAMI

FLORIDA HEART ASSOCIATION

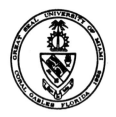

SELF ASSESSMENT IN CLINICAL CARDIOLOGY II

Edited by

Michael S. Gordon, M.D., Ph.D., F.A.C.P., F.A.C.C.
Clinical Associate Professor of Medicine;
Director, Annual Teaching Conference in Clinical Cardiology
University of Miami School of Medicine
Miami, Florida

YEAR BOOK MEDICAL PUBLISHERS, INC.
35 East Wacker Drive • Chicago

Copyright © 1976 by Year Book Medical Publishers, Inc. All rights reserved.
No part of this publication may be reproduced,
stored in a retrieval system, or transmitted, in any form or by any means,
electronic, mechanical, photocopying, recording, or otherwise,
without prior written permission from the publisher.
Printed in the United States of America.

Library of Congress Catalog Card Number: 74-77256

International Standard Book Number: 0-8151-3801-6

TO LEE AND DORÉE

JOAN

DAVID, KEVIN, AND CATHY

PREFACE

The acceptance of our first effort has stimulated the writing of Self Assessment in Clinical Cardiology II. Again, the work has evolved from the Teaching Conference in Clinical Cardiology held each spring for the last 8 years at the University of Miami. We hope it will continue to be valuable to medical students, house officers and practicing physicians.

It is nearly impossible to please "all of the students all of the time." The book, however, does cover a broad range of topics from basic principles in bedside diagnosis, a core curriculum in electrocardiography and practical drug therapy, to advances in electrophysiology, the hemodyanmics of cardiogenic shock and cardiac scintigraphy. The section on echocardiography is extensive by design: it is an extremely important non-invasive technique deserving wide application. Throughout, we have tried to be teachers - to clarify the old and simplify the new - and relate our efforts to clinical patient care.

As stated in the preface to the first volume, "The deadline we faced for our conference means that the book may not be 'polished.' I believe it does, however, accurately state where we are in most of the important areas of clinical cardiology and it does allow the reader to assess his abilities and knowledge in the practical aspects of caring for cardiac patients - an important feature in these days of recertification as a means of improving patient care. It does so at a low cost in dollars, but possibly at a high cost in terms of alienation of colleagues.

If you want to get a visiting professor to hate you, just ask him, two months in advance of his talk, for a comprehensive but succinct "abstract" of his presentation which really says something - not just an outline - but real information. Add to that a request for selected references, graphs and figures, in addition to well thought out questions and answers. Then keep reminding him of the deadline. Finally, take his work and edit it, most often without an opportunity for his further approval. The result is before you. If there are errors, they are my own, born of an urgency that wants to teach what is new new - the kind of urgency that will get this book to the printer within the hour."

Thanks to our guest faculty for their superb teaching and becoming my friends. Thanks to Proc Harvey for teaching me and stimulating me to teach. Thanks to Emanuel Papper for always nurturing innovation in education. Thanks to Vi, Pam, Susan and Pat for their support. And special thanks to Judith Greve whose intelligence and patience have made this book a reality.

M.S.G.

GUEST CONTRIBUTORS

Lawrence S. Cohen, M.D., Professor of Medicine, Chief of Cardiology, Yale University School of Medicine

Gordon Ewy, M.D., Professor of Medicine, Director, CCU and Diagnostic Cardiology, Arizona Medical Center

Robert A. O'Rourke, M.D., Associate Professor of Medicine, Director, Clinical Cardiology, University of California, San Diego

William C. Roberts, M.D., Chief, Section of Pathology, National Heart and Lung Institute, Professor of Pathology and Medicine, Georgetown University

James Ronan, M.D., Assistant Professor of Medicine, Georgetown University, Co-Director, Division of Cardiology, Washington Adventist Hospital

H.J.C. Swan, M.D., Ph.D., Professor of Medicine, UCLA School of Medicine, Director of Cardiology, Cedars-Sinai Medical Center

Andrew G. Wallace, M.D., Professor of Medicine, Chief, Division of Cardiology, Duke University

Hein J.J. Wellens, M.D., Professor of Cardiology, University of Amsterdam, Head, Department of Cardiology, Wilhelmina Gasthuis, Amsterdam

UNIVERSITY OF MIAMI CONTRIBUTORS

Benjamin Befeler, M.D., Associate Professor of Medicine, Chief, Cardiovascular Laboratory, Veteran's Hospital

Robert J. Boucek, M.D., Professor of Medicine

Agustin Castellanos, M.D., Professor of Medicine, Chief, Clinical Electrophysiology, Jackson Memorial Hospital

Nabil El-Sherif, M.D., Assistant Professor of Medicine, Chief, Coronary Care Unit, Veteran's Hospital

Michael S. Gordon, M.D., Ph.D., Clinical Associate Professor of Medicine

Stuart Gottlieb, M.D., Assistant Professor of Radiology and Medicine, Head, Ultrasound and Cardiovascular Units, Division of Nuclear Medicine, JMH

Gerard Kaiser, M.D., Professor of Surgery, Chief, Division of Thoracic and Cardiovascular Surgery

Nilza Kallos, M.D., Instructor of Radiology (Nuclear Medicine and Ultrasound, Jackson Memorial Hospital)

Ralph Lazzara, M.D., Associate Professor of Medicine, Chief of Cardiology, Veteran's Hospital

Louis Lemberg, M.D., Professor of Clinical Cardiology

James R. LePage, M.D., Associate Professor of Radiology, Chief, Cardiac and Vascular Radiology Section, Jackson Memorial Hospital

Stephen M. Mallon, M.D., Assistant Professor of Medicine, Chief, Cardiovascular Laboratory, Jackson Memorial Hospital

Joan Mayer, M.D., Clinical Associate Professor of Medicine

Alvaro Mayorga-Cortes, M.D., Assistant Professor of Medicine, Director, Coronary Care Unit, Jackson Memorial Hospital

Robert J. Myerburg, M.D., Professor of Medicine, Director, Division of Cardiology

Eliseo Perez-Stable, M.D, Professor of Medicine, Chief, Medical Service, Veteran's Hospital

David S. Sheps, M.D., Assistant Professor of Medicine, Director, Exercise and Non-Invasive Laboratory, Jackson Memorial Hospital

Manuel Viamonte, Jr., M.D., Professor and Chairman, Department of Radiology, Director of Radiology, Jackson Memorial Hospital and Mt. Sinai Hospital

Willis H. Williams, M.D., Assistant Professor of Surgery

TABLE OF CONTENTS

Preface	vii
Contributors	ix

BEDSIDE DIAGNOSIS AND AUSCULTATION

Review of Cardiac Anatomy and Physiology. Robert A. O'Rourke, M.D.	1
Pathology of Aortic and Mitral Valve Disease William C. Roberts, M.D.	7
Bedside Diagnosis - Without Auscultation Michael S. Gordon, M.D.	14
Bedside Diagnosis - Auscultation, Michael S. Gordon, M.D.	22
Synthesis of the Physical Examination Michael S. Gordon, M.D.	24
The Clinical Evaluation of Patients with Aortic and Mitral Valve Disease Michael S. Gordon, M.D.	31
The Physical Examination of the Acute Cardiac Patient Michael S. Gordon, M.D.	39
The Cardiomyopathies, Lawrence S. Cohen, M.D.	47
The Radiologic Approach to Valvular Heart Disease Manuel Viamonte, Jr., M.D.	49
Surgical Considerations in Valvular Heart Disease Willis H. Williams, M.D.	57

ELECTROCARDIOGRAPHY CORE CURRICULUM

Axis Determination, Hemiblocks and Bundle Branch Blocks Joan Mayer, M.D.	63
Ischemia, Injury, and Infarction Patterns, Including Non-Specific ST-T Wave Abnormalities Robert J. Myerburg, M.D.	69
Ventricular Hypertrophy, Stephen M. Mallon, M.D.	73
Arrhythmias - An Overview, Joan Mayer, M.D.	77
Supraventricular Arrhythmias, Hein J.J. Wellens, M.D.	80

Ventricular Arrhythmias, Andrew G. Wallace, M.D.   85

His Bundle Studies and Pacemakers   88
Benjamin Befeler, M.D., Agustin Castellanos, M.D.

ELECTROCARDIOGRAPHY - ADVANCES

Rhythm and Conduction Disturbances in Adolescents   91
and Young Adults, Robert J. Myerburg, M.D.

Diagnosis and Medical Management of Pre-Excitation   93
Syndromes, Hein J.J. Wellens, M.D.

Surgical and Pacemaker Therapy of Supraventricular   98
Tachyarrhythmias, Andrew G. Wallace, M.D.

Tachycardia and Bradycardia Dependent Conduction   100
Disorders, Nabil El-Sherif, M.D.

Current Status of Stress Testing and Cardiac   104
Rehabilitation, David S. Sheps, M.D.

CORONARY ARTERY DISEASE

Coronary Artery Disease and Myocardial Infarction   111
An Overview, H.J.C. Swan, M.D.

Pathology of Sudden Cardiac Death and Acute Myocardial   113
Infarction, William C. Roberts, M.D.

A Clinical View of Coronary Pathology   118
Robert J. Boucek, M.D.

Angina Pectoris - Clinical Presentation   122
Robert J. Myerburg, M.D.

Prognosis in Angina Pectoris, Andrew G. Wallace, M.D.   123

The Intermediate Coronary Syndrome, Lawrence S. Cohen, M.D.   125

Acute Myocardial Infarction - The First 24 Hours   126
Andrew G. Wallace, M.D.

Bundle Branch Block and Myocardial Infarction   128
Hein J.J. Wellens, M.D. and K.I. Lie, M.D.

The Hemodynamically Unstable Myocardial Infarction   130
Patient, Alvaro Mayorga-Cortes, M.D.

Acute Pump Failure - Bedside Correlation with Hemodynamic   135
Measurements, H.J.C. Swan, M.D.

Acute Pump Failure - Practical Management   137
H.J.C. Swan, M.D.

Coronary Angiography, Benjamin Befeler, M.D. — 139

Surgery for Coronary Artery Disease, Gerard Kaiser, M.D. — 144

PRACTICAL THERAPY

Digitalis and Diuretics, Robert A. O'Rourke, M.D. — 146

Arrhythmias, James A. Ronan, Jr., M.D. — 148

Medical Treatment of Angina Pectoris
Robert A. O'Rourke, M.D. — 152

Cardiac Failure, Gordon Ewy, M.D. — 155

Cardiopulmonary Resuscitation, Ralph Lazzara, M.D. — 159

HYPERTENSION

Pathology of Hypertension, William C. Roberts, M.D. — 162

The Physical Examination in Patients with
Hypertension, Michael S. Gordon, M.D. — 163

Workup of the Newly Discovered Hypertensive Patient
Eliseo Perez-Stable, M.D. — 165

Radiologic Evaluation of Hypertension
James R. LePage, M.D. — 170

Practical Therapy of Hypertension
Eliseo Perez-Stable, M.D. — 173

ADVANCES IN DIAGNOSIS

The Echocardiogram in Cardiac Diagnosis
Stuart Gottlieb, M.D. — 177

Radioisotope Cardiography (Cardiac Scintigraphy)
Stuart Gottlieb, M.D., Nilza Kallos, M.D. — 203

SELF-ASSESSMENT QUESTIONS — 208

Bedside Diagnosis and Auscultation — 209

ECG Core Curriculum — 251

ECG - Advances — 269

Coronary Artery Disease — 274

Practical Therapy, Hypertension, Advances in Diagnosis — 319

SELF-ASSESSMENT ANSWERS — 338

BEDSIDE DIAGNOSIS AND AUSCULTATION

REVIEW OF CARDIAC ANATOMY AND PHYSIOLOGY

Robert A. O'Rourke, M.D.

A brief discussion of the functional anatomy of the cardiovascular system is a necessary prelude to further instruction concerning the diagnosis and treatment of cardiac disease. Differences in anatomy between the right atrium and right ventricle which return unoxygenated blood to the low resistance pulmonary circulation should be compared to the left atrium and left ventricle which function respectively as a receiving chamber for oxygenated blood and a thick walled high pressure chamber for pumping blood against the systemic vascular resistance.

A diagramatic representation of pressure tracings recorded within the right and left-sided cardiac chambers and great vessels together with simultaneous electrocardiogram and phonocardiogram are shown in Figure 1. The diagonal cross-hatched areas labeled ISOV represent the isovolumic phases of left ventricular contraction and relaxation. Isovolumic right ventricular contraction and relaxation is represented by double cross-hatching. M_1 and T_1 represent sounds produced by closure of the mitral and tricuspid valves respectively. A_2 and P_2 are sounds produced by closure of the aortic and pulmonic valves while OT and OM represent sounds produced by opening of the tricuspid and mitral valve, respectively. PEP represents the pre-ejection period from the onset of the Q wave on ECG to the opening of the aortic valve. LVET is the left ventricular ejection time.

As the physician cares for his patients, he should be thinking of these hemodynamic relationships, as they form the foundation for understanding and practicing cardiology at any level. As his sophistication increases, more practical data is added, e.g., the volume curve of the left ventricle, the jugular venous pulse, the apex cardiogram, and today, even echocardiographic movement of the valves.

An understanding of the anatomy of the mitral valve and its functional components (annulus, leaflets, chordae tendineae, papillary muscles, left atrium and left ventricle) is important in understanding the causes and consequences of acute or chronic mitral regurgitation (Figure 2). With this understanding there follows an appreciation of why "mitral regurgitation begets mitral regurgitation," i.e., when the mitral valve leaks, the left atrium is volume or preloaded, delivers this extra volume to the ventricle during the next diastole, chronically enlarging the ventricle, which pulls on the papillary muscles and results in further unseating of the valve in systole and more regurgitation. Similarly, alteration in the continuity or geometry of any one or combination of these structures can produce severe mitral regurgitation and markedly elevated pulmonary venous pressure. This sequence depends particularly on the compliance characteristics of the left atrium, i.e., in acute severe mitral regurgitation, the left atrium is small and relatively non-compliant and ventricular pressures are hence reflected back into the pulmonary circulation. Finally, thickening of the mitral leaflets, fusion of the commissures and shortening of the chordae produce mitral stenosis with or without coincident mitral regurgitation in many patients with rheumatic heart disease.

Both semilunar valves (pulmonic and aortic) usually have three leaflets, but some patients have a bicuspid aortic valve. With time, significant aortic stenosis and/or aortic regurgitation develop in many of these patients, and a congenital bicuspid aortic valve, frequently calcified, is the most common cause of isolated aortic valve disease.

Knowledge of the anatomy of the coronary circulation and the distribution of the left anterior descending, left circumflex and right coronary arteries to the left and right ventricular myocardium, the papillary muscles of the mitral valve, the ventricular septum, the SA and AV nodes, and the branches of the trifascicular conduction system is a prerequisite for understanding the various complications of severe coronary artery disease and acute myocardial infarction (Figures 3 and 4).

The relationship between the left ventricular stroke volume and the left ventricular filling pressure or end-diastolic volume is shown in Figure 5. In the normal ventricle, the volume of blood ejected from the left ventricle is related to the volume of blood distending the left ventricle at end diastole (ventricular function curve). In patients with a reduced left ventricular performance, the curve relating cardiac output to left ventricular end-diastolic fiber length is shifted downward and to the right so that a higher left ventricular filling pressure is necessary to maintain a normal cardiac output and the cardiac output resulting from any given left ventricular filling pressure is reduced. This relationship should be kept in mind when using a variety of cardiac drugs, e.g., digitalis and diuretic therapy in patients with congestive heart failure.

Selected References

1. Silverman, M.D., and Schlant, R.C.: Anatomy of the Cardiovascular System, in The Heart (3rd Edition). Edited by J.W. Hurst, McGraw Hill Publishing Company, New York, pp. 20-33.

2. James, T.M.: The Coronary Circulation and Conduction System in Acute Myocardial Infarction, Prog. in Cardiov. Dis., 10:410, 1968.

3. Ross, J., Jr., and O'Rourke, R.A.: Indirect Methods of Examination of the Heart, Harrison's Principles of Internal Medicine (7th Ed). McGraw-Hill Publishing Company, 1974, pp. 1092-1098.

FIGURE 1

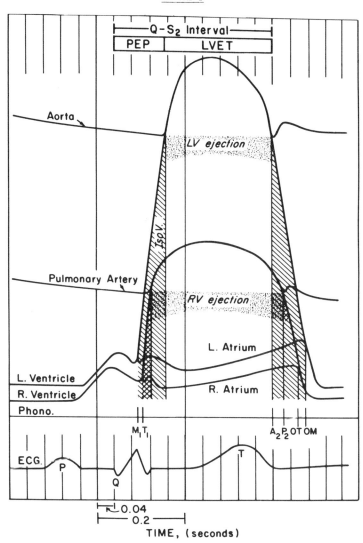

The first third of systole and diastole are the periods of rapid ejection and filling during which two-thirds of the stroke volume leaves or enters the ventricle. Hence murmurs related to flow and turbulence alone are heard early in their respective phases of the cardiac cycle.

The S3 and S4 diastolic filling sounds are heard as blood rapidly decelerates after initial rapid filling, and again as it decelerates in presystole after rapid filling from atrial contraction.

FIGURE 2

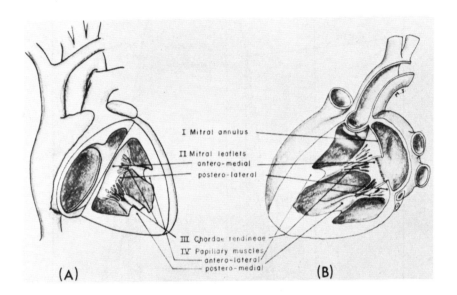

The mitral valve is the most complex of the cardiac valves. Its leaflets are unequal in size: one is continuous with the left atrial endocardium and the other with the aorta. The valve contains about 120 chordae tendineae connecting the leaflets to myocardial pillars (papillary muscles), which in turn are continuous with the left ventricular free wall. It has only a partial annulus fibrosis (only at the base of the posterior mitral leaflet). Since the mitral valve connects with the left atrial wall via the mural endocardium, conditions affecting this chamber also may affect mitral function.

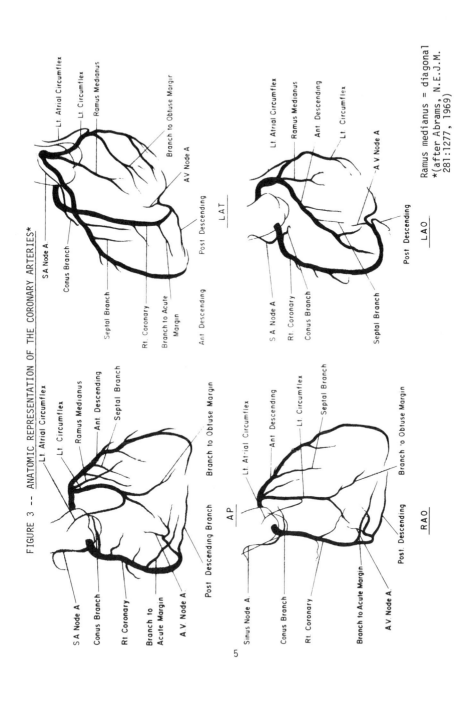

FIGURE 3 -- ANATOMIC REPRESENTATION OF THE CORONARY ARTERIES*

Ramus medianus = diagonal
*(after Abrams, N.E.J.M. 281:1277, 1969)

FIGURE 4

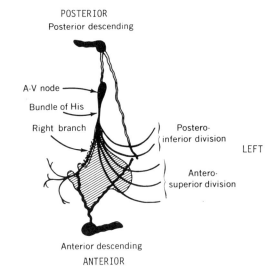

The A-V conduction system as seen from above. Note that in this view the posteroinferior division appears to be above the anterosuperior division.

FIGURE 5

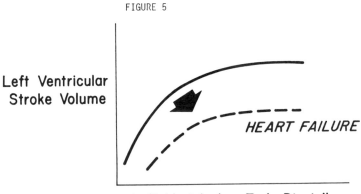

PATHOLOGY OF AORTIC AND MITRAL VALVE DISEASE

William C. Roberts, M.D.

Aortic Valve

It is now clear that isolated valvular aortic stenosis (with or without associated aortic regurgitation) is nearly always non-rheumatic in origin, and most commonly represents a congenital malformation of this valve. Isolated valvular aortic stenosis is the most common cause of fatal valvular dysfunction in patients over 14 years of age. Of 543 patients with severe (functionally Class III or IV, New York Heart Association classification) fatal valvular cardiac disease, 182 or 34% had aortic valvular stenosis. Mitral stenosis is the second most common fatal valvular lesion, and is only half as frequent as aortic stenosis. In patients with clinically isolated valvular aortic stenosis, the mitral valve is normal anatomically in 90% of them. In contrast, of patients with clinically isolated mitral stenosis (with or without regurgitation), only about 55% of them have anatomic involvement limited to the mitral valve.

It is helpful to subdivide patients with valvular aortic stenosis into three groups according to age: 1) Patients less than 15 years old; 2) Patients 15 to 65 years old; and 3) Patients older than 65 years.

Table I

CONFIGURATION OF AORTIC VALVE IN ISOLATED AORTIC STENOSIS IN RELATION TO AGE

	No. valve cusps	age 15 years	Age 15-65	age 65 years
1	1	60%	10%	0
2	2	20%	60%	10%
3	3	15%	25%	90%
4	Uncertain	5%	5%	0

Little anatomic information is available in the group less than 15 years of age. The data available tends to indicate that the aortic valve in these young individuals is either unicuspid or bicuspid and only occasionally tricuspid. In the group aged 15 to 65 years, the aortic valve is congenitally malformed in about 60% of them. Of the patients older than 65 years of age, the aortic valve is tricuspid in more than 90% and congenitally malformed (bicuspid) in less than 10%.

Although it frequently involves a congenitally malformed aortic valve, valvular aortic stenosis is usually not congenital but acquired, the result of fibrosis and calcification of the malformed cusps. Thus, acquired valvular aortic stenosis is fundamentally of two types: 1) that involving a previously congenitally malformed, but initially normally functioning valve, and 2) that involving a previously normal valve.

Several types of congenitally malformed aortic valves occur. Each type is determined by its number of cusps and commissures. At least two types of unicuspid aortic valves exist. In one, the orifice is centrally located and the cusp is devoid of lateral attachments to the wall of the aorta (simple dome or acommissural valve.) This type of valve is usually the one underlying valvular pulmonic stenosis. A second type of unicuspid valve is the unicommissural one. This valve is characterized by an eccentrically located orifice with only one lateral attachment to the aortic wall and that at the level of the orifice. From above, this valve has the appearance of an exclamation point. This is the most frequent malformation found in fatal valvular aortic stenosis in children less than one year of age (Fig. 1).

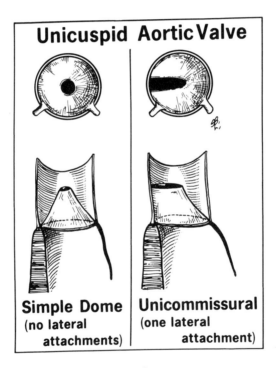

Fig. 1

The most frequent malformation of the aortic valve is the presence of only 2 cusps. The bicuspid valve is basically of 2 types. In one the cusps are located right and left, the commissures anteriorly and posteriorly; a raphe or false commissure, if present, is always in the right cusp, and a coronary artery arises from behind each cusp. In the second type, the cusps are located anteriorly and posteriorly, the commissures right and left; a raphe, if present, is always in the anterior cusp and both coronary arteries arise in front of the anterior cusp. These 2 types are divided about equally among patients with congenitally bicuspid aortic valves (Fig. 2).

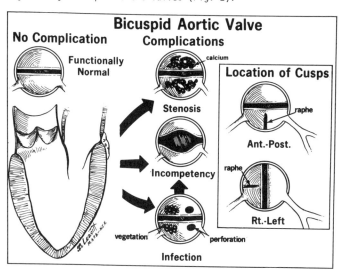

Fig. 2

Of 107 patients over 14 years of age with congenitally bicuspid valves studied personally at necropsy, 75 had aortic stenosis, 17 had pure aortic regurgitation, and 15 had functionally normal valves. The 15 patients with normally functioning congenitally bicuspid valves were found during routine examination of 1600 hearts at necropsy, none of which had dysfunctioning cardiac valves or shunts. How many patients with bicuspid valves at birth develop complications (stenosis, regurgitation, infection) and how many never develop any of these complications during an entire lifetime is unknown. The bicuspid condition of the aortic valve appears to be the most common congenital malformation of the heart or great vessels; possibly as many as 2% of births have this anomaly. Stenosis, not infection, is by far the most common complication of the congenitally bicuspid aortic valve.

Occasionally a tricuspid aortic valve is malformed. When this occurs, the cusps may be of unequal size. Minor differences in cuspal size are frequent, but major differences appear to constitute congenital malformations. There may be some basis for believing that contact of unequal sized cusps with one another can lead to focal cuspal fibrosis with eventual calcification and stenosis. A quadricuspid aortic valve may, on rare occasions, be stenotic. Most quadricuspid valves, however, function normally.

Function of the malformed aortic valves at birth is variable. The fewer the the number of cusps and commissures the greater the likelihood that the valve is stenotic at birth. The acommissural and unicommissural unicuspid valves are stenotic from birth; the orifices of these valves are small and there is little opportunity for that valvular orifice to alter its size during either phase of the cardiac cycle. Most patients with unicuspid aortic valves have precordial murmurs from birth, whereas this is probably not the case in patients with congenitally bicuspid aortic valves. Whether or not the bicuspid aortic valve is ever stenotic at birth is unclear. Probably most often this valve becomes stenotic only as it thickens and calcifies.

Acquired stenosis of a 3-cuspid aortic valve is common. Of patients aged 15 to 65 years with clinically isolated aortic stenosis (with or without regurgitation) studied personally at necropsy, 37% had tricuspid valves, and among the patients over 65 years, 93% had tricuspid valves. In the 15 to 65 year age group, about half with clinically isolated aortic stenosis had diffuse fibrous thickening of the mitral leaflets as well. The associated diffuse mitral thickening in them is strong evidence that the etiology of the aortic stenosis is rheumatic. Of the group of patients between 15 and 65 years with anatomic disease of the mitral valve as well as valvular aortic stenosis, about 70% had positive histories of acute rheumatic fever, whereas only 6% of the group with anatomically normal mitral valves had positive histories. The etiology of aortic stenosis in patients with anatomically normal mitral valves is unsolved. Possibly, as mentioned earlier, minor abnormalities in cuspal size from birth set the stage for abnormal leaflet contact with resulting fibrosis and finally stenosis.

Stenosis of the aortic valve in patients greater than age 65 is usually characteristic. The valves are usually tricuspid, nodular calcific deposits are rather uniformly distributed on the aortic aspects of each cusp, and the commissures are not fused. Obstruction results from the calcific deposits which prevent the cusp from retracting adequately during ventricular systole. Because the commissures are usually not fused, associated aortic regurgitation is infrequent (Fig. 3).

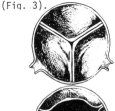
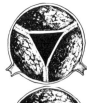
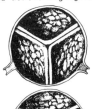

Diastole

TRICUSPID AORTIC VALVE

Systole

Normal   Aortic Valve Stenosis with Fused Commissures   Aortic Valve Stenosis without Commissural Fusion

Fig.3

The cause of aortic stenosis in elderly patients is uncertain, but simple wear and tear or degeneration appears to be the most reasonable explanation. The presence in the same hearts of other wear and tear lesions such as calcified mitral anuli, calcified coronary arteries, and focal thickening of other valve leaflets supports this contention.

Mitral Valve

Obstruction at the mitral orifice can either be acquired (commonest), congenital, or caused by the interposition of nonleaflet tissue within the left atrial cavity. Of the nine single or combined cardiac valve lesions (excluding tricuspid regurgitation and papillary muscle dysfunction) severe enough to be fatal, mitral stenosis, in my experience, ranks second. Of 543 patients over 14 years with functional severe (Classes III or IV) valvular cardiac disease whom I studied at necropsy, 206 (37%) had mitral stenosis. Only valvular aortic stenosis was commoner. Mitral stenosis occurred alone in 94 patients and in combination with other functional valvular lesions in the other 112 patients. Mitral stenosis was rheumatic in origin in all 206 patients.

A valve may function normally and yet be anatomically abnormal. Only 57% of the 94 patients with isolated mitral stenosis (with or without mitral regurgitation) had anatomic involvement limited to the mitral valve. In contrast, 87% of the 182 patients with clinically isolated aortic stenosis (with or without regurgitation) had anatomic disease of the aortic valve only.

Rheumatic heart disease may be viewed as a disease of the mitral valve; other valves may also be involved both anatomically and functionally, but anatomically the mitral valve is always involved. To my knowledge, Aschoff bodies have never been found in hearts without anatomic disease of the mitral valve. Twelve of the 543 patients with severe valvular heart disease whom I studied at necropsy had Aschoff bodies, and all had mitral valve disease both anatomically and functionally.

In all patients with rheumatic mitral stenosis, the leaflets are diffusely thickened, either by fibrous tissue or calcific deposits, or both. The commissures are usually fused, and the chordae tendineae are shortened and usually fused to some degree. The greatest obstruction to this funnel-shaped valve occurs at its apex, which is within the left ventricular cavity. The primary orifice, located at the level of the anulus, is far less narrowed. Fusion may involve one or both commissures. When only one is fused or one fused more than the other, the stenotic orifice is eccentrically located. A centrally located orifice indicates symmetrical commissural fusion. In rheumatic mitral stenosis the chordae tendineae are occasionally so retracted that the leaflets appear to insert directly into the papillary muscles. When this occurs, the stenosis is always severe because the interchordal spaces are virtually entirely obliterated. Sometimes chordae inserting into one papillary muscle are well preserved, whereas those inserting into the other papillary muscle are completely fused. Mitral commissurotomy on a valve in which the leaflets insert almost directly into the papillary muscle(s) usually must include a splitting of the papillary muscle(s) as well as the leaflet commissure(s). If there are normally about 120 third-order chordae and about 24 first-order chordae, in mitral stenosis these numbers are usually halved and, on occasion, even reduced to just one for practical purposes.

The amount of calcium in the leaflets of stenotic mitral valves varies considerably. Generally, men have more calcium than women, and older patients have more calcium than younger patients. The rapidity with which calcification progresses also varies considerably.

A new, acquired cause of mitral stenosis, the rigid-frame prosthetic valve, was introduced in 1960. Since the natural mitral valve is within the left ventricle, a prosthetic mitral valve is also located within this cavity. The prosthesis must be small enough for the contracting left ventricular wall not to interfere with the prosthetic poppet or disk. When the prosthesis is too large for the cavity into which it was inserted, the poppet may be prevented from moving adequately and may therefore obstruct left atrial emptying. The latter state is far commoner than obstruction to left ventricular emptying by the prosthesis. Thrombus formation on a mitral prosthesis also may obstruct left atrial emptying.

Congenital obstruction to left atrial flow falls into three categories: 1) Congenital mitral stenosis (obstruction at valvular level caused by congenitally abnormal leaflets and chordae), the parachute mitral valve, or supravalvular stenosing ring; 2) Cor triatriatum; and 3) Congenital pulmonary-vein stenosis. Congenital mitral stenosis means that the obstruction is at the orifice itself - that is, within the leaflets or their chordal support. Cor triatriatum is caused by a partition within the left atrial cavity; the mitral valve and its chordal apparatus are normal. Pulmonary vein stenosis (very rare) is remote from the mitral orifice and left atrium.

The commonest cause of congenital mitral stenosis is the parachute mitral valve, or single papillary muscle syndrome. In addition to mitral stenosis, these patients usually have other cardiovascular anomalies: supravalvular mitral ring, which in itself may cause stenosis; subaortic stenosis; valvular aortic stenosis, usually superimposed on a congenitally malformed valve; and coarctation of the aortic isthmus.

Still another form of obstruction to left atrial flow is left atrial myxoma. The myxomas may be small, thus not interfering with left atrial emptying, and may be found incidentally at necropsy. On the other hand, they may completely obstruct left atrial outflow, causing sudden death or a variety of other symptoms. Tumors of similar sizes may cause symptoms in some patients and none in others, depending on the location of the stalk. Small tumors may cause symptoms in some patients, and large tumors may not in others, again depending on the location of the stalk. The key is the site of attachment of the tumor to the atrial wall. If the left atrial tumor contacts the mitral leaflets too vigorously for too long, the leaflets may become thickened.

Although some early writers described difficulties in distinguishing left atrial myxoma from left atrial thrombus, the differences between them are great; there are many more differences than similarities between the two. The myxoma is attached to the atrial wall by a pedicle, the diameter of which is far smaller than the largest diameter of the myxoma. A thrombus is virtually never attached by a pedicle but is instead attached to atrial endocardium over a large area. The myxoma resembles a ping-pong ball floating in a glass of water; as the water level drops (blood descending from left atrium to left ventricle), the ping-pong ball descends. Since the myxoma more or less floats in the atrial cavity, injection of contrast material into the cavity "lights up" the entire surface of the tumor. Contrast material in the left atrial cavity containing a thrombus in its body shows an area of no filling, and the borders of the thrombus are usually not well outlined. The surface of the myxoma is smooth and shiny; that of the thrombus is often ragged. With rare exception, neither thrombus nor myxoma in the left atrium interferes with pulmonary venous drainage. Although thrombi occur in left atrial appendages in a variety of conditions (usually those associated with severely depressed cardiac output), thrombi occur in the body of the atrium only in patients with mitral stenosis. In other words, relatively severe stasis of blood is required for thrombus formation in the atrial body. Thrombi virtually never occur in the bodies of left atria in patients with pure mitral regurgitation, presumably because their atrial cavities are constantly being "washed out" during both phases of the cardiac cycle, thus preventing stasis. In contrast, myxomas occur entirely within the bodies of atria, never in atrial appendages, and the "valvular obstruction" totally disappears after excision of the neoplasm. Both thrombi and myxomas tend to form in atria that are of normal size or, at most, are moderately dilated. The huge left atrium rarely contains a thrombus.

Although thrombi and myxomas are the commonest cause of filling defects in the left atrium, other neoplasms and infected masses may occur in this chamber and interfere with left atrial emptying. In contrast to thrombus and myxoma, however, the other filling defects also usually interfere with pulmonary venous return.

Selected References

1. Roberts, W.D.: Valvular, Subvalvular, and Supravalvular Aortic Stenosis: Morphologic Features. Cardiovas. Clin. 5:98-126, 1973

2. Roberts, W.C. and Perloff, J.L.: Mitral Valvular Disease. A Clinico-Pathologic Survey of the Conditions causing the Mitral Valve to Function Abnormally. An. Int. Med., 77:939-975, 1972

BEDSIDE DIAGNOSIS - WITHOUT AUSCULTATION
Michael S. Gordon, M.D.

The title of this paper emphasizes the importance of the non-acoustic aspects of the cardiac physical examination. The "5 Finger" approach to patient evaluation outlined below by Drs. Harvey and Perloff cannot be improved upon, and will be followed in our discussion. It is important to note that the diagnostic laboratory is relegated to the little finger of clinical diagnosis - invasive procedures are most often not necessary to make sophisticated bedside diagnoses. Note also that auscultation is relegated to a similar position in assessing physical signs - acoustic events must be judged in the context of the "company they keep" on the rest of the examination.

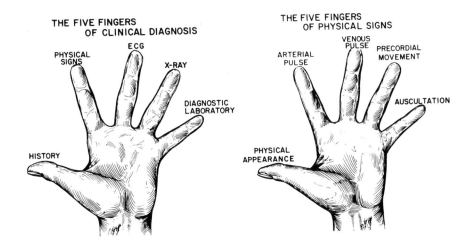

With this approach, and with an understanding of the hemodynamic curves outlined on p. 3, the clinician can predict pathophysiology at the bedside with great accuracy. This is more true today than ever before, due to a renewed interest in bedside diagnosis engendered by non-invasive echocardiography, often coupled with phonocardiography.

The Physical Appearance

The physical appearance of the patient may be considered in two categories:
1. The physical appearance resulting from the state of the circulation.
2. The physical appearance as it reflects a disease which also involves the heart.

Examples in each category are numerous. Several have been selected and are listed below.

1. The physical appearance resulting from the state of the circulation.
    a. Cyanosis or clubbing as a clue to reversal of a central shunt
    b. Excessive sweating due to peripheral vasodilatation and increased "run-off" in aortic regurgitation
    c. The so-called "pink cheek on a pallid face" of tight mitral stenosis
    d. The shock syndrome, where the patient's cold clammy skin, confused sensorium and dusky cyanosis are striking reflections of the seriously compromised circulation.

2. The physical appearance as it reflects a disease which also involves the heart
    a. Acquired
        1) The eye findings in hyperthyroidism associated with a hyperdynamic circulation and supraventricular arrhythmias
        2) The skin findings in a variety of disease states, e.g., scleroderma associated with cardiomyopathy and cor pulmonale
        3) The "flushing" attacks in carcinoid tumors associated with right heart valvular lesions
        4) The joint manifestations of rheumatoid arthritis associated with aortic root disease and aortic regurgitation
    b. Congenital
        1) The Marfan's habitus as a clue to mitral apparatus disease with mitral regurgitation or aortic root disease with aneurysm and/or aortic regurgitation
        2) The Holt Oram syndrome with upper extremity bony abnormalities (especially the "fingerized thumb") associated with atrial septal defect.
        3) The "Elfin facies" of supravalvular aortic stenosis
        4) Mongolism (trisomy 21) associated with endocardial cushion defects and Turner's syndrome associated with coarctation of the aorta.

Finally, the straight back syndrome is an often missed variation in body habitus which can cause "pseudo heart disease."

In the straight back syndrome there is a lack of normal dorsal curvature of the spine and the heart may be pushed forward so that certain normal findings are exaggerated or modified, and cardiac disease simulated as outlined below. However, there is an increased incidence of associated mitral apparatus disease (the click-murmur syndrome) apparently due to a mesenchymal abnormality of the mitral apparatus, and possibly of the pulmonary valve. The PA and lateral chest X rays define the diagnosis with the straight back syndrome ratio being less than 40%.*

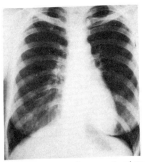 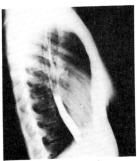

*Ratio $\dfrac{\text{anterior-posterior}}{\text{transthoracic}} \dfrac{(\text{Ant T8 to post sternum})}{(\text{at diaphragms})} = <40\%$

EXAMINATION

1. Palpable left parasternal systolic impulses
2. Loud delayed tricuspid closure
3. Exaggerated respiratory splitting of second heart sound
4. Pulmonic ejection murmur

ELECTROCARDIOGRAM

1. Vertical axis
2. rSr' in leads V1 or aVr

X-RAY

1. Prominent pulmonary arteries
2. Levo displacement of the heart
3. "Pancake" cardiac configuration simulating cardiomegaly

DIFFERENTIAL DIAGNOSIS

1. Atrial septal defect
2. Mild pulmonary stenosis
3. Idiopathic dilatation of the pulmonary artery

The Venous Pulse

The venous pulse can be evaluated either by inspection of the external or internal jugular veins. The latter is generally more reliable in that it more directly reflects right atrial dynamics. There are two types of information which can be obtained from the venous pulse: mean central venous pressure, and wave form (physiologic reflections of right atrial dynamics).

Mean Central Venous Pressure (CVP)
The most important principle is to place the patient in the proper position. While the veins are often described at a $30°$ or $45°$ angle with such terms as "engorged" or "flat," it is a simple matter to estimate the CVP exactly. If the CVP is high, then the patient should be more upright, and if low, lying more flat. A mechanical bed or examining table is a great help, and the patient should lie comfortably without any sharp angle caused by undue elevation of the head on a pillow. One can then see the undulating venous wave form moving the sternocleidomastoid and identify it by timing with the carotid or the heart sounds. The following steps will result in an accurate assessment of the CVP: 1) Identify the sternal angle of Louis across from the second rib. It is 5 cm. higher than the mid-right atrium (which is the arbitrary zero reference point). 2) Measure the vertical height at which the veins can be seen to pulsate (with a little practice, one can mean the individual waves readily). 3) Add 5 cm. to this figure (remember the sternal angle is at a level of 5 cm. CVP) and the result is an accurate estimation of the CVP in cm. of H_2O (which is approximately the same as mm. of Hg.)

Wave Form
The normal venous waves include: 1) The positive "a" wave reflecting atrial contraction and occurring just before the carotid pulse and first heart sound; 2) The negative "x" descent following the "a" wave and reflecting atrial relaxation, which is interrupted by: 3) The positive "c" wave (more often recorded than seen) which is a transmitted movement from the carotid pulse; 4) The positive "v" wave due to passive filling as blood from the periphery enters the right atrium in the latter part of ventricular systole, and; 5) The negative "y" descent inscribed as the tricuspid valve opens and blood enters the right ventricle from the right atrium.

Several observations and abnormalities of venous wave form may be seen including: 1) Giant "a" waves occur whenever it is more difficult for the contracting right atrium to empty into the right ventricle, e.g., any cause of poor compliance of the right ventricle or tricuspid stenosis; 2) Pathologic "c-v" waves occur with tricuspid regurgitation due to a "ventricularization" of the right atrial pressure curve, and may occur before a murmur can be heard; 3) Kussmaul's sign or inspiratory increase in mean venous pressure seen in constrictive pericarditis as well as a variety of restrictive myocardial diseases.

It is this observer's opinion that while arrhythmias can be well reflected in the neck veins and as such abnormal patterns are instructive, the ECG is obviously far superior, and neck vein judgments in arrhythmias only rarely are helpful in making clinical decisions.

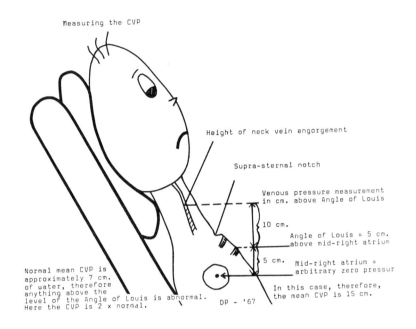

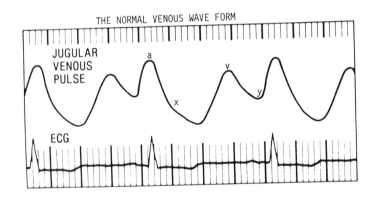

The Arterial Pulses

The carotid arterial pulse should be lightly palpated just inside the sternocleidomastoid, assessing its upstroke, peak and downstroke. It is my habit to feel the left carotid while watching the right internal jugular or listening to the heart for timing. All arterial pulses should be examined subsequently with the brachial and femoral palpated simultaneously to detect diminution or delay in the latter as a clue to coarctation.

In simple terms, the carotid may be small, large or bifid.

A small (hypokinetic) pulse is due either to severe pump failure or obstruction. The obstruction can be at a number of levels: The great vessels, aortic valve, mitral valve, pulmonary circulation (severe pulmonary hypertension) and occasionally the right-sided valves.

A large (hyperkinetic) pulse is due either to a high output (anxiety, thyrotoxicosis, anemia, etc) or due to a decreased resistance to left ventricular ejection, which increases the velocity of contraction, e.g., aortic and mitral regurgitation and some shunt lesions. Occasionally both mechanisms are operative.

A bifid pulse is found in aortic regurgitation with or without aortic stenosis, and in IHSS.

Other more specific abnormalities of the arterial pulse include pulsus tardus et parvus, dicrotic, anacrotic, bisferiens, bigeminal and paradoxicus. They will be discussed in greater detail subsequently.

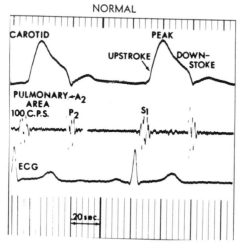

Precordial Movement

Precordial movement should be evaluated at the apex, left mid-parasternal edge, upper left and right parasternal edges, and ectopic area.

On examination of the normal chest wall, one can only feel a brief dime-sized apical tap of the left ventricle in the fifth intercostal space at the midclavicular line, occurring in early systole as the aortic valve opens and the ventricle begins to eject. The impulse is best felt with the patient on his left side. There is normally a zone of "septal" retraction medial to the impulse. Precordial movements should be evaluated in terms of their location, size, systolic duration and diastolic motion.

When the ventricle is volume loaded (preloaded) as in mitral or aortic regurgitation, the impulse is often displaced laterally, more diffuse and brief. When it is pressure loaded (afterloaded) as in aortic stenosis and hypertension, it is most often not displaced, but is enlarged and sustained. Filling sounds (S3 and S4 or ventricular and atrial diastolic gallops) are commonly felt, even when not audible, due to their low frequency.

Impulses at the mid left sternal edge and occasionally in the subxiphoid area are usually caused by right ventricular contraction and hence movements analagous to those of the left ventricle may occur. Occasionally a very large right ventricle may occupy the apex and no septal retraction is then seen.

Impulses at the upper left and right parasternal edge are usually due to a dilated pulmonary artery and aorta respectively.

Impulses in the ectopic area located between the apex and sternum are usually due to anatomic or physiologic aneurysms of the left ventricle.

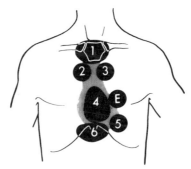

1. Sternoclavicular Area
2. Aortic Area
3. Pulmonary Area
4. Right Ventricular Area
5. Apical Area
6. Epigastric Area
7. Ectopic Areas (location variable)

NORMAL APEXCARDIOGRAM

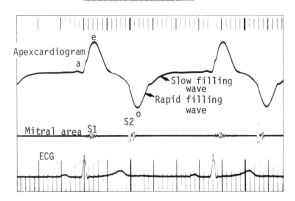

The recorded waves include:

-- The small "a" wave representing presystolic ventricular filling associated with left atrial contraction. The fourth heart sound when present is its audible equivalent.
-- The "e" point representing the normal brief palpable apical impulse and occurring at the time of the first heart sound.
-- The "o" point at the time of mitral valve opening.
-- The rapid and slow filling waves representing these two phases of ventricular diastole. A third heart sound may be felt and heard in some patients between the two waves.

Selected References

1. Glossary of Cardiologic Terms Related to Physical Diagnosis and History. Committee on Standardized Terminology, American College of Cardiology and American Heart Association. AJC, 20:385, 1967; AJC, 21:273, 1968; AJC, 24:444, 1969, AJC, 27:708, 1971.

2. Physiologic Principles of Heart Sounds and Murmurs. Ed., Leon, D. and Shaver, J., American Heart Association Monograph #46, 1975.

3. Examination of the Heart, Parts I-IV, American Heart Association Series, 1972.

4. Hurst, J.W., ed.: The Heart, Hurst and Logue, McGraw-Hill, Inc., 1972.

AUSCULTATION

Michael S. Gordon, M.D.

The following is a brief outline and definition of cardiac auscultatory events. Greater detail will be found in papers discussing specific disease states.

Heart sounds are discrete, short auditory vibrations of varying intensity and frequency. Their genesis has recently been clarified by echo- phonocardiographic studies.

The first sounds indicate the onset of systole and are due to mitral and tricuspid valve closures. They are normally split, as left ventricular contraction begins just before right ventricular contraction. The sounds are relatively high frequency and are best heard at the apex (mitral) and left sternal edge (tricuspid) with firm pressure on the diaphragm. Splitting is best heard at the tricuspid area.

The second sounds indicate the onset of diastole and are due to aortic and pulmonary valve closures. Normal splitting is due to an inspiratory drop in intrathoracic pressure with greater venous return to the right ventricle, pooling of blood in the lungs, and less venous return to the left ventricle. Hence, right ventricular ejection is prolonged and left ventricular ejection is reduced, resulting in first aortic, then pulmonary closure during inspiration. Abnormal splitting includes: 1) Unusually wide splitting on inspiration which persists during expiration, e.g., when right ventricular ejection is prolonged as in pulmonary stenosis or RBBB; 2) Wide splitting that does not vary with respiration, e.g., when both ventricles fill equally in both phases of respiration as in atrial septal defects, and; 3) Splitting that appears or increases on expiration (paradoxic splitting), e.g., when left ventricular ejection is prolonged as in aortic stenosis and LBBB. The second sounds are also relatively high frequency and are best heard at the upper right (aortic) and left (pulmonary) sternal edges with firm pressure on the diaphragm. Splitting is best heard in the pulmonary area.

The third sound is a filling sound and lower in frequency than S1 and S2. As blood accelerates into the ventricle during the rapid filling phase and then abruptly decelerates, vibrations of the mitral apparatus cause the S3. If ventricular filling is accelerated, as in the dynamic circulation of children, or in mitral regurgitation, or if deceleration is enhanced as with the stiff non-compliant failing ventricle, an S3 is heard. A pericardial knock is a higher frequency earlier third sound heard in pericardial constriction.

The genesis of the fourth heart sound is similar to the third sound, but it occurs in presystole related to active ventricular filling from atrial contraction. The S4 indicates an alteration in ventricular compliance, although it is not clear if an S4 invariably implies heart disease in the older patient. Since the S3 and S4 are low in frequency, they are best heard with light pressure on the bell. They are heard at the apex when generated from the left ventricle and at the mid left sternal edge when from the right ventricle. When an S3 and S4 are both present and heart rate increases, they may fuse in mid diastole to become a single loud "summation gallop."

Additional heart sounds include: 1) The opening snap of the mitral valve heard in mitral stenosis and occurring at the time of abrupt termination of the opening movement of the valve; 2) The ejection sound of the semilunar valve heard in valvular stenosis and regurgitation and with dilatation of the root of the great vessels, occurring when the valve reaches its fully open position; 3) Systolic clicks occurring at the time of mitral prolapse in patients with the click-murmur syndrome.

All of these acoustic events can be best appreciated by careful review of the hemodynamic curves found on p. 3.

Murmurs may be systolic, diastolic or continuous. By definition, the latter continues through the second sound. Murmurs are described in terms of their intensity, frequency, quality, configuration and duration.

The intensity of a murmur may be graded according to the Levine-Harvey method as follows: A grade 1 murmur is so faint that it can be heard only with special effort. A grade 2 murmur is faint but can be recognized readily. A grade 3 murmur is moderately loud. A grade 4 murmur is so loud that it may be palpated (a thrill felt). A grade 5 murmur can be heard with only the edge of the stethoscope on the chest. A grade 6 murmur is so loud it is heard with the stethoscope just removed from the chest. The frequency of a murmur varies from low to high. The classic low frequency murmur is that of mitral stenosis heard at the apex with light pressure on the bell. The classic high frequency murmur is that of aortic regurgitation heard at the left sternal edge with firm pressure on the diaphragm. The quality of murmurs has been variously described as musical, blowing, rumbling, etc. Configurations (shapes) include crescendo, diamond shaped and sustained. The duration of a murmur may be long or short and may be described in terms of its onset and termination as early, late, mid and holosystolic or diastolic. Examples of various murmur will be found in subsequent papers.

Selected References

1. Craig, E.: On the Genesis of Heart Sounds: Contributions Made by Echocardiographic Studies. Circ., 53:207, 1976.

2. Also see previous article references.

SYNTHESIS OF THE PHYSICAL EXAMINATION
(bringing the five fingers together to form a fist)

Let us use the common systolic murmur to illustrate how effectively one can correlate all the bedside findings to arrive at the correct diagnosis. We are essentially discussing mitral regurgitation and aortic stenosis, although certainly other systolic murmurs are occasionally encountered. In fact, in the younger patients an innocent early, short, pulmonary diamond-shaped murmur at the upper left sternal edge is the most frequently heard.

Systolic murmurs have been divided into ejection and regurgitant types, (the preferred terms today are crescendo-decrescendo, and holosystolic which are purely descriptive and do not imply hemodynamic cause). The first figure shows the typical "ejection" murmur of aortic stenosis, best heard at the upper right sternal edge and radiating into the neck. By examination of the left ventricular and aortic pressure contour, the characteristics of the murmur are readily understood. In contrast, the second figure shows the classic systolic "regurgitant" murmur of mitral regurgitation, best heard at the apex and radiating into the axilla. Reference to the pressure contour explains the reason for the murmur beginning at the first sound and sometimes going through the aortic second sound.

The basic differentiation between ejection and regurgitant murmurs as described by Leatham is valid. However, there are important exceptions; some have been recently recognized. To enumerate a few: (1) The classic papillary muscle dysfunction murmur of mitral regurgitation is often "ejection" in configuration. (2) Aortic stenosis is not infrequently heard very well at the apex and occasionally heard best at the apex. (3) Mitral regurgitation, especially that due to abnormalities of the posterior leaflet, may be heard best at the base and radiate into the neck, due to the anteriorly directed jet of blood. (4) Sounds considered to be extracardiac in the past, such as honks and clicks, have been shown in most cases to be due to mitral valve disease and, more specifically, disease of the paravalvular apparatus, i.e., the chordae and papillary muscles.

How then can one be certain from which valve the murmur is generated? There are two methods: First, and most important, the company the murmur keeps on physical examination, especially (a) the carotid pulse and (b) the chest wall evaluation, and second, certain interventions which may be used to selectively increase or decrease the murmur. These interventions include giving vasoactive drugs, postural changes, the Valsalva maneuver and isometric hand grip. One of the major mechanisms of these interventions involves a change in peripheral resistance or afterload. For example, when afterload is reduced as with amyl nitrate, forward flow is enhanced and hence, generally aortic outflow obstruction murmurs are increased and mitral regurgitation murmurs decreased.

The Carotid Vessel: Let us start with evaluation of the company the murmur keeps and look first at the carotid vessel. The normal carotid pulse contour is divided into three simple areas, upstroke, peak and downstroke, ending with the dicrotic notch as was shown previously.

The patient with significant aortic stenosis has a slow rising pulse, often with a shudder superimposed (Fig. 3). If significant aortic insufficiency is associated with aortic stenosis, the arterial pulse will rise rapidly, have two systolic peaks, and fall off rapidly during diastole, the so-called bisferiens pulse (Fig. 4). Figure 5 shows the pulse contour of a patient with idiopathic hypertrophic subaortic stenosis, with which mitral regurgitation may be associated. In this disease, due to a dynamic muscular outflow tract obstruction, a virtually diagnostic pulse contour, characterized by a rapid upstroke and two systolic peaks in the absence of an accentuated downstroke, is frequently observed. Figure 6 shows the carotid pulse of a patient with mitral regurgitation, characterized by a rather rapid upstroke. This feature correlates with the more rapid velocity of ventricular contraction seen in mitral regurgitation, due to the fact that mean resistance to contraction is reduced when blood flows into the low resistance left atrium during systole.

The Chest Wall: By palpating a thrill more pronounced at the base or apex, one obtains the tactile equivalent of inching over the chest wall with the stethoscope to decide where the murmur is loudest. If the thrill is loudest at the base and radiates into the neck, one generally, but not always, can assume that the murmur is due to aortic stenosis. If the thrill is maximal at the apex, it is more likely due to mitral regurgitation.

The apexcardiogram is a clinically useful reflection of precordial movement. Its major practical value, as is true of phonocardiography in general, is in the timing of hemodynamic events. It is of inestimable value in the teaching of bedside cardiology. A normal left ventricular apexcardiogram was presented previously.

An interesting chest wall movement which occurs in some patients with mitral regurgitation is the left atrial rock. In this condition the left sternal border rises much as it would with right ventricular hypertrophy. More careful timing during palpation reveals that the left ventricular thrust at the apex, which begins with isometric contraction, precedes the lift of the right ventricle. Hence, a rocking motion is imparted to the chest wall and to the palpating hand. With acute expansion of the left atrium, it is possible for the atrium to throw the right ventricle forward and give "pseudo right ventricular hypertrophy".

Another nearly diagnostic chest wall finding occurs in idiopathic subaortic stenosis in which two systolic apical impulses may be felt. Left bundle branch block and Barlow's (systolic click-murmur) syndrome may mimic this. In idiopathic hypertrophic subaortic stenosis, filling sounds are frequently palpable, and it is possible to palpate presystolic and mid-diastolic expansion at the apex; hence, three and even four apical impulses are felt at the apex (Fig. 7).

Another chest wall movement which may suggest a murmur due to mitral insufficiency is that occurring in what has been called the ectopic area, located between the usual left and right ventricular areas of the chest wall, and due to an aneurysm of the left ventricle. Due to the association of papillary muscle dysfunction with ventricular aneurysms, mitral regurgitation may be a concomitant finding; and in the presence of a left ventricular aneurysm an associated systolic murmur may be due to mitral insufficiency. Figure 8 shows the classic chest wall and acoustic findings in papillary muscle dysfunction in a patient with atherosclerotic heart disease. The palpable movement is typical of recent onset mitral regurgitation and rare in longstanding rheumatic valvular regurgitation wherein the baggy thin, compliant atrium does not generate enough "kick" to accelerate blood into the ventricle and cause an S4. The murmur starts after S1 as the papillary muscles do not begin to dysfunction until the aortic valve opens and ejection begins.

Finally, it is often possible to tell the difference between a diastolic (volume) and a systolic (pressure) overloaded ventricle. A stronger, more sustained apical impulse occupying a somewhat larger area than normal, but not very dynamic, is consistent with aortic stenosis. A left ventricular impulse which is dynamic, widely palpable and displaced downward and to the left should be considered more consistent with mitral regurgitation.

Selected References

1. Gordon, M.S.: The Bedside Evaluation of Common Systolic Murmurs - Brief Review of Current Concepts. J. Fla. Med. Assoc., 56:839, 1969.

2. See also selected references from 2 previous articles.

MID-SYSTOLIC EJECTION MURMUR

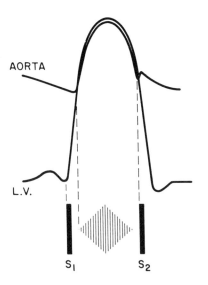

Fig. 1. The classic mid-systolic ejection murmur occurs during the period of ventricular ejection. As a result, the onset of the murmur is separated from the first sound by the period of isometric contraction, and the murmur, which is crescendo-decrescendo in nature, stops before the respective semilunar valve closure.

PANSYSTOLIC REGURGITANT MURMUR

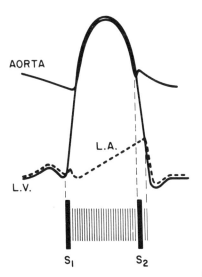

Fig. 2. The classic pansystolic regurgitant murmur of mitral insufficiency begins with, and may replace, the first heart sound. This murmur continues up to and through the aortic closure sound, since at that time ventricular pressure continues to exceed left atrial pressure.

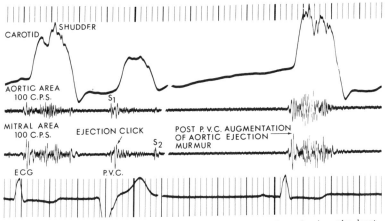

Fig. 3. Carotid tracing in moderate aortic stenosis. During the beat following an extrasystole, the murmur is louder due to enhanced flow across the aortic valve. This is the result of the fall in aortic root pressure which occurs in the long post extrasystole diastolic filling period. The reverse obtains during the extrasystolic beat, resulting in a diminution of the murmur.

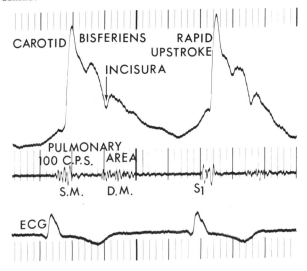

Fig. 4. Carotid tracing in aortic regurgitation with mild aortic stenosis. Note the rapid rise and double systolic impulse. The short early systolic murmur indicates the mild nature of the aortic stenosis. In fact, pure aortic insufficiency is frequently associated with a short early systolic "flow" murmur.

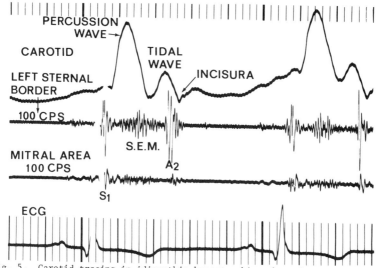

Fig. 5. Carotid tracing in idiopathic hypertrophic subaortic stenosis. Note the bifid pulse with percussion and tidal waves, and the ejection quality systolic murmur maximum at the left sternal border though well heard at the apex.

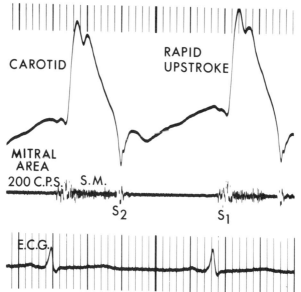

Fig. 6. Carotid tracing in mitral insufficiency. Note the rapid upstroke which is correlated with rapid left ventricular ejection in this disease.

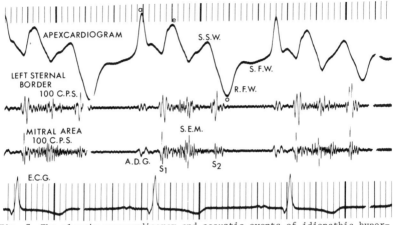

Fig. 7. The classic apexcardiogram and acoustic events of idiopathic hypertrophic subaortic stenosis. Note the triple apical impulse with prominent "a" wave and two systolic waves. The second systolic wave often occurs at the peak of the murmur, but may be slightly delayed.

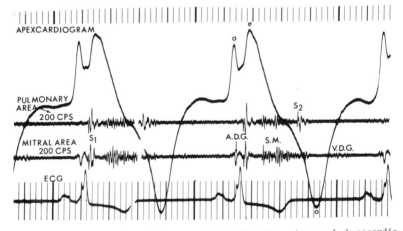

Fig. 8. The syndrome of papillary muscle dysfunction. Apex and phonocardiogram. Note the prominent "a" wave associated with an atrial gallop sound and the ejection quality apical mitral systolic murmur.

CLINICAL EVALUATION OF PATIENTS WITH AORTIC AND MITRAL VALVE DISEASE

Michael S. Gordon, M. D.

Aortic Valve

When considering disease of the aortic valve, the concept of "aortic outflow tract disease" must be stressed. Obstruction (with or without associated regurgitation) may occur above the valve, at the valve, or below the valve, where it may be muscular and dynamic as in IHSS, fibrous and fixed, or even related to anatomic abnormalities of the mitral apparatus. (Figure 1)

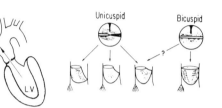

Figure 1. Anatomic features of left ventricular outflow obstruction.

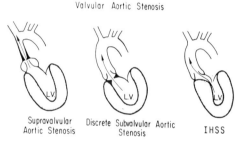

(after Glancy and Epstein Prog. Cardiov. Dis. 14:153, 1971)

It now seems likely that the majority of patients with isolated aortic valve stenosis, in fact, have congenital biscuspid valves which progressively fibrose and calcify. In the elderly, such calcified stenosed valves appear to be due to neither rheumatic nor congenital disease, but rather are due to degenerative disease, much as degenerative disease of the conduction system has been recently recognized as a significant cause of heart block.

Historically, patients with aortic stenosis present with the rather classic triad of effort syncope, angina, and dyspnea. Patients usually first become symptomatic when the valve orifice size is reduced to less than 1/3 of its normal size of approximately 3.0 cm^2. Pressure work (increased afterload) is very costly in terms of oxygen consumption, and once critical stenosis has occurred (orifice size less than .7 cm^2 or greater than 75 mm. gradient with normal cardiac output), there is a real risk of sudden death.

Failure is the most serious and usually the latest appearing symptom (except in the elderly when it may be the first symptom, apparently because their reduced physical activity reduces the likelihood of effort syncope and angina.) The natural history of patients with aortic regurgitation is less grave, at least one reason for which is the fact that volume work (preload) is not very costly in terms of oxygen consumption. Even patients with severe regurgitation may be asymptomatic for a decade or more.

On physical examination, guidelines for estimating severe aortic valvular stenosis include: carotid pulse - slow upstroke, small; chest wall - sustained but not necessarily displaced left ventricular impulse, palpable fourth sound; auscultation - long (not necessarily loud) murmur, fourth sound, paradoxically split S_2 or inaudible A_2; blood pressure - narrow pulse pressure. Left ventricular strain on ECG similarly correlates with severe stenosis.

Clinically, aortic stenosis in the elderly is characterized by several features that are either absent or more prominent than in younger subjects with this valvular lesion, as outlined on Table 1 below and in Figure 2.

Table 1. AORTIC STENOSIS IN THE ELDERLY

History:

    May present with failure before effort syncope or angina.

Physical Examination:

Blood pressure:	May have wide pulse pressure due to systolic hypertension.
Rhythm:	Atrial fibrillation in approximately 1/3.
Carotid:	May not be small. Bruits may relate to local disease.
Chest wall:	Chest configuration masks impulse. If enhanced impulse present, could relate to atherosclerotic heart disease.
Auscultation:	Atrial sound common in this age group. Chest configuration, 'spray' effect (lack of commissural fusion decreased jet) and failure decrease basalar murmur. Apical murmur due to calcified annulus (2/3 of patients) and/or papillary dysfunction mitral regurgitation.

Pathology:

    Tricuspid calcified aortic valve (Etiology degenerative?)
    Commissural fusion rare.

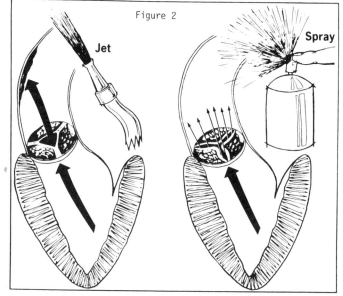

Figure 2

Jet   Spray

Diagram illustrating the auscultatory differences between fixed orifice (left) and non-fixed orifice (right) valvular aortic stenosis. A jet lesion appears to occur when severe fixed stenosis is present but is not apparent when there is a spray effect in non-fixed stenosis.

from Roberts Et.al.
A.J.C. 27:504, 1971

The tricuspid, originally normal valve, with degenerative fibrosis and calcification without commissural fusion is the type often seen in the elderly. There are several reasons why the basal murmur is less intense in this group: (1) the spray effect results in a relatively mild degree of turbulence of ejected blood, (2) the patients are frequently in failure with decrease in cardiac output, and (3) older persons tend to have increased upper thoracic chest dimensions.

The physical examination in moderate to severe aortic regurgitation includes: carotid pulse - rapid upstroke, possibly bifid; chest wall - displaced dynamic left ventricular impulse; auscultation - (listen for four murmurs) diastolic decrescendo murmur along left sternal edge (if loudest to right of sternum, suspect non-rheumatic etiology), systolic crescendo - decrescendo flow murmur across the aortic valve (may be loud but it is usually short), apical systolic murmur of papillary dysfunction mitral regurgitation, apical diastolic "Austin Flint" murmur due to diastolic vibration of the anterior mitral leaflet; blood pressure - wide pulse pressure.

It is important to emphasize that non-acoustic bedside findings often make the determination of the dominance of obstruction or regurgitation and may best estimate severity. The differential diagnosis of aortic regurgitation is extensive, but here again it is likely that congenital bicuspid valves account for a higher percentage than had been appreciated in the past.

An outline of the Differential Features of Left Ventricular Outflow Obstructions follows. (Table 2 - from Glancy and Epstein, Prog. Cardiov. Dis. 14:153, 1971)

Table 2. Differential Features of Left Ventricular Outflow Obstructions

	Congenital Aortic Stenosis			Acquired Aortic Valvular Stenosis		Hypertrophic
	Valvular	Subvalvular	Supravalvular	Nonrheumatic	Rheumatic	Subaortic Stenosis
History						
Onset of murmur	Birth	Birth	Birth	Early to late adulthood	Late childhood to early adulthood	Early childhood to late adulthood
Hx of rheumatic fever	Absent	Absent	Absent	Absent	Common	Absent
Neonatal renal insufficiency and/or hypercalcemia	Absent	Absent	Rare, but diagnostic if present	Absent	Absent	Absent
Family history of heart murmur	Rare	Rare	Common	Rare	Occasional	Common
Family history of sudden death in childhood	Absent	Absent	Occasional	Absent	Absent	Common
Angina or syncope after cessation of exercise	Absent	Absent	Absent	Absent	Absent	Common
Worsening of Symptoms						
With digitalis	Absent	Absent	Absent	Absent	Absent	Occasional
With nitroglycerin	Rare	Rare	Rare	Rare	Rare	Common
Physical Exam						
General appearance	Normal	Normal	Often characteristic	Normal	Normal	Normal
Carotid pulse	Slow upstroke, sustained peak	Slow upstroke, sustained peak	Right carotid rapid upstroke, left carotid-slow upstroke	Slow upstroke, sustained peak	Slow upstroke, sustained peak	Brisk upstroke; double peak usually recorded
Pulse volume on post-PVC beat	Increases	Usually increases	Increases	Increases	Increases	Decreases
Aortic ejection sound	Usual	Rare	Rare	Uncommon	Uncommon	Rare

	Second right interspace	Second right interspace	First right interspace or suprasternal notch	Second right interspace	Second right interspace	From lower left sternal edge to apex
Maximal thrill and murmur						
Intensity of Murmur						
During Valsalva	Decreases	Decreases	Decreases	Decreases	Decreases	Often increases
With squatting	No change or increase	No change or increase	No change or increase	No change or increase	No change or increase	Usually decreases
Murmur of aortic insufficiency	Common	Common	Uncommon	Common	Common	Rare
Chest X ray						
Aortic valvular calcium	Related to age	Absent	Absent	Common	Common	Absent
Dilatation of ascending aorta	Absent to marked	Absent to mild	Absent	Mild to marked	Absent to mild	Rare
Enlarged right heart	Absent unless other anomalies present	Absent unless other anomalies present	Absent unless other anomalies present	Absent	Absent unless mitral disease present	Common
Electrocardiogram						
Atrial fibrillation	Rare	Rare	Rare	Rare	Dependent upon severity of mitral valvular disease	Present in about 10% of patients
Abnormal Q waves in standard and left precordial leads	Absent	Absent	Absent	Absent	Absent	Common
Delta waves	Absent	Absent	Absent	Absent	Absent	Present in about 15% of patients
Catheterization						
Systemic arterial pulse pressure on post-PVC beat	Increases	Usually increases Rarely decreases	Usually increases	Increases	Increases	Decreases
Outflow pressure gradient during Valsalva	Decreases	Decreases	Decreases	Decreases	Decreases	Increases

Mitral Valve

A major advance in our understanding of abnormal hemodynamics has been the definition of the mitral apparatus, consisting of: (1) the papillary muscles, (2) the chordae tendineae, (3) the valve, and (4) the valve ring. The components of the mitral apparatus may become diseased and/or malfunction alone or in combination resulting in an entire spectrum of disease states. (See Figure 2. p. 4)

Papillary muscle dysfunction murmurs are commonly seen every day in the physician's office in patients with atherosclerotic heart disease. Normal valve closure and the mechanism of papillary muscle dysfunction are described below.

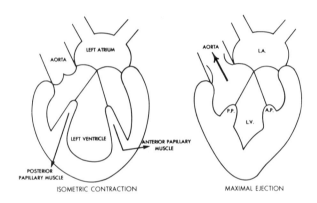

Figure 3. Normal mitral valve close. The mitral apparatus has been simplified to show one chordae from each papillary muscle to one leaflet only, after Burch. During isovolumetric contraction, the leaflets are tightly sealed by rising left ventricular pressure and tension development in the chordae-papillary muscle complex. During ejection, the papillary muscles shorten as the ventricle becomes smaller, maintaining the proper position of the leaflets. The dome of the valve does not ascend above the plane of the annulus. When the papillary muscles dysfunction, the leaflets approximate during isovolumetric contraction, hence the first sound is intact. During ejection, impaired contraction of the involved myocardium allows leaflet separation and regurgitation, hence the murmur begins after the first sound and has a crescendo-decrescendo configuration. If the papillary muscles are significantly shortened by fibrosis, or if the ventricle is significantly dilated, or if a significant aneurysm is present at the point of attachment of the papillary muscles, they are displaced laterally and downward from the ring permitting leaflet separation during both isovolumetric contraction and ejection, resulting in the classic holosystolic murmur as heard in rheumatic valvular regurgitation.

The systolic click-murmur syndrome is also commonly seen, especially in thin young females in association with straight backs, but is being recognized in many different settings. Possibly in its purest expression, it represents a congenital mesenchymal abnormality and might be thought of as a "forme fruste Marfan" syndrome replete with redundant chordae and a floppy posterior mitral leaflet.

Acute severe mitral regurgitation (the small left atrium, high pulmonary artery pressure syndrome) has also become better defined. The basic pathology lies in the suspensory apparatus rather than in the leaflets. The syndrome is best explained by the fact that the elastic relatively thick walled and forcefully contracting left atrium does not dilate significantly, and left ventricular pressures are reflected into the left atrium and hence into the pulmonary circulation. (Table 3, Figure 4)

The classic findings in moderate to severe chronic mitral regurgitation in the absence of severe failure include: carotid - rapid upstroke; chest wall - displaced and diffuse left ventricular impulse, possible palpable thrill and S_3; auscultation - absent fourth sound, holosystolic apical murmur, prominent third sound with associated diastolic flow rumble.

Table 3. Acute vs. Chronic Mitral Regurgitation

(from Ronan, et al: A.J.C. 27:289, 1971)

	Chronic	Acute
Sex	Both	men
Age	Youth	over 45
Murmur Course	Many years	Recent
	Heart Failure Late	Heart Failure Early
Rhythm	A. F. usual	Sinus usual
Murmur	Holosystolic	Decreases in late systole, to base
S3	Present	Present
S4	Absent	Present
L.A. size	Large	Small
Pulmonary hypertension	Mild to mod.	Mild to severe

The valve ring may also be diseased, and degenerative calcific diseases of the ring are being recognized especially in elderly females (we have seen the same disease in teenagers).

The classic findings in moderate to severe mitral stenosis with sinus rhythm include: jugular venous pulse - likely elevated central venous pressure with possible giant "a" wave or pathologic c-v wave if tricuspid regurgitation is present; carotid - small; chest wall - right ventricular impulse at the left sternal edge and small apical impulse (right ventricle occupies the apex and no septal retraction is seen), possible apical diastolic thrill, palpable P_2 and O.S.; auscultation - loud S_1, loud P_2, O. S. close to A_2, long (not necessarily loud) diastolic rumble with presystolic accentuation.

Figure 4. The
Syndrome of Mitral
Regurgitation.

(from Roberts and
Perloff, Ann. Int.
Med., 77:951, 1972)

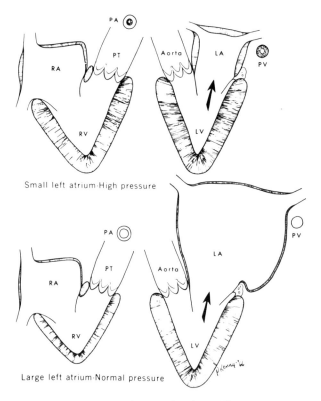

The two extremes of the spectrum of pure mitral regurgitation. When severe mitral regurgitation appears suddenly in individuals with previously normal or near-normal hearts, the left atrium (LA) is relatively small, and the high pressure within it is reflected back into the pulmonary vessels and right ventricle (RV). The anatomic indicator of this latter physiologic event is severe hypertrophy of the left atrial and right ventricular walls and marked intimal proliferation and medial hypertrophy of the pulmonary arteries (PA), arterioles, and veins (PV). In the other extreme, the left atrial cavity is of giant size, and its wall is thin. It is thus able to "absorb" the left ventricular (LV) pressure without reflecting it back into the pulmonary vessels or right ventricle. As a consequence, the pulmonary vessels remain normal, and the right ventricular wall does not thicken. PT = pulmonary trunk; RA = right atrium.

Selected References

1. Roberts, W.C., and Perloff, J.K.,: Mitral valve disease. Ann. Int. Med. 77:939, 1972

2. Reichek, N., Shelburne, J.C., and Perloff, J.K.: Clinical aspects of rheumatic valvular disease Prog. Cardiov. Dis.: 15:491, 1973

THE PHYSICAL EXAMINATION OF THE ACUTE CARDIAC PATIENT,
INCLUDING THE ASSESSMENT OF VALVULAR HEART DISEASE
PRESENTING AS AN ACUTE EMERGENCY

Michael S. Gordon, M.D.

The following discussion emphasizes the acutely ill patient. However, the bedside diagnostic findings of many of the important cardiac disease states are outlined, as most heart disease can present in the emergency setting. The same orderly "five finger" approach will be utilized.

I. PHYSICAL APPEARANCE - The physical appearances of patients with severe pump failure, anemia and acute vascular occlusion are helpful guides in their emergency care. The other examples mentioned below are interesting, but uncommon to rare.

Cardiogenic shock is diagnosed by signs of reduced tissue perfusion which can be detected at the bedside. When a fall in cardiac output activates sympathetic reflexes, certain vascular beds are intensely constricted, including those to skeletal muscle and skin. As a result, the patient is most often pale, cold, clammy and cyanotic, peripheral pulses weaken or disappear, and auscultatory blood pressure may become inaudible. This vasoconstriction may result in maintenance of normal or even elevated intraatrial pressure. Hence, a reduction of cuff pressure does not always mean hypotension, though certainly cuff blood pressure and pulse pressure are general indicators of cardiac output. In the setting of acute myocardial infarction, cardiogenic shock occurs with massive cardiac tissue destruction, most often greater than 40% of total ventricular muscle, and the amount of tissue destroyed is directly correlated with mortality. Similarly, the obviously dyspneic patient in pulmonary edema due to an acute myocardial infarction has had significant tissue destruction, with a mortality approaching 50% as compared to 75%+ in patients with frank shock. As such, the physical appearance of the patient alone is an important indicator of prognosis and correlates well with sophisticated hemodynamic measurements in patients with pump failure due to acute myocardial infarction.

Patients may present with an acute increase in congestive failure and ischemic cardiac pain precipitated by anemia, which can be appreciated on general inspection. The skin color and temperature changes beyond an occluded artery or proximal to an occluded vein are also obviously helpful in assessing the patient by general inspection.

Occasionally, the acute cardiac patient presents with findings on general inspection which are clues to the etiology of the patient's cardiac disease, especially the connective tissue disorders associated with diffuse inflammation. Examples include the pericarditis associated with systemic lupus erythematosus, rheumatoid arthritis and rarely gout, and the pancarditis of acute rheumatic fever. Non-inflammatory connective tissue diseases such as Marfan's and Ehler's-Danlos syndromes have been associated with acute aortic root dissection. The skin manifestations in acute endocarditis are rarely helpful in assessing acute cardiac patients. The several described lesions, e.g., Osler's nodes and Janeway lesions, were apparently more common in longstanding smoldering sub-acute endocarditis in years past, and splinter hemorrhages are found in other disease states, and even in normal people. Other exceedingly rare examples of acute cardiac lesions with clues from the patient's appearance include heart block associated with rheumatoid spondylitis, tamponade from pericardial effusion in myxedema, and tricuspid and pulmonary valve disease associated with carcinoid. Finally, some abnormalities of venous and arterial pulsation and chest wall movement described below are so exaggerated that they can be seen on general inspection of the patient.

II. ARTERIAL PULSE - The arterial pulse may be absent, small, enhanced, bifid, alternating or vary excessively with respiration.

Probably the most compelling example of the importance of assessing the arterial pulse is during cardiac arrest. In the first place, the assessment of any patient who has an apparent arrest should begin by palpating the femoral or carotid pulse to be sure it is absent. Occasionally patients with seizures or a stroke will collapse in or near a hospital or emergency facility, and will be promptly set upon with fists to the chest, etc. The fact that the arterial pulse is present obviously precludes the diagnosis of cardiac arrest. In the second place, during resuscitation, the adequacy of peripheral perfusion is assessed by feeling the arterial pulse. Finally, an occasional patient is apparently successfully resuscitated as evidenced by ECG complexes moving across the oscilloscope. However, the lack of an arterial pulse at that time reveals that while the patient's myocardium has electrical activity, there is no excitation-contraction coupling, and hence, no cardiac output. Other urgent situations in which the absence or marked diminution of peripheral arterial pulsations are of obvious importance, include emboli and dissecting aneurysm.

The commonest cause of a small arterial pulse is low cardiac output, e.g., left ventricular failure in myocardial infarction, cardiomyoapthy, and cardiac tamponade or constrictive pericarditis. A small arterial pulse associated with a crescendo-decrescendo upper right sternal border murmur radiating into the neck may be found in patients with aortic stenosis who may present acutely with ischemic cardiac pain or syncope. Severe obstruction at the mitral valve associated with a diastolic rumbling apical murmur may also result in a small arterial pulse, and such patients may present with emboiic sequelae of atrial fibrillation, acute pulmonary edema, or hemoptysis. In coarctation of the aorta, delay of the femoral pulse may be as important as diminution of the pulse in defining the diagnosis.

The arterial pulse may be enhanced in a variety of acute causes of aortic regurgitation, including trauma, dissection and infective endocarditis. Ruptured Sinus of Valsalva aneurysm centrally or a traumatic A-V fistula distally may also result in a hyperkinetic pulse. In all these situations, there is an increased stroke volume of the left ventricle, a wide pulse pressure, and a decrease in peripheral resistance. In complete heart block with bradycardia, the increased stroke volume may also produce a hyperkinetic pulse.

A bifid or twice beating pulse may be seen in patients who have aortic regurgitation, combined stenosis and regurgitation, or subvalvular muscular obstruction (idiopathic hypertrophic subaortic stenosis.) These patients may present acutely with neurologic symptoms including syncope, chest pain, and occasionally congestive failure.

Pulsus alternans refers to a regular pulse in which there is alternation of the height of the pulse pressure. It is associated with LV failure and is caused by regular alteration in left ventricular contractile force.

Finally, pulsus paradoxicus (which is paradoxically not paradoxical, but rather is an exaggeration of the normal decline in systolic blood pressure during inspiration), may be found associated with several cardiac and pulmonary diseases. Normally, with inspiration, there is a drop in systolic pressure of up to 10 mm. Hg. due to a pooling of blood in the lungs. If this normal drop is exceeded, the pulse is referred to as pulsus paradoxicus. In obstructive lung disease, wide fluctuations in intrathoracic pressure are probably transmitted to the aorta and great vessels and may cause a greater than normal respiratory variation in pulmonary vascular volume. In patients with pericardial disease (tamponade, constriction), the inspiratory tensing of the pericardium as it is pulled down by the diaphragm may interfere with cardiac filling, or alternatively the enhanced filling of the right heart during inspiration may compress the left ventricle which is limited in its distensibility by the pericardium.

III. VENOUS PULSE - Assessment of both the central venous pressure and the venous wave form may be important in the evaluation of the acute cardiac emergency. The wave form may have exaggerated positive waves ("a" and "v") or negative waves ("x" and "y").

The method of assessing the central venous pressure has already been presented. It should normally be less than 8 cm. (or less than 3 cm. above the sternal angle). Abnormal elevation of the central venous pressure may be seen in any cause of right ventricular failure. The most important of these in the acute setting is pulmonary embolism with pulmonary hypertension, due either to showers of small emboli or occasionally a massive embolism in a large pulmonary vessel. Cardiac tamponade is another acute situation in which venous pressure is commonly elevated, and in addition, Kussmaul's sign may be seen. The latter (often found in patients with pulsus paradoxicus) is a truly paradoxical increase in venous distension during inspiration due to inspiratory tensing of the pericardium which raises the intrapericardial pressure and obstructs venous return to the heart.

The venous wave form may also provide clues to the diagnosis of an acute cardiac emergency. The venous "a" wave due to atrial contraction, may become very large or "giant" when the right atrium is contracting against an increased resistance as in acute pulmonary embolism. The "v" wave may also become "giant" due to ventricularization of the right atrial (and hence jugular venous) wave form with systolic expansion of the veins in the neck. These are also called pathologic "c-v" waves. This wave form indicates tricuspid regurgitation which may be acute in onset, as with trauma to the chest or infective endocarditis. The latter is classically seen in heroin addicts with associated septic staphylococcal vegetations embolizing to the lungs. When tricuspid regurgitation is severe, the large "v" waves may cause the earlobe to "dance" with each pulsation - which less commonly occurs with hyperdynamic carotid pulsations. Finally, the venous wave form in constrictive pericarditis may have very prominent negative waves (the "x" and "y" descent) followed by a precipitous rise in pressure. This is due to the marked lack of compliance of the constricted right atrium and ventricle, so that blood filling these chambers after atrial contraction ("x" descent) and after opening of the tricuspid valve ("y" descent) encounters little elasticity of the receiving chamber, resulting in rapid rising pressures as filling occurs. This wave form has been described as "M" shaped, and may also be seen in restrictive myopathies with rigidity of the atrial and ventricular wall.

IV. PRECORDIAL MOVEMENT - An outline of normal and abnormal chest wall movement has been presented. Our discussion will first consider the apical impulse.

For example, a patient presenting with acute onset aortic regurgitation from trauma, dissection, or infective endocarditis is likely to have a forceful but non-sustained impulse due to the hyperdynamic circulation. This is due to increased contractility associated with the increased preload (Starling effect) as well as to an increased velocity of contraction due to the reduced afterload. The impulse may not be displaced when the preload is of recent onset, but as the ventricle enlarges to accommodate the additional volume, it most often becomes displaced to near the anterior axillary line. In contrast, the patient with outflow obstruction at the aortic valve who might present with syncope or angina, has a non-displaced, enlarged, nearly holosystolic sustained apical impulse. This is due to hypertrophy as well as to the prolonged ejection associated with the afterloaded ventricle. Patients with subvalvular muscular obstruction who may present in an identical fashion clinically often have two systolic apical impulses, the second apparently due to a thrusting out of the left ventricle as it encounters the dynamic muscular obstruction in mid-systole.

Finally, and possibly most important, filling sounds (third and fourth sounds or ventricular and atrial diastolic gallops) are commonly felt, even when not audible, due to their low frequency. In many clinical settings, the third heart sound and to a lesser extent, the fourth sound, are indicators of left ventricular failure, and are felt in early and late diastole (presystole) respectively. Patients with coronary artery disease presenting with chest pain are especially likely to have these palpable pathologic filling sounds due to poor compliance or stiffness of the left ventricle, which does not readily accept the rapidly accelerated blood entering the chamber during these filling periods in diastole. As the blood is rapidly decelerated, the mitral valve and paravalvular apparatus generate low sound frequencies which may be either felt or heard over the area of the left ventricle at the apex. In mitral regurgitation of acute onset, often presenting with acute left ventricular failure and pulmonary edema, a palpable (and audible) fourth sound is of diagnostic importance. In contrast to patients with long-standing mitral regurgitation whose atria are large and stretched and not capable of much acceleration of blood flow into the left ventricle during atrial contraction, patients with recent onset mitral regurgitation have small contractile left atria, and hence the fourth sound is readily generated as blood is decelerated by the left ventricle following atrial contraction, and the mitral structures vibrate. The finding of a third heart sound in mitral regurgitation does not necessarily indicate left ventricular failure, as it may be a flow phenomenon related to the severity of the mitral regurgitation.

In patients with mitral stenosis, who may present with acute complications related to pulmonary edema or embolism, the left ventricle is "protected" by the stenosed valve, and hence the left ventricular impulse may not be present, and the right ventricle may occupy the apex.
A right ventricular impulse felt at the left mid-parasternal edge, is especially prominent in patients presenting with pulmonary hypertension from a variety of causes, the classic acute situation being pulmonary embolism. Sometimes the right ventricular impulse is delayed in patients with severe mitral regurgitation due to acute expansion of the left atrium in midsystole which thrusts the right ventricle forward, resulting in what has been called the "left atrial rock." Right-sided filling sounds (third and fourth sounds or gallops) may also be palpated at the left sternal border and are augmented during inspiration when right heart filling is enhanced.

Examples of other chest wall movements of pertinence to the physician evaluating the emergency cardiac patient include: the upper left sternal border impulse of the pulmonary artery, occasionally felt with pulmonary embolism; the upper right sternal border impulse occasionally felt with aortic aneurysm including dissection; and the impulse felt in the "ectopic" areas (just between the left sternal border and apex) in patients with ventricular aneurysm, who may present acutely with congestive heart failure, ventricular arrhythmia, or peripheral arterial embolism. During an episode of angina, patients with coronary artery disease may have "physiologic aneurysms" or dyskinetic areas which can be palpated, i.e., ischemic areas of the myocardium which bulge out during ventricular contraction and contract normally when not ischemic.

Finally, murmurs may be felt as thrills if they are grade 4 or more, and heart sounds may be palpated when intense, for example, the first heart sound in mitral stenosis, and the second heart sound in pulmonary hypertension. Occasionally the lack of precordial movement may also be of diagnostic importance, e.g., in tamponade.

V. AUSCULTATION - The evaluation of heart sounds should include an assessment of the first, second, third, and fourth sounds, pericardial knock, opening snap, ejection sound, midsystolic clicks and frictions. The evaluation of murmurs should include systolic, diastolic and continuous murmurs.

Heart sounds may give important diagnostic information in patients with acute cardiac emergencies. The first sound may be increased in mitral stenosis, and is decreased or at least "buried" in the early sounds of the murmur in mitral regurgitation. It is also reduced in the syndrome of acute onset aortic regurgitation as described below. The second aortic sound is often absent or diminished in calcific aortic stenosis due to the fact that the valve is rigid. It is often louder in aortic regurgitation and hypertension, where the dilated aortic root enhances the vibrations responsible for its generation. The pulmonary second sound is increased in the presence of pulmonary hypertension, as with acute pulmonary embolism. Splitting of the second sound may also be affected in acute cardiac disease. During ischemic cardiac pain, due to dyssynergic left ventricular contraction, the second sound may be paradoxically split, as it may be in the afterloaded ventricle with aortic ouflow tract obstruction. The common denominator here is prolonged ventricular ejection. Wide splitting may occur with severe right ventricular failure and pulmonary hypertension, due to prolonged ejection from pump dysfunction and increased afterload.

Third sounds occur with rapid filling and may be due to excess flow, as with significant mitral regurgitation, or more commonly are due to poor ventricular compliance and left ventricular failure with abrupt deceleration of early diastolic filling causing vibrations to occur in the mitral apparatus. Fourth sounds are so common in acute infarction (90% of patients admitted to the coronary care unit in normal sinus rhythm) that they are of little diagnostic importance in that setting, and do not indicate significant pump failure. In fact, some believe that the fourth sound is a normal finding with advancing age, reflecting a normal diminution of ventricular compliance with elderliness. The fourth sound is very important as an indicator of recent onset mitral regurgitation as described above under precordial movement. It is also of value in younger patients (less than 45 years old) with aortic stenosis. Its presence indicates a valve gradient usually greater than 75 mm. Hg. The pericardial knock is a special kind of third heart sound seen in patients with constrictive pericarditis. It occurs slightly earlier, and is somewhat higher in frequency than the usual third sound.

The opening snap of pliable valve mitral stenosis is of value in judging the severity of obstruction, as the greater the stenosis, the higher the left atrial pressure, and the earlier the valve opens after the aortic second sound. Right-sided ejection sounds may be heard in the acutely ill patient with pulmonary hypertension, and in that circumstance, the dilated pulmonary artery is a factor in its production. An ejection sound generated in the area of the aortic valve may be heard in aortic regurgitation which may present acutely in infective endocarditis and dissection. Midsystolic clicks are rarely associated with urgent cardiac presentations, as Barlow's Syndrome (systolic click-murmur syndrome or the floppy mitral valve), which is by far the commonest cause of these sounds, has a generally benign course. Friction rubs often have three components, one in systole and the other two in diastole at the time of the S3 and S4, and are diagnostic of pericarditis which is a fairly common cause of acute chest pain, especially in younger patients.

Murmurs may be systolic, diastolic, or continuous. The systolic crescendo-decrescendo murmur of aortic stenosis is usually best heart at the upper right sternal edge, radiating into the neck, and the rumbling low frequency diastolic murmur of mitral stenosis is best heart at the apex, often requiring the use of the bell of the stethoscope to appreciate. While patients with stenosed valves may present with acute illness, a patient with acute illness associated with the recent onset of a murmur almost always has a leaking valve, or more rarely an arteriovenous communication, and presents special diagnostic features in contrast to longstanding valve regurgitation or arteriovenous shunts.

Acute severe mitral regurgitation has the following special features: It is predominantly found in men over the age of 45 with the sudden onset of left ventricular failure, the murmur is loud, apical and holosytolic with a late systolic decrease. This late systolic decrease is due to the marked pressure rise (giant characteristic "v" waves) in the small, relatively undistended left atrium which may reach ventricular level in late systole. Acute tricuspid regurgitation as may be seen in heroin addicts is also associated with decrescendo systolic murmurs for the same reason. The murmur of acute severe mitral regurgitation frequently radiates towards the base, mimicking aortic stenosis, and is accompanied by third and fourth heart sounds. Physical findings of pulmonary hypertension are present. Left atrial enlargement and atrial fibrillation are conspicuous by their absence. Radiographically, there is evidence of severe pulmonary vascular congestion despite a heart of near normal size. The basic pathology lies in the suspensory apparatus of the valve, rather than the leaflets, e.g., ruptured chordae tendineae or papillary muscle dysfunction. Frank rupture of a papillary muscle is fatal in the great majority of patients. It occurs from two days to two weeks after infarction, especially with inferior wall infarction involving the more poorly perfused posterior papillary muscle, and must be distinguished from a ventricular septal defect occurring after myocardial infarction. Ventricular septal defects may follow either anteroseptal or inferoposterior infarction, and occur from two days to two months after the infarct. The murmur is best heard at the left sternal border, is holosystolic, and is often accompanied by a thrill. Radiation of the murmur to the right of the sternum, and elevation of the central venous pressure is said to be more common than in papillary muscle rupture. Right heart catheterization with a step-up in oxygen in the right ventricle is diagnostic, while in severe mitral regurgitation of any cause, the pulmonary wedge pressure reveals giant "v" waves.

Acute severe aortic regurgitation also presents a rather distinctive clinical picture. It usually occurs in males with the sudden onset of forceful heart action or dyspnea which is usually progressive over days to occasionally months. The left ventricular volume acutely and rapidly increases in diastole with diastolic pressures rapidly reaching up to

50 mm. Hg. resulting in premature (diastolic) closure of the mitral valve, and a soft first heart sound. The murmur may be short because of the rapid rise in diastolic left ventricular pressure, and may have a cooing quality, especially if due to a torn cusp. It is often heard best to the right of the sternum, indicating a nonrheumatic etiology. The peripheral signs of aortic regurgitation may be absent and the heart may not be enlarged despite pulmonary edema. The etiology is most often infective endocarditis, although dissection and spontaneous or traumatic cusp rupture may also occur. In the case of dissection, the classic patient is a middle-aged male with a history of hypertension, and hence often black. Chest, back, and abdominal pain, concurrent stroke or a pulseless extremity, the murmur of aortic regurgitation not previously present, and occasionally a rub due to pericardial rupture are classic features.

The acute onset of a continuous murmur is usually due to a ruptured Sinus of Valsalva aneurysm into the right atrium. It is characteristically found in a previously healthy young adult male who develops sudden chest pain and dyspnea, bounding pulses, and cardiac failure, with the murmur best heard over the mid-sternum.

Selected References

1. J. Willis Hurst, M.D., ed., The Heart, McGraw-Hill, 1974.

2. J. Ronan, M.D., et. al., The Clinical Diagnosis of Acute Severe Mitral Insufficiency., Am. J. Card. 27:284, 1971.

3. Physiologic Principles of Heart Sounds and Murmurs. Ed.: Leon, D. and Shaver, J. American Heart Assoc. Monograph #46, 1975.

THE CARDIOMYOPATHIES

Lawrence S. Cohen, M.D.

The cardiomyopathies are a heterogeneous group of disorders which have a variety of etiologies, clinical presentations, clinical courses and pathologic findings. Any attempt at classification carries certain problems, but in general, three major categories can be distinguished: 1) Congestive cardiomyopathy; 2) Hypertrophic cardiomyopathy (with and without obstruction; and 3) Restrictive cardiomyopathy.

Although estimates vary, a specific etiology for the diagnosis of cardiomaopathy can be found in only approximately 10% of patients with this diagnosis. Hence, at the present time we are ignorant of the specific causes in the vast majority of cases which we diagnose as cardiomyopathy. All of the secondary heart muscle disorders fall into the congestive cardiomyopathy group. It is extremely important to attempt to identify a specific cause if present, as therapy of the underlying disorder may be quite beneficial in reversing the myocardial aspects of the disease.

Specific Causes of Cardiomyopathy

1. Infective
   Viral
   Bacterial
   Rickettsial
   Fungal
2. Metabolic
   Thyrotoxic
   Myxedema
   Acromegaly
   Beri-beri
   Puerperal
3. Associated with Neuromuscular Disorders
   Muscular Dystrophy
   Friedreich's Ataxia
4. Ischemia
5. Infiltrative Diseases
   Amyloid
   Hemochromatosis
   Tumor
   Sarcoid
   Glycogen Storage Disease
6. Collagen Disease
   Lupus Erythematosus
   Polyarteritis Nodosa
   Rheumatoid Arthritis
   Scleroderma
   Dermatomyositis
7. Toxic
   Alcohol
   Cobalt
   Daunomycin

Specific treatment of either thyrotoxicosis or myxedema may improve cardiac function in a patient who may have either of these endocrinologic disorders. Similarly, there is evidence that specific treatment of hemochromatosis may reverse the cardiac dysfunction which is part of that disorder. Unfortunately, for the majority of patients with congestive cardiomyopathy, there is no specific therapy.

The clinical presentation of the patient with congestive cardiomyopathy is often insidious. The physical examination at the time that symptoms are present usually denotes serious left ventricular dysfunction. Sinus tachycardia is common and pulsus alternans may be present. The apical impulse is diffuse and displaced to the left. A diastolic filling gallop is virtually the rule and an atrial gallop is almost as common. A murmur of mitral regurgitation due to papillary muscle dysfunction may be quite prominent and can mislead the clinician into suspecting a rheumatic etiology. The second heart sound is usually normally split but may be paradoxically split if left bundle branch block is present.

The chest roentgenogram will often show a markedly enlarged heart with all four chambers dilated. Pulmonary venous congestion is common.

The electrocardiogram may display a variety of abnormalities such as left ventricular hypertrophy, left atrial hypertrophy, bundle branch block or fascicular block.

The course of congestive cardiomyopathy may be quite variable. A certain number of patients will follow a rapid inexorable deteriorating course and will die within weeks or months after the clinical onset of the disease.

More frequently there will be an initial improvement once digitalis and diuretics are begun. This remission may last for months to years, but failure may supervene and not be responsive to therapy. Occasionally the patient may follow a stable course for years and not discernibly deteriorate.

Certain complications are so common that they must be considered part of the natural history of the disease. These relate to both pulmonary and systemic embolization, dysrhythmias and conduction disturbances.

The hallmark of hypertrophic cardiomyopathy is ventricular hypertrophy, usually without dilatation. Although there is no uniformity of opinion, it is generally agreed that those patients who manifest left ventricular outflow tract obstruction have disproportionate hypertrophy of the interventricular septum. It is agreed that obstruction is due to coaptation of the anterior leaflet of the mitral valve with the hypertrophied septal muscle mass. Hypertrophic cardiomyopathy with obstruction was commonly referred to as idiopathic hypertrophic subaortic stenosis. This entity is of particular interest to hemodynamicists in that the obstruction is not a fixed but rather a dynamic one. Interventions which augment myocardial contractility such as digitalis or isoproterenol; decrease the size of the left ventricular end diastolic volume such as hypovolemia or assuming the erect position; or decrease the distending force of the left ventricular outflow tract such as hypotension all augment the gradient between the left ventricle and aorta.

Selected References

1. The Cardiomyopathies. Circulation Research 35: (Supplement 2), 1974

2. Goodwin, J.F.: Prospects and Predictions for the Cardiomyopathies. Circulation, 50:210, 1974.

A RADIOLOGIC APPROACH TO VALVULAR HEART DISEASE

M. Viamonte, Jr., M.D.

At our institution routine chest roentgenography for cardiovascular evaluation includes the following five films: 1) posteroanterior chest roentgenogram without barium; 2) left anterior oblique view at $45°$ without barium; 3) right anterior oblique view at $60°$ with barium; 4) a lateral view with barium; and, 5) a posteroanterior view overpenetrated with barium. Because the heart is a three-dimensional structure, all these views are essential for complete evaluation of chamber enlargement. Cardiac fluoroscopy, especially in infants and children and in women of child-bearing age, should be conducted using minimum exposure and employing maximum patient protection. It is our policy to analyze the chest roentgenograms prior to the fluoroscopic examination. A barium swallow is not always necessary.

The overall size of the heart is evaluated by means of the cardiothoracic ratio which is the maximum internal transverse diameter of the heart divided by the maximum internal transverse diameter of the chest. This ratio should be less than 50% except in extremely obese patients or in one whose diaphragm is elevated and whose heart consequently has adopted a horizontal position. Cardiomegaly may be misdiagnosed in the presence of a prominent pericardial fat pad. The latter is easily recognized by the relative translucency observed around the apex of the left ventricle and at the left cardiodiaphragmatic junction. A pericardial fat pad may also exist at the right cardiophrenic angle.

The Normal Cardiac Contour

In the postero anterior view, the right heart border has two arches. The cephalad one is the vascular arch, caused by the ascending aorta in adults, by the superior vena cava and right lobe of the thymus in infants and young children or by the superposition of the ascending aorta and the superior vena cava in certain individuals. The caudal arch of the right heart border is formed by the right atrium.

The upper position of the left heart border in the frontal projection is formed by the aortic knob (the junction of the transverse and descending portions of the thoracic aorta). The middle arch is formed by the left border of the pulmonary trunk (upper two-thirds), the left auricular appendage (lower one-third), and the proximal portion of the left branch of the pulmonary artery. The caudal arch of the left heart border is formed by the left ventricle.

The left anterior oblique projection separates the left heart chambers from the right. The latter occupies the anterior half of the heart. The posterior heart border is symmetrically convex, and appears separated from the left bronchus by a radiolucent area representing aerated lung parenchyma. The anterior half of the heart is occupied by the right atrium superiorly, and by the right ventricle inferiorly. A line extending the anterior border of the trachea divides the heart into almost equal halves, and usually indicates the plane of the interatrial and interventricular septa. The left anterior oblique projection is utilized during selective angiocardiography for the study of left-to-right shunts at the atrial or ventricular levels. If contrast medium which has been injected into any of the left heart chambers is seen to be directed anteriorly, a left-to-right intracardiac shunt is indicated. This view is also excellent for evaluating valvular, subvalvular or supravalvular aortic pathology. The left anterior oblique projection unfolds the thoracic aorta. Left ventricular outflow tract obstructions are best analyzed in this projection. This is the projection of choice for selective injection of the right and left coronary arteries. The right coronary artery is directed anteriorly, and the left coronary artery posteriorly. The anterior descending division of the left coronary artery crosses the mass of the heart in the left anterior oblique projection.

The right anterior oblique projection is the view that separates the atria from the ventricles. The right anterior oblique projection should be taken at $60°$, for this degree of rotation of the patient is that which separates the heart from the spine. The left and right atria are projected posteriorly, and the right and left ventricles are superimposed anteriorly. Selective ventriculography is essential to the evaluation of pathology of the atrioventricular valves. It is also very important for the evaluation of atrial enlargement.

The left lateral view of the heart separates the left atrium and left ventricle posteriorly, from the right ventricle and right atrium anteriorly. In the lateral projection of the heart taken after deep inspiration, one usually sees a vertical line crossing the angle formed by the posterior heart border (diaphragmatic portion of the left ventricle) and the left leaf of the diaphragm. This line corresponds to the posterior wall of the inferior vena cava. When the posterior heart border projects behind the caval line, left ventricular enlargement is usually indicated. The left lateral projection is important for the evaluation of heart size in the ventro-dorsal direction; for the evaluation of left atrial, left ventricular and right ventricular enlargement; for the diagnosis of obstructive airway disease (i.e., diffuse obstructive pulmonary emphysema); and for the recognition of thoracic-wall deformities such as sternal depression and the so-called straight-back syndrome. This is an excellent view for analyzing the size of the primary division of the pulmonary artery. The right pulmonary artery usually projects as an oval shadow just behind and below the tracheal bifurcation. The left pulmonary artery courses above and behind the left bronchus.

The overexposed frontal view of the heart is of value in the recognition of abnormal cardiac calcification, in the detection of an enlarged left atrium, in localizing the thoracic aorta, and in analyzing the esophagus-heart relationships.

Cardiac Configuration and Chamber Enlargement

The posteroanterior view of the heart is used for evaluating heart size in the frontal plane and for determining cardiovascular configurations. The heart is said to have an "aortic or left-ventricle configuration" when the left ventricular arch and the aortic knob are prominent. This determines relative narrowing of the waist of the heart (relative concavity of the middle arch of the left heart border). The "mitral configuration" is said to be present when the shadow of the aortic knob is small, when the middle arch of the left heart border appears to be straight or convex, and when the left ventricular arch is inconspicuous. The left heart border follows a straight line directed from the midline to the left hemi-diaphragm. A double density caused by left atrial enlargement and inversion of the pulmonary vasculature (upper medial pulmonary vessels appearing larger than the lower medial pulmonary vessels) complete the picture of the "mitral cardiovascular syndrome." The "left-to-right shunt configuration" is said to be present when there is marked convexity of the middle arch of the left heart border and uniform pulmonary vascular plethora. The "Fallot configuration" is said to be present when there is a prominent rounding of the left ventricular border which appears raised above the diaphragm, and when the middle arch of the left heart border appears concave. This heart configuration is usually associated with pulmonary hypovascularity (secondary to right-to-left shunt). This group of findings is not pathognomonic of Fallot's tetralogy. It may be seen with other anomalies such as tricuspid atresia and persistent truncus arteriosus. The so-called "water bottle configuration" is said to be present when the right and left heart borders appear rather symmetric. There is enlargement of the transverse diameter of the heart, and the pulmonary vasculature appears to be normal or decreased. This configuration is the consequence of massive pericardial effusion or of cardiac dilatation (primary and secondary myocardiopathies).

Of all the heart chambers, the left atrium is the easiest to analyze. It is farthest posterior and hence touches the esophagus. In the frontal projection, when the left atrium is enlarged, one may see a slight convexity of the lower third of the middle arch of the left heart border due to dilatation of the left auricular appendage. A disc-like density appears in the center of the heart, causes a double density on the right heart border, and occasionally accounts for a third arch at the right heart border (the middle one). The interbronchial angle may appear to be widened (greater than 70º) when enlargement of the left atrium is directed superiorly. In extreme left atriomegaly, the esophagus may appear displaced to the right or to the left of the midline. Rarely, one may see atelectasis of the left lower lobe secondary to obstruction of the left lower-lobe bronchus caused by a markedly enlarged left atrium.

In the left anterior oblique projection the enlarged left atrium will obliterate the clear infrabronchial space, and one may see elevation of the left main bronchus. In the right anterior oblique projection the esophagus no longer parallels the thoracic spine. Variable degrees of esophageal displacement may be encountered. Elongated, marked esophageal displacement indicates the marked left atrial enlargement usually seen with severe mitral insufficiency. A localized, slight esophageal displacement indicates mild left atrial enlargement and predominant mitral stenosis.

Right atrial enlargement is best evaluated by means of the left anterior oblique projection. Prominence of the superior aspect of the anterior heart border usually reflects enlargement of the right auricular appendage. In the frontal projection, the right atrial border may appear displaced to the right and cephalad. There may be cephalad displacement of point B (the junction of the right atrial border and the vascular arch). The right anterior oblique and the left lateral projections are not helpful for evaluating right atrial enlargement.

Enlargement of both ventricles will displace the apex of the heart caudally and toward the left. However enlargement of the right ventricle is suspected if there is convexity of the middle arch of the left heart border. Since the right ventricle is not a border-forming structure in the frontal projection, indirect evidence of right ventricular pathology is suspected whenever one observes convexity of the middle arch of the left heart border and abnormal pulmonary vascularity. Pulmonary valvular stenosis, left-to-right shunts and pulmonary arterial hypertension are the commonest causes of convexity of the middle arch of the left heart border. Rarely, the ascending aorta may occupy the middle arch of the left heart border (in corrected transposition of the great arteries, for example). In some instances abnormal convexity of the middle arch of the left heart border is related to herniation of the left auricular appendage through a partial pericardial defect, or to a nonvascular condition such as an enlarged thymus, tumor or adenopathy.

The left lateral projection of the heart is best for profile analysis of the right ventricle. The closeness of the anterior heart border to the sternum is not a good sign of right ventricular enlargement, as in patients with a narrowed antero-posterior chest diameter, the heart is close to or touching the sternum. The left and right anterior oblique projections are not helpful in assessing right ventricular enlargement.

The best view for evaluating left ventricular enlargement is the left anterior oblique projection. When the left ventricle is enlarged, it usually overlaps and may project beyond the thoracic spine. The angle formed between the left ventricle and the left hemidiaphragm may become obtuse. The right anterior oblique projection is not useful for evaluating left ventricular enlargement. In the frontal projection the shape of the left ventricular arch may reflect volume (broad, large arch) and pressure (rounding, short arch) hypertrophy.

Pressure hypertrophy of either ventricle may be radiographically silent. Physical findings and electrocardiography are usually more sensitive than conventional roentgenography for the establishment of right or left ventricular hypertrophy. However volume hypertrophy of either ventricle modifies heart size and configuration, and will exaggerate the convexity of the chambers.

Asymmetric enlargement of the ascending aorta may be seen with aortic valvular stenosis (post-stenotic dilatation) and with syphilis. When the aorta becomes dilated and tortuous, the descending aorta may project beyond the middle arch of the left heart border. In such instances the right superior mediastinum may show a convex density usually caused by a tortuous, dilated and/or displaced innominate artery. Arteriosclerosis dilates and at the same time elongates the thoracic aorta. Since the thoracic aorta has a fixed position at the level of the aortic valve and at the aortic hiatus of the diaphragm, elongation will occur and the aorta will be displaced anteriorly, cephalad, to the right and dorsally, beyond the thoracic spine.

Analysis of calcification at the level of the thoracic aorta is important. Dissecting hematoma, and lues (with ascending-aorta calcification) cause characteristic findings. Pericardial, coronary-artery and valvular calcification are best analyzed during fluoroscopy. The best view for separating mitral from aortic valvular calcification is the left anterior oblique. In this view, aortic calcification will project in the center of the heart and will have a cephalo-caudal (head-foot) motion. Mitral valvular calcification will project in the posterior third quadrant of the heart, and will have a reverse C-shaped motion.

(The schematic figures of the cardiac series of chest x-rays on pages 29-32 are taken from The Heart, Hurst and Logue, 2nd edition, 1970. McGraw Hill Publishers.)

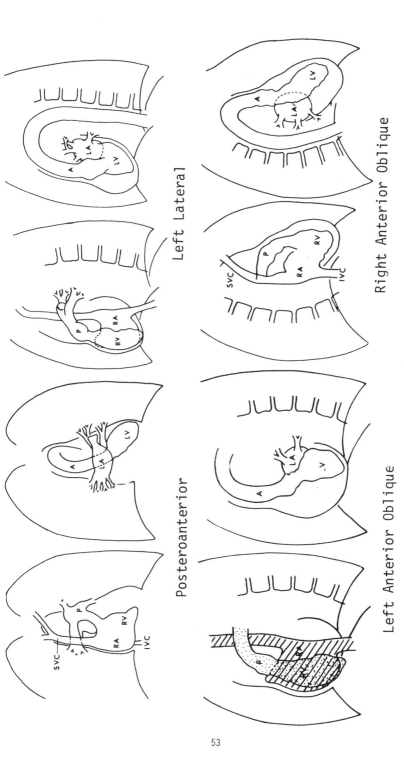

The Normal Cardiac Series – SVC, superior vena cava; IVC, inferior vena cava; RA, right atrium; RV, right ventricle; P, pulmonary artery; LA, left atrium; LV, left ventricle; A, aorta

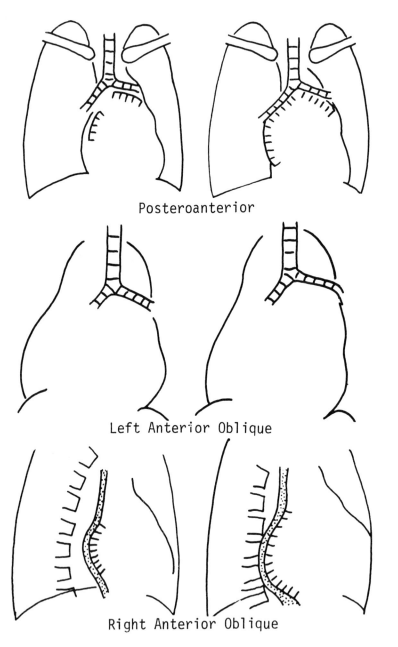

Left Atrial Enlargement, moderate (left) and marked (right) in three different views, displacing the left main bronchus and esophagus.

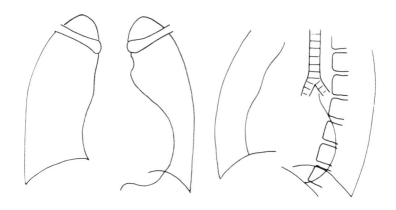

Left Ventricular Enlargement. PA (left) bulges down and to left, LAO (right) extends past the spine and downward.

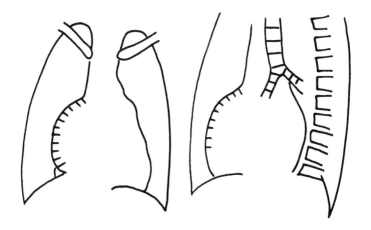

Right Atrial Enlargement. PA (left) bulges to the right, LAO (right) extends anteriorly toward the sternun ("shelving" sign).

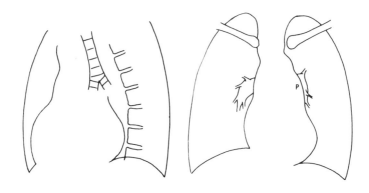

Right Ventricular Enlargement. LAO (left) bulges anteriorly toward the sternum, PA (right) indirect evidence reflected in enlarged pulmonary artery and main bronchus In the RAO (not shown) pulmonary outflow tract enlargement is also indirect evidence of right ventricular enlargement .

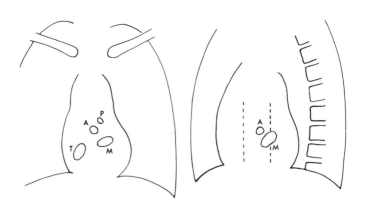

Heart Valve Position. PA (left) and LAO (right). The latter view is best to evaluate valve calcification using image intensification flouroscopy.

SURGICAL CONSIDERATIONS IN VALVULAR HEART DISEASE

Willis H. Williams, M.D.

Surgical management of coronary artery disease with its complications and the complete correction of congenital heart defects in infancy -- focal points of clinical investigation during the "70's" -- have offered new techniques and challenges in the treatment of cardiac valvular dysfunction. The "60's," although years of dramatic progress in the surgical treatment of valvular disease, left for this decade several frustrating problems in the development of a "perfect" human heart valve substitute. In part because of these problems, there has been revived enthusiasm for some of the more conservative reconstructive, "salvage," and plastic valvular operations, especially in young patients with valvular dysfunction. Judgments regarding surgical intervention must be made with the following questions in mind:

   I. When in the evolution of valvular dysfunction should surgical intervention with or without valve replacement be advised?

  II. If replacement of the valve seems preferable, which of the several available prosthetic and bioprosthetic substitutes should be selected?

 III. What predictions are justifiable concerning immediate operative mortality, longterm survival, complications, and potential for rehabilitation?

I. Guidelines for Surgical Intervention

Patients with <u>uncomplicated pure mitral stenosis</u> are candidates for simple mitral valvotomy or commissurotomy when their symptoms restrict them from ordinary activities (Functional Class II). The etiology is almost always rheumatic and these patients are often young and in otherwise good health. They should not be forced to spend years of restriction of their normal activity with gradual progression of symptoms to severe disability. Operation can be carried out without need for valve replacement and with a very low operative risk.

In several major centers, such patients are operated upon without cardiac catheterization and by the original "closed" technique without cardiopulmonary bypass. The majority of cardiac surgeons now prefer pre-operative study and carry out the commissurotomy under direct vision - an "open" operation performed on cardiopulmonary bypass - feeling that this is safer and allows more accurate incision of the commissures, examination of the left atrium for occult thrombus, and repair of residual regurgitation by annuloplasty if necessary. When a previous commissurotomy has been performed, the open technique is advisable for a second attempted commissurotomy.

When mitral stenosis is further complicated by mitral regurgitation, heavy calcification, immobile leaflets, fused and shortened chordae, left atrial thrombus, left ventricular failure, coronary artery disease, or associated dysfunction of other valves, pre-operative catheterization and an "open" operation are clearly advisable. Study and operation should be recommended before massive left atrial enlargement occurs, and, if possible, before the patient progresses to having symptoms with less than normal activity (Functional Class III and IV). At the time of operation the surgeon can decide between "salvage" of the patient's valve by commissurotomy with annuloplasty or total replacement of an unreconstructable valve. Intra-operative assessment of the tricuspid and aortic valves allows consideration of immediate versus future repair of associated dysfunction.

Mitral regurgitation without significant stenosis may be due to dilatation of the annulus, fenestration of a leaflet, papillary muscle dysfunction or ischemic origin, retraction of a leaflet, fusion and shortening of the chordae tendineae, rupture of chordae (or head of papillary muscle), or may follow previous commissurotomy. Risk of operation and likelihood for rehabilitation are poor when the disease has progressed to the stage of significant left ventricular failure. Operation should be advised for patients with moderate symptoms (Class II to III), and when left ventricular enlargement progresses, even if symptoms are minimal. Mitral valve disease is often insidious in its course, the patient progressively limiting his activities over many years without realizing how far from "normal" he has drifted until severe disease and its complications are present.

Current practice dictates total replacement of a structurally deformed valve with annuloplasty being reserved for the relatively normal valve made incompetent by annular dilatation. The use of a prosthetic ring and procedure devised by Carpentier has made annuloplasty a more objective and predictable operation for tricuspid and mitral incompetence with low hospital mortality. All of these procedures require total cardiopulmonary bypass. Should the surgeon be dissatisfied with the hemodynamic improvement achieved by annuloplasty, valve replacement may be carried out at the same operation.

While disease of the mitral valve is usually progressively symptomatic over many years, aortic valve dysfunction may be present and progressive for many years in a totally asymptomatic patient. Such a patient is at risk and the onset of symptoms usually indicates the beginning of rapid deterioration.

Aortic stenosis is usually congenital or rheumatic. Because of the risk of sudden death in this disease, asymptomatic patients with characteristic bedside findings of significant stenosis are advised to undergo cardiac catheterization. Operation is advised if the peak pressure gradient between the left ventricle and the aorta is 50 mmHg or greater. Patients with poor ventricular function and low cardiac output may have lower gradients even though the valve is stenosed. If the valve orifice size is calculated to be critically narrowed (usually less than 0.7 cm^2), then operation is indicated in spite of the greater risk associated with poor ventricular dysfunction. Coronary angiography should be carried out in all symptomatic patients, especially those with angina. We then perform simultaneous bypass grafts to appropriate vessels, as the additional risk is low.

Aortic commissurotomy (valvotomy) is usually reserved for the treatment of congenital aortic stenosis in infants and children or the young adult having pliable leaflets and no calcification. Most of these patients will require subsequent valve replacement as calcification and re-stenosis develop.

<u>Aortic regurgitation</u> may occur gradually over many years due to congenital rheumatic disease. It may also occur acutely in association with cystic medial necrosis and an aneurysm of the ascending aorta as a result of abrupt deceleration trauma, or from infective endocarditis. Acute severe aortic regurgitation should be treated by replacement of the the aortic valve or resuspension of the leaflets in association with repair of the aortic aneurysm with an interposition graft.

In contrast to patients with aortic stenosis, those with chronic aortic regurgitation are usually followed expectantly and advised to undergo operation only when symptoms develop and progress. However, whereas patients with mild aortic regurgitation may have a long and uncomplicated life expectancy, those with moderate to severe left ventricular enlargement by X ray, progressive left ventricular hypertrophy, and "strain" by electrocardiogram and a wide pulse pressure (systolic pressure over 140 mmHg, diastolic pressure less than 40 mmHg), are at great risk even if asymptomatic. The osnet of angina pectoris or symptoms of left ventricular failure in the patient with aortic incompetence demands early replacement of the valve. Even then, postoperative rehabilitation will be far less rewarding than in the patient operated upon before the disease reaches this "end-stage." Replacement of the aortic valve should be carried out whenever possible before the cardiothoracic ratio exceeds 0.60 even if the patient is asymptomatic. Under such circumstances large series of patients have been operated upon with a mortality approaching only 2%, and with late postoperative survival approaching that of the overall population when matched for age and sex.

Patients having signs and symptoms suggestive of <u>multiple valvular dysfunction</u> or with <u>associated coronary arterial occlusive disease</u> require more critical preoperative assessment by cardiac catheterization, and when indicated, coronary arteriography. In general, when relatively mild mitral disease is present in association with significant aortic disease, the mitral valve should be managed conservatively. In contrast, when relatively mild aortic disease is present in association with significant mitral disease, the aortic valve should be managed aggressively, as the results of surgery are poor when even mild aortic disease is left uncorrected.

<u>Tricuspid valve dysfunction</u> may be intrinsic, resulting from rheumatic involvement which usually produces both regurgitation and stenosis often associated with calcification. This lesion is rarely isolated, frequently

coexisting with mitral and/or aortic disease. Tricuspid valve replacement is appropriate in such situations, commissurotomy usually producing more severe regurgitation. Pure tricuspid regurgitation, on the other hand, may result from annular dilatation secondary to severe mitral valve disease, with pulmonary and right ventricular hypertension. As is the case with mild mitral regurgitation in the presence of severe aortic disease, mild to moderate tricuspid regurgitation secondary to mitral disease will often improve if nothing is done other than to replace the mitral valve or otherwise correct the mitral pathology. When the functional tricuspid regurgitation is severe, the Carpentier ring annuloplasty offers the simplest and most predictable result without the production of undesirable tricuspid stenosis and risk of emboli associated witb prostheses.

II. Choice of a Substitute for the Human Heart Valve

The Starr-Edwards caged-ball prosthesis has remained, through numerous modifications, the standard of performance against which all other valve substitutes have been compared. The "track record" of this valve has been excellent in both mitral and aortic positions and it has gained widespread acceptance. As with all prosthetic valves, poppet wear, thromboembolism and hemodynamic function have been persistent challenges. Improved alloys and manufacturing standardization have all but eliminated the older problem of poppet wear - so-called "ball variance" - in the round poppet with its infinite surface and ever-changing points of contact.

Efforts to minimize the incidence of thromboembolism have included the covering of exposed non-moving parts of the prosthesis with porous cloth, allowing fibrous ingrowth to form a natural autologous surface. Well-controlled anticoagulation with warfarin offers the best control of thromboembolism to date, but with the added risks complicating this mode of therapy. The relatively low incidence of thromboembolic complications, less than 5%, reported with the newer cloth-covered model Starr-Edwards prostheses (the 6400 mitral and 2400 aortic), are encouraging; the point may be approaching when the embolic risk will be less than the risk of anticoagulation complications.

A variety of low profile valves have been designed for insertion into smaller ventricular cavities, although problems with wear at points of contact have not been resolved.

The "ideal" flow dynamics of the normal human valve have prompted attempts to use biologic substitutes -- homologous and heterologous, fresh and preserved in a variety of ways, with or without mounting stents.

The bioprosthetic valve enjoying the most widespread clinical acceptance has been the gluteraldehyde-preserved porcine heterograft mounted on a flexible stent by Hancock Laboratories. Unacceptable obstruction to forward flow has occurred when the smaller sizes of this valve were placed in the aortic position. Although durability has been good during the seven years of this valve's use, concern still exists as to the durability and stiffening or calcification after several years of implantation, especially in the stressful mitral position. Risk of thromboembolism is low even without anticoagulation; the silent function is appealing to patients even if the porcine origin of the valve is psychologically bothersome to some.

III. Longterm Results

Numerous excellent reviews and individual reports describe the longterm survival, usually in actuarial form, and the complications for each of the many available valves. In the best of surgical hands, using the Starr-Edwards or an equivalent valve substitute in a patient who has not progressed to the high risk categories described earlier, isolated valve replacement should be performed with a 2-4% operative mortality. Longterm survival should be little different from a comparable normal population. Excellent symptomatic improvement can be expected. This ideal statistical circumstance is rarely achieved, unfortunately. As Dr. Richard Ross of the Johns Hopkins Hospital stated concerning coronary artery disease in his opening address to the American College of Cardiology in 1975,

"Surgical mortality figures...prove that a surgeon can select any mortality figure he wishes by selecting his patients."

Good technique and postoperative management must not be underrated.

Overall, with available valve substitutes and the state of the cardiovascular surgical art, an optimistic attitude toward surgical correction of valvular dysfunction seems justified.

Selected References

1. Behrendt, D.M., and Austen, W.D.: Current Status of Prosthetic Valves for Heart Valve Replacement, pp. 275-307, in Valvular Heart Disease, ed. by Sonnenblick, E.H., and Lesch, M., Grune and Stratton, Inc., New York, 1974.

2. Kirklin, J.W., and Karp, R.B.: Surgical Treatment of Acquired Valvular Heart Disease, Chap. 46, pp. 971-983, in The Heart, 3rd edition, ed. by Hurst, J.W., Logue, B.R., Schlant, R.C., and Wenger, N.K., McGraw-Hill Book Company, New York, 1974.

3. Pluth, J.R., and McGoon, D.C.: Current Status of Heart Valve Replacement, Mod. Conc. of Cardiov. Dis., 43:65-70, 1974.

FIGURE I

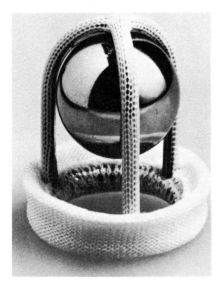

Starr-Edwards aortic prosthesis Model 2400. The metallic poppet, in contrast to the older silastic plastic derivative, has essentially eliminated the problem of poppet wear. The cloth covering of exposed non-moving parts allows fibrous ingrowth to form a natural autologous surface, thus reducing the incidence of thromboembolism.

FIGURE II

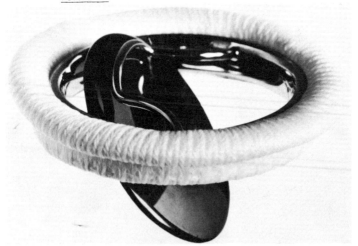

Bjork Shiley tilting disc eccentric monocusp valve prosthesis which preserves the concept of semi-central flow and low profile for insertion into small ventricles.

ELECTROCARDIOGRAPHY - CORE CURRICULUM

ELECTROCARDIOGRAPHIC INTERPRETATION -- AXIS DETERMINATION HEMIBLOCKS AND BUNDLE BRANCH BLOCKS

Joan Mayer, M.D.

AXIS DETERMINATION

The ventricular electrical axis in the frontal plane can be located in four quadrants: superior right, superior left, inferior right and inferior left. The electrical axis can be determined from the QRS deflections in the six standard leads. The normal range of the electrical axis is from $-30°$ to $+90°$. Between $-30°$ and $-90°$ is an abnormal superior left deviation of the electrical axis.

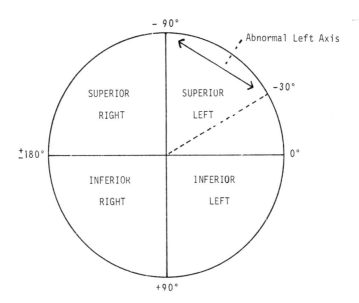

If the QRS in leads I and II shows a major positive deflection, the electrical axis is normal. If the major deflection is positive in leads I and aVF, the axis is between $0°$ and $90°$, and is located in the inferior left quadrant. If the major deflection is negative in lead I and positive in aVF, the electrical axis is located in the inferior right quadrant. If both leads I and aVF show a major negative QRS deflection, the electrical axis is located between $\pm180°$ and $-90°$, and is located in the superior right quadrant.

HEMIBLOCKS

The main left bundle branch subdivides into two fascicles: the anterior superior division and the post inferior division. It is possible for conduction to be blocked in only one of these fascicles, causing only half of the left bundle to be blocked, i.e., hemiblock. When hemiblock occurs, there are still normal conduction pathways to the ventricles. Therefore, there is no delay in conduction. The hemiblocks cause shifts in the electrical axis.

Left Anterior Hemiblock (LAH)

Abnormal superior and left deviation of the electrical axis is diagrammed in the following figure.

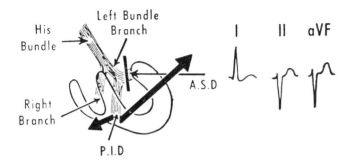

FRONTAL PLANE VIEW

ASD = anterosuperior division of left bundle branch

PID = posteroinferior division of left bundle branch

There are several mechanisms by which an abnormal superior and left axis occurs. The first of these is pure LAH or block of the superior anterior division of the left bundle. The typical electrocardiogram follows. Note there is an "r" wave in leads II and aVF.

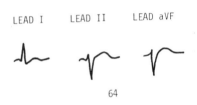

LEAD I   LEAD II   LEAD aVF

The second is an extensive inferior wall myocardial infarction. Note there is a Qr in leads II and aVF. The Q wave reflects the inferior infarction.

LEAD I   LEAD II   LEAD aVF

The third mechanism is coexisting left anterior hemiblock and inferior wall myocardial infarction. Note only a Q deflection in leads II and aVF. Hence this patient had LAH and a superimposed inferior infarction which resulted in loss of the initial small R and development of the Q wave.

LEAD I   LEAD II   LEAD aVF

The fourth mechanism is moderately severe pulmonary emphysema.

LEAD I   LEAD II   LEAD aVF

Type B Wolff-Parkinson-White, a pacemaker in the apex of the right ventricle, and moderately severe K excess are less frequently occurring causes of abnormal left superiorly directed electrical axis.

LEAD I   LEAD II   LEAD aVF   LEAD I   LEAD II   LEAD aVF

TYPE B WOLFF-PARKINSON-WHITE   MODERATELY SEVERE K INTOXICATION

LEAD I   LEAD II   LEAD aVF

PACEMAKER APEX RIGHT VENTRICLE

Left Posterior Hemiblock (LPH)

Inferior and right deviation of the electrical axis means that it is located between $90°$ and $±180°$. The most frequent cause of this type of axis is right ventricular hypertrophy (RVH). The second important mechanism for this type of axis is left posterior hemiblock.

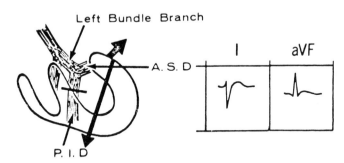

Because activation occurs through only the anterior superior division, the initial forces are shifted superior and to the left, giving the small r in lead I and the q in aVF. The main force then shifts inferiorly and to the right. These forces produce large R waves on leads II and aVF, resulting in a right inferior axis.

These changes are the same as those seen in RVH. The electrocardiogram alone is not enough to differentiate between RVH and left posterior hemiblock. Additional clinical, X ray, and pathological information is needed. Other important causes of right axis deviation are chronic lung disease, W-P-W type A, right ventricular pacing in the outflow tract, dextrocardia, extensive lateral wall myocardial infarction, and hyperkalemia.

LATERAL WALL INFARCTION

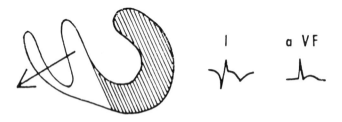

Extensive lateral wall infarction and LPH can coexist:

COEXISTING LATERAL WALL INFARCTION AND LPH

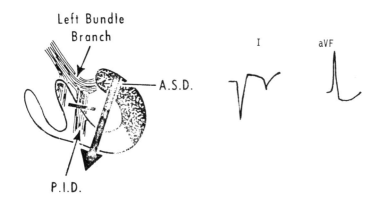

BUNDLE BRANCH BLOCKS

When conduction disturbances occur along one of the main branches of the bundle of His, either left or right bundle branch block is seen on the electrocardiogram.

Normal septal depolarization occurs from left to right, anteriorly, and superiorly in the semivertical heart. This vector becomes inferiorly oriented in the horizontal heart. These forces give rise to the normal .02 sec. q waves seen in left ventricular leads (I, V_6, sometimes aVL).

Left Bundle Branch Block

When there is a lesion which slows conduction down, the left bundle septal depolarization is reversed and takes place from right to left. This causes loss of the normal .02 sec. q wave in the left ventricular leads, and is diagnosed as any of the following synonymous terms: ILBBB, septal fibrosis or abnormal septal depolarization.

LEAD I, aVL or V_6

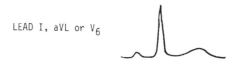

If the main left bundle is completely blocked, the depolarization wave travels down the intact right bundle only and the left ventricle is indirectly activated through arborization branches in the septum. The normal septal q wave is lost in the left ventricular leads, since the septum now depolarizes from right to left (reversal of normal), and there is a medial delay in the QRS that is positive in all left ventricular leads. Secondary T wave changes are also present in these leads.

LEAD I or V_6

The total QRS duration is .12 seconds or greater.

Right Bundle Branch Block (RBBB)

If the main right bundle is blocked, the septum depolarizes in the normal fashion, i.e., left to right, but the right ventricle is activated after the left. This causes no changes in the initial QRS depolarization, but shows right ventricular activation for the first time since it is not overshadowed by the left in this case. A preterminal delay, positive in the right ventricular leads (i.e., V_1), and negative in the left ventricular leads occurs.

LEAD V_1 LEAD V_6

The difference between incomplete and complete RBBB is merely a matter of time. Incomplete is diagnosed if the QRS duration is .10 to .12 seconds. Complete occurs if the QRS is .12 or greater in duration. Secondary T wave changes occur in the right ventricular leads.

Selected References

1. Castellanos, A., and Lemberg, L.: Programmed Introduction to Electrical Axis and Action, Potential Tampa Tracings, Tarpon Springs, Florida

2. Lipman, B.S., and Massie, E.: Clinical Scalar Electrocardiography, 5th ed., Year Book Medical Publishers, Chicago, 1965.

ISCHEMIA, INJURY AND INFARCTION PATTERNS
INCLUDING NON-SPECIFIC ST-T WAVE ABNORMALITIES

Robert J. Myerburg, M. D.

Ischemic processes in the heart may produce changes in depolarization as manifested by alterations of the QRS complex and changes in repolarization as manifested by ST-T wave changes. The triad of T-wave inversion indicating ischemia, ST-segment elevations indicating injury, and pathologic Q-waves indicating infarction are the cardinal signs of an acute ischemic process on the electrocardiogram. Depending upon the stage, sequence, and extent of the process, any one, two, or three of these findings may be present on a single tracing. The location will be determined by the site of the ischemic process, the reciprocal changes may be present in those leads which are oriented opposite to the site of the ischemic process. It is important, and often difficult, to differentiate the reciprocal changes in an acute inferior wall myocardial infarction from the changes indicating a true posterior wall myocardial infarction.

The importance of recognizing the less obvious and less specific electrocardiographic signs of acute myocardial infarction has become evident in recent years because of the very high risk of serious arrhythmias in the early stages of an acute ischemic process. The earliest changes of an acute ischemic process, whether transmural or intramural, are the so-called "hyperacute T-waves" in the leads reflecting activity in the involved area. These are recognized initially as an upward straightening of the ST-segment into a peaked T-wave, which later becomes progressively taller, and this may be followed by an elevation of the ST-segment with terminal inversion of the T-wave. Elevation of the ST-segment in a single precordial lead in the transitional zone may not be indicative of an acute myocardial infarction, but conversely may be the earliest sign. If the clinical picture is at all suggestive, such a localized electrocardiographic finding must be considered serious until proven otherwise. Primary T-wave inversions in anterior or inferior leads in the absence of ST-segment or QRS changes may indicate a non-transmural acute injury process or a non-transmural infarct. Serial electrocardiograms and enzyme studies are necessary to determine the ultimate significance of such changes.

ST-segment elevations without reciprocal depressions or T-wave changes may indicate pericarditis, or may be a normal stable variant. As the pericarditis progresses, if this is the cause, ST-segments usually return to the baseline, and this is followed by inversion of T-waves. In an acute infarction, the inversion of T-waves usually occurs coexistent with the ST elevation.

Secondary ST-segment changes, such as seen in the strain patterns or intraventricular conduction abnormalities, are characterized by a downward sloping ST-segment, merging into an asymmetrically inverted T-wave. A primary change, as stated earlier, is characterized by symmetrical T-wave inversion. The downward coving of the ST-segment seen in the presence of digitalis effect is a fairly non-specific finding and may be seen in early left ventricular strain patterns or as an indication of ischemia. The most reliable evidence of chronic ischemia is the horizontal ST-segment depression often seen in the precordial leads, as well as low T-wave voltage or minor T-wave inversion. Acute ST-segment elevations during chest pain, which return to the baseline at the end of an anginal episode, are the hallmark of the Prinzmetal variant of angina pectoris. It is important to differentiate this from the ST-segment elevations of acute myocardial infarction or pericarditis.

Examples of the above ST-T variations are shown in the diagrams which follow on the next page.

Knowledge of the anatomic location of an infarction allows the physician to anticipate complications. Occlusion of the left anterior descending branch of the left coronary will produce an anteroseptal infarction. The leads that reflect these changes are leads VI thru V3 and the reciprocal changes will be seen in leads II, III and aVF. Occlusion of the circumflex branch of the left coronary will produce anterolateral changes and will be shown in leads I, V4-V6 and aVL with reciprocal changes in VI, II, III and aVF. Occlusion of the main trunk of the left coronary may cause infarction in the anterior and lateral wall of the left ventricle with changes in I, aVL and all the V leads.

Occlusion of the right coronary artery will produce inferior wall myocardial damage with changes in leads II, III and aVF with reciprocal changes in leads I and aVL. If the distal branch of the right coronary is the sole supply of the posterior wall, occlusion of this will cause death of tissue here and can only be seen by the reciprocal changes noted in the opposite leads, i.e., VI-V3, since there is no standard electrode which looks directly at the posterior wall of the left ventricle. In the presence of a posterior wall myocardial infarction, there is an increase in the amplitude of the R wave with depression of the ST segment and J point with tall peaked T waves during the evolutionary stages.

Selected References

1. Hurst, J. W., Myerburg, R. J.: Introduction to Electrocardiography, McGraw Hill Book Co., New York, 1973.

2. Lipman, B. S., Massie E., Kleiger, R. E.: Clinical Scaler Electrocardiography, Year Book Medical Publishers, Chicago, 1972.

ST AND T WAVE CHANGES

1. NORMAL ST AND T WAVE CONFIGURATION

2. NORMAL VARIANT J POINT ELEVATION "EARLY REPOLARIZATION"

3. ACUTE MYOCARDIAL INFARCTION WITH Q WAVE, ST ELEVATION, AND TERMINAL T WAVE INVERSION

4. EARLY ACUTE MYOCARDIAL INFARCTION WITH "HYPERACUTE" T WAVE. THIS CAN BE A NORMAL VARIANT IN THE TRANSITION ZONE OF THE PRECORDIAL LEADS. SIMILAR T WAVES MAY BE SEEN IN HYPERKALEMIA.

5. PRIMARY T INVERSION OF NON-TRANSMURAL INFARCTION

6. ACUTE PERICARDITIS WITH DOWNWARD COVING OF ELEVATED ST SEGMENT.

7. SECONDARY ST-T SEGMENT CHANGES OF
    LEFT VENTRICULAR STRAIN WITH DOWN-
    SLOPING ST SEGMENT MERGING INTO
    ASYMMETRICALLY INVERTED T WAVE.

8. DIGITALIS EFFECT WITH DOWNWARD
    COVING OF ST SEGMENT MERGING INTO
    AN UPRIGHT T WAVE.

9. NON-SPECIFIC ST-T CHANGE OFTEN SEEN
    IN CHRONIC ISCHEMIC HEART DISEASE
    WITH HORIZONTAL ST DEPRESSION AND
    LOW VOLTAGE T WAVE.

10. PRINZMETAL VARIANT ANGINA WITH ST
    ELEVATION DURING PAIN WHICH RETURNS
    TO THE BASELINE AT THE END OF THE
    EPISODE.

11. ANGINA PECTORIS (USUAL FORM) WITH
    HORIZONTAL OR DOWNSLOPING ST SEGMENT
    DURING EXERCISE.

12. HYPOKALEMIA WITH FLAT T WAVE MERGING
    INTO PROMINENT U WAVE.

VENTRICULAR HYPERTROPHY

Stephen M. Mallon, M. D.

To electrocardiographically identify ventricular hypertrophy, look especially at the precordial leads. The standard limb leads are less specific and chiefly reflect alterations of the cardiac position within the thorax related to chamber enlargement.

The left ventricle normally contributes three-fourths of the potentials that produce the QRS deflection. The effective electrical localization of the left ventricle is posterior, to the left, and superior. The effective electrical orientation of the right ventricle is to the right, anterior, and may be either inferior or superior. The interventricular septum is situated almost, but not completely parallel to the frontal plane in the body.

Activation of the interventricular septum is initiated in the middle third of the left side of the septum and proceeds from the left toward the right, followed by activation of both ventricular walls. Because of expedient conduction occurring via specialized conducting tissue, activation of the septal mass, despite its thickness, progresses rapidly and generally produces forces of relatively small magnitude. When septal activation occurs abnormally, septal forces are capable of generating potentials of large magnitude, as we shall see. During later stages of activation of the outer layers of the ventricular walls, a significant magnitude of electrical voltage is produced and recorded (the R wave). The magnitude of the generated electrical forces is dependent upon the richness of the Purkinje network and the thickness of the ventricular wall, as well as other factors such as the relationship of the recording electrode to the heart muscle, chest wall characteristics, etc.

Left Ventricular Hypertrophy (LVH)

Because of the poor specificity of voltage criteria in the diagnosis of left ventricular hypertrophy, Estes has developed a point system to diagnose left ventricular hypertrophy. A score of 5 or more points is diagnostic of LVH, and a score of 4 points indicates that there is probable LVH. The maximum number of points available is 10. This system is as follows:

1) If the largest <u>voltage</u> of the R or S wave in the limb leads is 20 mm or more, or if the largest S wave in V1, V2 or V3 is 25 mm or more, or if the largest R wave in V4, V5 or V6 is greater than 25 mm, then 3 points are given.

2) If the <u>ST segment</u> is opposite in direction to the QRS, provided that the patient is not receiving any digitalis, 3 points are

given. If the patient is receiving digitalis, this typical "strain" pattern receives only 1 point.

3) If the <u>intrinsicoid deflection</u> is .04 seconds or more in the left chest leads, 1 point is given.

4) If the <u>QRS duration</u> is .09 seconds or more, 1 point is given.

5) If the <u>axis</u> is to the left of minus 15 degrees, 2 points are given. When the axis exceeds -30 degrees, it is likely that LVH alone is not the cause, e.g., left superior hemiblock or inferior infarction may be the etiology.

(Some electrocardiographers will allow points toward the diagnosis of LVH if <u>left atrial enlargement</u> criteria are met.)

The so-called pattern of "ventricular strain," a terminology suggested by Katz and others, will tend to appear in the left precordial leads or in leads AVL or AVF, depending on heart position. Electrocardiographers tend to eschew this term because it has a mechanical rather than electrical connotation. I think, as a clinician and a hemodynamicist, that the term is an attractive one, and is "physiological."

Sodi and some other electrocardiographers have attempted to differentiate various types of LVH based on a relationship to different anatomic lesions. The pattern of pressure overloading of the left ventricle such as seen in valvular aortic stenosis or hypertension is characterized by a normal or even vertical QRS axis (the heart shadow is not enlarged on X ray in these cases). The diastolic or volume overloading variety, as seen in aortic or mitral regurgitation, associated with both ventricular dilatation and hypertrophy, tends to produce leftward electrical axis. Systolic overloading tends to have a major effect on repolarization, which is prolonged, and this produces a negative T wave in V5 and V6, and in the limb leads facing the left ventricle. Diastolic overloading has a propensity to produce delay in the intrinsicoid, prolonged intraventricular conduction, and frequently upright T waves in the leads overlying the left ventricle.

Right Ventricular Hypertrophy (RVH)

The diagnosis of RVH based on limb lead patterns is not very helpful. The precordial leads are also more reliable in differentiating right axis deviation due to positional change compared to right axis deviation due to RVH.

A normal right ventricular epicardial complex, exemplified by V1, with a small R wave and deep S wave reflects the normal preponderance of left ventricular forces over the right. In RVH, the increased bulk and thickness of the right ventricular wall tends to reverse this relationship. Therefore, the characteristic features of RVH are best seen in the right precordial leads, particularly V1, V2 or V4R. Because of the nearly ten-fold increase in predominance of left ventricular forces over the right, a large magnitude of RVH is necessary to overbalance or abolish the dominance of left ventricular forces.

Criteria for RVH
A. Precordial leads (best for diagnosis)
 1. R wave greater than S wave in V1 or V3R. (R/S ratio >1.0)
 2. qR pattern in V1 or V3R
 3. Ventricular activation time greater than 0.03 seconds in V1 or V3R
 4. Persistent S waves greater than 5 mm in V5 and V6
 5. ST segment depression and/or T wave inversion in V1 or V3R
B. Extremity leads
 1. Tall R in AVR (unless accompanied by precordial lead criteria not indicative of RVH).
 2. Tall R with depressed ST and inverted T in AVF (not diagnostic pattern unless confirmed by precordial leads).
C. Standard leads
 1. Right axis deviation (+100° or more)
 2. Depressed ST segment and inverted T waves in leads II and III.
(Right atrial enlargement may also be used as a criterion for RVH.)

In RVH, varying degrees of change in QRS configuration or voltage occur in proportion to the degree and type of hypertrophy much more reliably than in LVH. The so-called concentric or pressure overloading hypertrophy of the right ventricle (as exemplified physiologically by valvular pulmonary stenosis), tends to offset left ventricular forces in a more distinctive manner than hypertrophy of the basal portions of the right ventricle such as seen in volume overloading conditions (as exemplified by atrial septal defect). Pressure overloading of the right ventricle tends to produce tall R waves in the right chest leads, whereas volume overloading of the right ventricle tends to produce rsR' patterns in these leads.

The accompanying table gives useful guidelines in differentiating different types of RVH.

Combined Ventricular Hypertrophy

The electrocardiographic diagnosis of ventricular hypertrophy of all types is far from perfect. Autopsy correlations with electrocardiograms have revealed that an electrocardiographic diagnosis of left ventricular hypertrophy can be made in 85% of cases using the criteria described. The same criteria also produce a false positive diagnosis in 10 to 15% of the cases. In right ventricular hypertrophy, particularly in patients with congenital heart disease, autopsy correlation is more reliable, but the correlation ranges from 23% to 100% in large series. Combined ventricular hypertrophy is seldom diagnosed electrocardiographically and the autopsy correlation is only 8% to 26%. The most reliable criteria for the presence of biventricular enlargement are those of left ventricular hypertrophy in the precordial leads with a frontal plane axis of more than +90°. This is particularly true when there have been serial progressive changes in the frontal plane axis toward the right in the presence of left ventricular hypertrophy in the precordial leads.

Selected References

1. Lipman, B. S., Massie, E., and Kleiger, R. E.: Clinical Scalar Electrocardiography, 6th Ed., Year Book Medical Publishers, 1972, pp. 93-137.
2. Schlant, R. C., and Hurst, J. W. (eds.): Advances in Electrocardiography, Grune and Stratton, Inc., New York, 1972. (Extensively referenced)

ECG DIFFERENTIATION OF THE TYPES OF RVH

	PRESSURE OVERLOAD	VOLUME OVERLOAD	EARLY MITRAL STENOSIS	CHRONIC LUNG DISEASE
ETIOLOGY	1. Pulmonary stenosis 2. Primary pulmonary hypertension 3. Secondary pulmonary hypertension, e.g., - repeated pulmonary emboli - late mitral stenosis - late A.S.D.	1. A.S.D. 2. Anomalous venous damage 3. Pulmonary or tricuspid regurgitation		
AXIS	Right	Vertical or Right	Vertical or Right	Mild: Vertical Moderate: Abnormal LAD Severe: Right (and superior)
ATRIUM	Right Atrial Enlargement with normal sinus rhythm (except in mitral stenosis - left atrial enlargement or atrial fibrillation)	Right atrial enlargement occasionally	Left atrial enlargement or atrial fibrillation	Right atrial enlargement
LEAD V1				

ARRHYTHMIAS - AN OVERVIEW

Joan Mayer, M.D.

The goal of this exercise is to provide experience for the practicing physician in the recognition of common arrhythmias. A systematic approach to arrhythmias is suggested. First, some general rules:

1. Analyze the P waves - what is depolarizing the atrium?
   A. Shape and direction of the P
   B. Rate of the P
   C. Regularity of the P

2. Analyze the QRS complex - where is the origin of ventricular depolarization?
   A. Shape; normal, aberrant, or bizarre
      Impulses arising in the ventricles (rather than supraventricular) are not transmitted through normal conduction pathways. As a result, depolarization of ventricular musculature usually occurs slowly with delay. The initial portion of the QRS, at least in some leads, will differ from that of the normal QRS even if the total QRS width is not increased. Impulses arising from supraventricular foci may depolarize the ventricle in normal fashion or, if they occur too early before complete repolarization has occurred, they will show some aberrancy of conduction. This aberrany affects the last 2/3 of the complex and is usually of the right bundle branch block type. The initial 1/3 of the complex is identical to the normal complex in all leads.
   B. Rate
   C. Regularity

3. Analyze the relationship between P wave and QRS complex, specifically, PR interval length and constancy

The following specific criteria are suggested:

SINUS RHYTHMS:
1. P wave upright in lead II; inverted in AVR
2. P wave rates range between 40-60 to 160-180
3. Supraventricular QRS with a constant PR interval

SUPRAVENTRICULAR ARRHYTHMIAS

Junctional Rhythms
1. P wave inverted in lead II; upright in AVR
2. Rate range: 40-100 Junctional rhythm
             100-180 Junctional tachycardia
3. P may be before, after, or lost in QRS
4. Supraventricular QRS

SUPRAVENTRICULAR ARRHYTHMIAS (Continued)

Atrial Tachycardia
1. P wave upright or inverted in lead II
2. Straight baseline exists between P's if other complexes irradicated
3. P rate 160-180 to 240-260
4. QRS shape normal or aberrant
5. QRS rate may be same as P or if some are not conducted, block exists
Note atrial tachycardia with block is classically associated with digitalis toxicity

Atrial Flutter
1. f wave rate 240-260 to 350
2. Undulating or saw-toothed baseline
3. QRS shape normal or aberrant
4. QRS rate usually less than P - most commonly there is a 2 to 1 conduction ratio, although it may vary
Note atrial flutter with block is usually not due to digitalis toxicity

Atrial Fibrillation
1. Atrial impulses so rapid that a definite P wave can no longer be seen. Morphology deteriorates and no P wave rate can be obtained
2. Ventricular response always irregular. A-V node bombarded with impulses of varying strength at varying times in cycle.

VENTRICULAR ARRHYTHMIAS

Premature Ventricular Contractions (PVC's) - General Characteristics
1. Occur early
2. QRS complex different from patient's normal complex
3. Interval between the preceding sinus beat and the PVC remains fixed or constant if the PVC's are arising from the same focus

PVC's - Parasystolic
1. QRS complex different from patient's normal complex
2. Interval between preceding sinus beat and ventricular beat is not constant
3. Interval between ventricular parasystolic beats is either constant or a whole number multiple of set distance

Ventricular Tachycardia (V.T.)
1. 3 PVC's or more in a row
2. Ventricular rate greater than 60
3. 2 Types
   a. Slow V.T. (non-paroxysmal VT) ventricular rate between 60-100 initiated by late PVC
   b. Fast V.T. (paroxysmal VT) ventricular rate greater than 100 initiated by early PVC - on or close to T wave of previous beat

HEART BLOCK

First degree atrioventricular (A-V) block
1. Sinus impulse delayed in reaching ventricle
2. Result of pathology above or below His bundle
3. PR interval greater than .20 sec
4. Each P wave followed by QRS complex

Second degree A-V block
1. One or more sinus impulses fail to activate the ventricles
2. Two types

Wenckebach - Type I	Mobitz - Type II
a. Lesion at A-V node - supra-Hisian	Lesion in Bundle Branch System: infra-Hisian
b. Associated with inferior wall myocardial infarction, digitalis toxicity, chronic conduction system lesions	Associated with anterior wall myocardial infarction, chronic lesions conduction system
c. Described as ischemic, reversible and transient	Described as necrotic in nature
d. Dropped QRS preceded by progressive prolongation of P-R	Dropped QRS preceded by a fixed P-R interval
e. Regular P-P intervals	Regular P-P intervals
f. Usually responds well to pharmacological intervention	Usually non-responsive to pharmacological intervention-requires pacing

Advanced A-V block - Occasional A-V capture by sinus P waves

Third degree A-V block
1. All of the sinus impulses fail to activate the ventricle
2. No fixed relationship between P wave and QRS complex
3. Can occur as end result of Type I or Type II second degree A-V block
4. Regular P-R interval
5. Regular R-R interval
6. Following Wenckebach, controlling rhythm usually junctional
7. Following Mobitz II block, controlling rhythm usually idioventricular

Arrhythmias become potentially life-threatening under three conditions:
1. When they originate in the ventricles
2. When they result in critically slow ventricular rates
3. When they result in critically fast rates

SUPRAVENTRICULAR ARRHYTHMIAS

Hein J.J. Wellens, M.D.

Supraventricular arrhythmias can be the result of incidental (extrasystoles) or sustained (tachycardia) ectopic activity at the supraventricular level. All arrhythmias with a site of origin in or proximal to the predivisional part of the common bundle (bundle of His) are called supraventricular. This includes the sinus node, atrium, A-V node, and bundle of His. Frequently, incidental supraventricular ectopic activity is provoked by such factors as nervousness, alcohol, tobacco, etc., is benign, and requires no therapy. Sometimes it is an expression of organic heart disease like infectious disease, coronary heart disease or (frequently age related), fibrotic changes. To determine the significance of supraventricular extrasystoles, a thorough history and physical examination is therefore essential. This becomes crucial in patients suffering from sustained supraventricular ectopic activity. Again, apart from the tachycardia, no other cardiac abnormalities may be present, but the tachycardia may also be provoked or seriously complicated by concomitant heart disease.

DIAGNOSIS

History - Complaints of irregular beating of the heart are common. Paroxysms of rapid rhythms are usually recognized by the patient. The experience of an attack of rapid beating of the heart frequently frightens the patient, he perspires, and may start to hyperventilate. The latter symptom is a common reason for misdiagnosing patients as hyperventilators or neurotics. In fact, 30% of 200 patients referred to our department with electrocardiographically documented supraventricular tachycardia were initially diagnosed by the general practioner as neurotics. In some, several years elapsed before the correct diagnosis was made. When heart rate is high, the resulting decrease in cardiac output may result in dizziness or rarely, loss of consciousness. Anginal complaints may develop during tachycardia, especially in patients with coronary heart disease. One should realize, however, that during high heart rates (over 200/min), anginal pain can occur in young patients without coronary heart disease. On termination of tachycardia, patients may experience dizziness or syncope, depending upon the time required for an escape pacemaker to take over the cardiac rhythm. It is a typical complaint of patients suffering from the so-called brady-tachycardiac syndrome. Physical and psychological stress may trigger tachycardia. Events preceding tachycardia should be discussed and possible contributing mechanisms identified.

Physical Examination - Apart from determining the rate and rhythm of the tachycardia, during the episode particular attention should be given to:

1) The first heart sound
2) Pulsations of the jugular veins, and
3) The arterial blood pressure.

If, during a regular tachycardia, changes are present in the loudness of the first heart sound, height of the jugular vein pulsations and systolic blood pressure of successive beats, dissociated activity of the atrium and ventricle can be diagnosed and a ventricular origin of the tachycardia made likely at the bedside. Expansive pulsations in the jugular veins with the same frequency as the tachycardia indicate atrial contraction against a closed tricuspid valve, and demonstrate activation of the atrium just prior to, or within ventricular systole. This phenomenon can be seen in A-V nodal tachycardia, atrial tachycardia with prolonged PQ time, and supraventricular tachycardia in patients with pre-excitation and a short ventriculo-atrial conduction time.

Electrocardiographic Diagnosis - Table 1 schematically represents the rate and rhythm of the atrium and ventricle in the different types of supraventricular tachycardia. Carotid sinus massage can be of great help in diagnosis and treatment. Proper execution is essential (Table 2). It should be done with great caution in: 1) The elderly patient; 2) When digitalis intoxication is suspected; and 3) In acute myocardial infarction.

Diagnosis of the site of origin can be extremely difficult if widened QRS complexes are present during the tachycardia. Then one has to differentiate between a supraventricular tachycardia with aberrant conduction and a ventricular tachycardia. Rate, rhythm, and QRS width are not helpful in making a correct diagnosis. Configuration of the QRS complex is, however, of great significance. In the presence of right bundle branch block shaped QRS complexes, an RSR' configuration in lead V_1 is highly suggestive for aberrant conduction, especially when combined with an intermediate QRS axis in the frontal place. An R or QR configuration in lead V_1 favors a ventricular origin, especially when combined with QS complexes in the left precordial leads. In the presence of left bundle branch block shaped QRS complexes, left axis deviation in the frontal plane with QS complexes in leads II and III is highly suggestive of a ventricular origin of the tachycardia. Examples of different supraventricular arrhythmias are shown in Table 3.

Selected Reference

1. Marriott, H.J.L., Sandler, I.A.: Criteria, old and new, for differentiating between ectopic ventricular beats and aberrant ventricular conduction in the presence of atrial fibrillation, Progr. Cardiovas. Dis., 9:18, 1966.

TABLE 1

	Atrial Rhythm	Ventricular Rhythm	Relation atrial to ventricular rhythm	Effect CSM
Sinus Tachycardia	100-200/min, regular	100-200/min, regular	1 to 1	Gradual slowing
Atrial Tachycardia				
No digitalis	120-260/min, regular	120-260/min, regular	Usually 1 to 1	Termination, no effect or increase in AV block
With digitalis	120-260/min, regular	60-260/min, regular	Frequently 2nd degree AV block	Increase in AV block
AV Nodal Tachycardia				
Paroxysmal	120-260/min, regular	120-260/min, regular	Usually 1 to 1	Termination or no effect
Non-Parosyxmal	70-150/min, regular or irregular	70-150/min, regular or irregular	Frequently A/V dissociation	No effect or slowing ventricular rate
SVT in Pre-excitation	120-260/min, regular	120-260/min, regular	1 to 1	Termination or no effect
Atrial Flutter	250-350/min, regular	125-350/min, regular or irregular	Usually 2nd degree AV block	No effect or increase in AV block
Atrial Fibrillation	350-600/min, irregular	150-180/min, irregular	High degree AV block	No effect or increase in AV block
Ventricular Tachycardia	70-250/min, regular or irregular	100-250/min, regular or irregular	1 to 1, 1 to 2, or A/V dissociation	No effect

Abbreviations: AV = Atrioventricular, CSM = Carotid sinus massage, SVT = Supraventricular tachycardia

TABLE 2 - RULES FOR CAROTID SINUS MASSAGE (CSM)

Precautions:

1) Try to exclude stenosis of one of the carotid arteries by palpation and auscultation.
2) Register the effect of CSM with the help of an electrocardiogram; if not available, listen to the heart with the stethoscope during carotid massage.
3) Realize that patients with tachycardia and especially the older patient may respond with a long period of cardiac arrest.

Proper Positioning:

1) Patient flat on his back with his head falling backward (either by placing the physician's left arm or a small pillow under the patient's shoulders).
2) Patient's head turned to the left during massage of the right carotid sinus, and vice versa.

Correct Massaging:

1) On the bifurcation of the carotid artery just below the angle of the jaw
2) Massage one side at a time
3) Start by slight pressure (some, especially elderly, patients are very sensitive). Thereafter, firm pressure should be applied with a massaging action.

SUPRAVENTRICULAR ARRHYTHMIAS

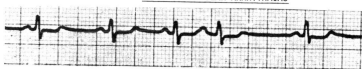

ISOLATED APC - The P wave of the fourth beat falls on the previous T wave and has a longer than normal P-R interval. There is no full compensatory pause.

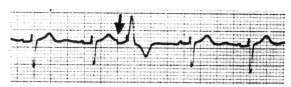

APC WITH ABERRANCY (Lead V1) - The arrow shows the early P wave followed by the aberrantly conducted beat which has an RBBB configuration.

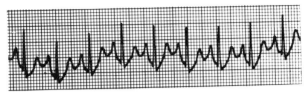

SINUS TACHYCARDIA - The rate is 140. The P wave and P-R interval are normal.

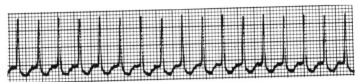

PAROXYSMAL ATRIAL TACHYCARDIA at a very rapid rate of 250. P waves are discernible before each QRS. The arrhythmia begins and ends abruptly and is regular.

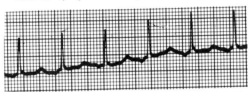

JUNCTIONAL TACHYCARDIA (Lead II) - Inverted P wave with short P-R interval at a relatively slow rate of 110.

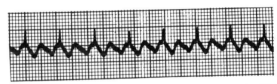

ATRIAL FLUTTER WITH 2:1 AV CONDUCTION. The atrial rate is 270 and the ventricular rate 135. Classic "sawtooth" flutter waves are easily identified.

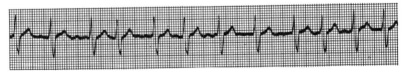

ATRIAL FIBRILLATION WITH INTRAVENTRICULAR CONDUCTION DELAY. Fibrillation waves can be seen and the ventricular response is absolutely irregular.

VENTRICULAR ARRHYTHMIAS

Andrew C. Wallace, M.D.

Ventricular rhythms comprise all those instances in which the impulse leading to ventricular contraction originates from below the AV node or AV junctional tissues. Beats originating from below the AV junction can occur as an isolated instance, intermittently, periodically, or they may be sustained for longer periods of time. When a ventricular beat or beats arise because of default (sinus arrest) or because of AV block, they are often referred to as passive or escape beats. When they arise prematurely or in a rapid sustained manner, some active mechanism is invoked. These latter active mechanisms include:

1) Enhanced automaticity
2) Reentry
3) Repetitive firing of depressed or depolarized myocardial fibers.

Current evidence suggests that only Purkinje fibers are capable of enhanced normal automaticity, while repetitive firing can occur either in depressed Purkinje or muscle fibers. Reentry of course requires within the reentry circuit, participation by myocardial elements with a markedly depressed conduction velocity.

Abnormal rhythms resulting from impulse formation below the AV junction can be classified in the following manner:

1) Isolated or Intermittent Rhythms
   a. Ventricular escape beats
   b. Ventricular premature beats
   c. Bigeminy
   d. Trigeminy
   e. Parasystole

2) Sustained Rhythms
   a. Idioventricular rhythm
   b. Accelerated ventricular rhythm
   c. Ventricular tachycardia
   d. Ventricular flutter and fibrillation

All ventricular rhythms are characterized by widening of the QRS complex to 120 msec. or greater (with rare exceptions). Beats with a widened QRS complex, however, do not always arise from below the AV junction. Examples of beats with a widened QRS arising from within or above the AV junction include:

1) Bundle branch block
2) Supraventricular beats or tachycardia with aberration of ventricular conduction
3) Pre-excitation or the Wolff-Parkinson-White Syndrome.

The distinction between ventricular rhythms and supraventricular rhythms with aberration is important from a diagnostic, prognostic and therapeutic point of view. Important criteria for distinguishing between ventricular beats and supraventricular beats with aberration include:

1) QRS morphology in sinus rhythm
2) QRS morphology of the beat or beats in question
3) Atrial activity (P wave) preceding the beat in question
4) Widening only following a long-short PR sequence
5) The presence or absence of fusion beats

These criteria are useful in most instances but occasionally, His bundle recordings are needed to make the distinction between ventricular rhythms and supraventricular rhythms with aberration.

A detailed discussion of the prognostic importance and implications of ventricular rhythms is not within the scope of this paper. Suffice it to say that escape beats represent a normal response to sinus slowing or AV block. Isolated PVC's may and do occur in many individuals with no demonstrable underlying pathology - they may occur as a consequence of drug toxicity - but in general, the prognosis is determined more by the cause of the PVC's than by the PVC's per se. Accelerated ventricular rhythm is observed most frequently in the acute phase of posterior or diaphragmatic infarction, is usually transient (hours to 1 or 2 days), and does not seem to forewarn of more catastrophic problems. Ventricular tachycardia occurs only rarely in an otherwise normal heart, and while rare patients do well despite recurrences, this rhythm nearly always constitutes a basis for aggressive therapy. Serious ventricular rhythms can be suppressed (or reduced) in a majority of instances, but while the benefit of therapy in acute settings is well-supported, efficacy of long-term antiarrhythmic therapy in an outpatient setting has been more challenging to establish.

VENTRICULAR ARRHYTHMIAS

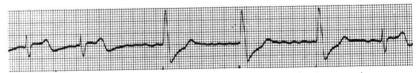

VENTRICULAR ESCAPE BEATS IN ATRIAL FIBRILLATION - These beats occur by "default" as the degree of junctional block is so great.

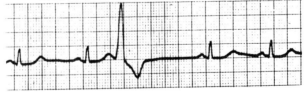

ISOLATED VPC - The third beat is early, wide, and there is a full compensatory pause.

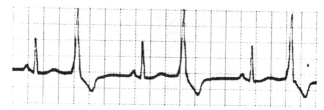

VENTRICULAR BIGEMINY - Every other beat is a VPC.

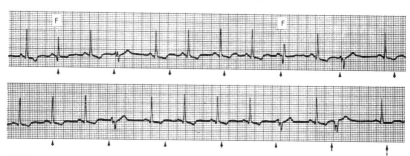

VENTRICULAR PARASYSTOLE - The interval from the normal beat to the VPC's is variable. Fusion beats are marked "F", and the interectopic interval measures exactly as marked by the arrows.

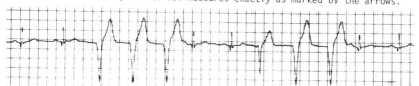

ACCELERATED VENTRICULAR RHYTHM (Slow ventricular tachycardia). The ventricular rate is 80 and the rhythm is initiated by a late VPC.

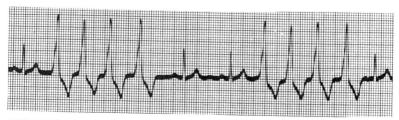

SHORT RUNS OF VENTRICULAR TACHYCARDIA. The rate is 130.

Selected Reference

1. Lindsay, A.E., and Budkin, A.: The Cardiac Arrhythmias, Year Book Medical Publishers, Inc., Chicago, 2nd edition, 1975, pp. 89-113.

HIS BUNDLE STUDIES AND PACEMAKERS

Benjamin Befeler, M.D.
Agustin Castellanos, M.D.

The classic ladder of Lewis which is frequently used in the analysis of cardiac arrhythmias has three steps which represent three levels of impulse conduction: atrial, AV nodal, and ventricular. A fourth step has been added as a result of the development of His bundle recordings. This new dimension in electrocardiography has permitted greater accuracy in evaluation of arrhythmias and conduction abnormalities.

The technique of His bundle recordings involves the transvenous introduction of a bipolar or tripolar catheter usually from the femoral vein, and its placement under fluoroscopic control in the area of the tricuspid valve. Recording the His deflections during the time when the surface electrocardiogram is electrically silent, i.e., PR interval, permits temporal measurements and identification of conduction times between the SA node, low atrial areas, AV node, and His-Purkinje system.

The following terminology is currently used for the deflections recorded on His bundle electrograms: A = atrial depolarization; H = His bundle deflections; V = ventricular depolarization; AH = AV nodal conduction; HV = His-Purkinje conduction. The normal value for AH or AV nodal conduction is 50 to 100 msec, and for HV or His-Purkinje conduction is 35 to 50 msec.

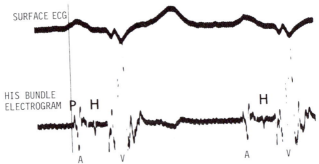

Different investigators have held different opinions as to the value of His bundle electrograms in clinical cardiology. Certainly, all would agree that this technique has clarified the interpretation of routine surface electrocardiograms, and that in selected individual patients, it is of significant clinical value.

His bundle electrocardiograms are useful in the accurate identification and evaluation of the following: 1) atrial, junctional and ventricular arrhythmias; 2) reciprocating tachycardias; 3) accessory pathways of AV conduction; 4) AV conduction abnormalities; 5) sick sinus syndrome. Antiarrhythmic drugs can now be tailored to individual requirements on a rational level not previously possible.

There are many types of pacemakers available today. The demand ventricular is, by far, the most frequently used. It has both a stimulating and sensing mechanism. The patient's own beats are recognized (sensed) by the intracavitary electrode and result in an inhibition of the pacemaker spike, i.e., it only fires on demand after a set interval during which no patient depolarization spike is sensed. Indications include AV block and electrical overdriving. The hazards of a ventricular pacemaker spike falling on the vulnerable period of the patient's own t wave and inducing repetitive firing led to the development of the demand pacemaker shown below.

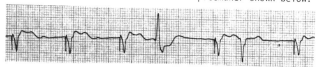

Continuous atrial pacing may be indicated in sinus arrest, S-A block and to electrically overdrive arrhythmias, as long as AV conduction is intact. It has the virtue of maintaining the atrial contribution to cardiac output and is shown below.

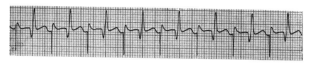

When AV conduction is not intact and in a clinical setting where atrial contraction is felt to be an important contribution to cardiac output, an atrioventricular (bifocal demand) pacemaker may be used as shown below.

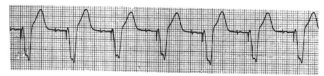

The following is a modification of the classification proposed by Schoenfeld and Bhardwaj of the indications for cardiac pacing. His bundle study may be helpful in several categories.

   A. Pacing for bradycardias

      1. Sick sinus node syndrome. Assessment of sinus node recovery after overdrive suppression may be helpful. Study is mostly for objective demonstration of SA node dysfunction, if data is not available from the surface ECG.

      2. Acquired heart block. When intermittent in a patient with syncope, His studies may uncover delay of His-Purkinje conduction if the QRS complex is normal.

B. Pacing with normal heart rates

In "bilateral bundle branch block" with intermittent "normal" A-V conduction in a patient with chronic disease, His bundle study may uncover further underlying disease.

C. Pacing for acute tachyarrhythmias

1. Supraventricular
2. W-P-W
3. Ventricular
His studies are useful and can be performed at the time of pacer insertion.

D. Acute myocardial infarction

In the presence of AV block with a slow ventricular rate, pacing is indicated in anterior infarction. In inferior infarction, pacing may or may not be necessary. In the presence of new right bundle branch block and either right or left axis deviation (left posterior and left anterior hemiblock respectively) pacing is desirable. There is controversy as to whether or not to pace patients with bifascicular block after acute infarction. Information is appearing which suggests that when the HV interval is prolonged under these circumstances, sudden death due to paroxymal A-V block may be prevented by permanent pacing. If this is the case a conduction study might provide very valuable information.

REFERENCES

1. Castellanos, A., Castillo, C.A., Agha, A.S., Befeler, B., Myerburg, R.J.: Functional properties of accessory AV pathways during premature atrial stimulation. Brit. Heart Journal. 35:578-584, 1973.

2. Fisch, C., Zipes, D.P.: His bundle electrocardiography. Am. Heart J. 86:289-291, 1973.

3. Narula, O.S.: Advances in Clinical Electrophysiology: Contribution of His bundle recordings. pp. 331-384. In Cardiac Pacing, Editor P. Samet. Grune and Stratton. New York, 1973.

4. Iyengar, R., Castellanos, A., Spence, M.E.: Continuous monitoring of Ambulatory patients with coronary disease. Prog. Card. Dis. 13:#4:392-404, 1971.

ELECTROCARDIOGRAPHY - ADVANCES

RHYTHM AND CONDUCTION DISTURBANCES IN ADOLESCENTS AND YOUNG ADULTS

Robert J. Myerburg, M.D.

Many of the rhythm and conduction abnormalities that occur with advancing age in the presence of ischemic or degenerative heart disease may also occur in adolescents and young adults. In addition, there are a group of disturbances, often of a relatively benign character, which are particularly prone to occur in younger individuals. The significance of any of these disturbances is determined, for the most part, by the setting in which they occur relative to underlying heart disease. In adolescents and young adults, a higher percentage of rhythm or conduction abnormalities are not associated with other evidence of organic heart disease. Frequently, abnormalities which are considered serious in older individuals carry a better prognosis in this age group. The recognition of specific disturbances and the determination of prognosis are important because they dictate the approach to management.

Supraventricular Arrhythmias

The supraventricular tachyarrhythmias as a group are among the most common rhythm disturbances in this population. In the overwhelming majority of patients these disturbances represent either a secondary reaction to a systemic problem or a primary cardiac rhythm disturbance which is disturbing, but not necessarily dangerous. However, in a few patients, the rate and associated symptoms are serious enough to warrant aggressive management. The differential diagnosis of rapid supraventricular tachycardias in the young include:

1) Sinus tachycardia
2) Paroxysmal supraventricular tachycardia
3) Paroxysmal atrial fibrillation
4) Ectopic atrial tachycardia
5) Atrial flutter.

The differential diagnosis may be made on the basis of an analysis of the combination of heart rate, atrial wave form morphology, and the response to carotid sinus massage or intravenous Tensilon. For example, paroxysmal supraventricular tachycardia (atrial or junctional) is a reentry or reciprocating rhythm where the impulse travels down through the junction, activating the ventricle and then reenters the supraventricular tissue, stimulating the next beat, i.e., due to varying conduction properties in dual electrical pathways, a reciprocating and self-perpetuating cycle is established so that a premature beat reenters the atrium at an early time, and is then conducted antegrade, producing another early ventricular beat. As such, carotid massage, by increasing vagal tone at the A-V node, will stop the arrhythmia (or have no effect), but will not merely slow the ventricular response. Ectopic atrial tachycardia (sometimes called PAT with block) is due to a protected irritable atrial focus which repetively discharges and drives the ventricles and hence, as in flutter and atrial fibrillation, carotid massage may slow the ventricular response, but not abolish the arrhythmia.

Paroxysmal supraventricular tachycardia and paroxysmal atrial fibrillation are the most common and the most likely to be benign. Paroxysmal supraventricular tachycardia requires a consideration of the presence of an abnormal bypass tract (Wolff-Parkinson-White syndrome or its variants). It may respond to nothing more than rest, sedation, and/or carotid sinus massage. In some instances digitalis or antiarrhythmic therapy may be required. Less common in the young otherwise normal adult is atrial flutter with 2:1 or 1:1 conduction. The latter is extremely rare, and anytime a supraventricular tachycardia at a rate of 150 is seen, the former (that is atrial flutter with 2:1 conduction) should be seriously considered. Depending upon the patient's response to the tachycardia, antiarrhythmic therapy or cardioversion may be considered. Ectopic atrial tachycardia in the absence of cardiac disease and/or digitalis therapy is unusual in young individuals. Rapid sinus tachycardia usually results from a secondary response to extra-cardiac or cardiac disease, but occasionally a tracing that appears to be a sinus tachycardia is in reality an ectopic atrial tachycardia or the more rare syndrome of sinus node reentry.

Ventricular Arrhythmias

Ventricular tachycardia in adolescents and young adults is unusual, but when it does occur, may carry a favorable prognosis, especially in women. There is a form of this arrhythmia in which there is continuous repetitive ventricular tachyarrhythmia in young individuals which is suppressed by increases in sinus rate, but is resistant to antiarrhythmic therapy. If it co-exists with organic heart disease, it is more serious. However, the problem may continue for many years without complications in the absence of organic heart disease. Premature ventricular contractions are usually benign in the absence of organic heart disease, even if they are frequent. The mechanism may be parasystolic or fixed coupling. Both premature beats and runs of ventricular tachycardia must be considered more serious in the presence of other cardiac abnormalities, especially cardiomyopathy or premature atherosclerotic heart disease in this age group.

Conduction Disturbances

Among the conduction disorders seen in adolescents and young adults, the Wenchkebach phenomenon in the A-V node is relatively common. It may occur in the presence or absence of organic heart disease in this age group. It may be associated with acute febrile illness, with or without actual cardiac involvement, as may first degree A-V block. When it is not a reflection of cardiac disease, it frequently disappears with changes in position. Intracardiac conduction abnormalities may be related to viral myocarditis, and more rarely to specific viral involvement of the specialized conducting system. These abnormalities may be quite serious and require long-term pacing. Sino-atrial block in the young does not carry the same connotation as it does in the elderly, in which setting it usually reflects underlying sinus node disease. In the young, it may be related to an autonomic imbalance transiently noted when digitalis is used, or may occur in pericarditis. In young children, it occasionally occurs as an isolated finding.

Selected Reference

1. Marriott, H. J. L., Myerburg, R. J.: Recognition and Treatment of Cardiac Arrhythmias and Conduction Disturbances, Hurst, et. al., The Heart, McGraw Hill, New York, 1974

DIAGNOSIS AND MEDICAL MANAGEMENT OF PRE-EXCITATION SYNDROMES

Hein J.J. Wellens, M.D.

Types of Pre-Excitation

The four possible pathways short-circuiting the specific atrioventricular conduction system and their electrocardiographic characteristics are listed in Table 1. It is not possible to give absolute values for the P-delta interval or QRS width for the different types of pre-excitation because these values will depend upon the site of impulse formation in the atrium, the site of take-off of the accessory connection, the length of the accessory connection, and its site of insertion into the ventricle.

The presence of an accessory pathway has two important consequences:

1) It frequently (all but Type 3 of Table 1) short-circuits part or all of the A-V node which in the case of a short refractory period of the accessory pathway, can lead to very high ventricular rates if atrial fibrillation or atrial flutter occur.

2) Together with the normal A-V conduction system, it may constitute a pathway for a rapidly circulating (reciprocating) impulse, resulting in tachycardia.

The introduction of programmed electrical stimulation of the heart enables us:

1) To classify pre-excitation according to type.

2) To study the properties of the accessory pathway.

3) To study mechanisms of tachycardia, and

4) To study the effect of drugs on 2 and 3 above.

From these studies we learned that as far as pre-excitation in an atrioventricular direction is concerned, a true accessory atrioventricular pathway (a Kent bundle) is the most common form of pre-excitation (125 of 131 patients with pre-excitation consecutively studied). Symptomatic Mahaim (junction ventricular) fibers are rare (5 of 131 patients). True A-V nodal bypass tracts are extremely rare (1 of 131 patients).

In approximately 40% of our patients with a Kent bundle, this structure had, in the A-V direction, a shorter refractory period than that of the A-V node. The length of the refractory period of the Kent bundle is an important determinant of the ventricular rate if atrial fibrillation occurs. By measuring the length of the refractory period of the Kent bundle, it is therefore possivle to identify patients at risk when atrial fibrillation supervenes.

The most common mechanism of tachycardia in pre-excitation is a circus movement with antegrade conduction over the A-V node - His pathway and retrograde conduction over the extra connection. This circus movement tachycardia is usually initiated by a premature beat which creates unidirectional block in one pathway, is exclusively conducted over the other pathway, followed by return to the chamber of origin of the premature beat via the pathway which was blocked at its other end. Perpetuation of this movement results in tachycardia.

Effect of Drugs on Pre-Excitation

In patients with the WPW syndrome, the effect of several drugs on the electrophysiologic properties of atrium, A-V node, H-V interval, accessory pathway and ventricle has been studied (Table 2). During these studies, it has become clear that although general conclusions can be made as to the acute effect of a certain drug on the electrophysiologic properties of the different parts of the tachycardia circuit, the outcome on the arrhythmia can vary considerably in the individual patients.

Factors which play a role are:

1) The size of the tachycardia circuit.

   When a circus movement tachycardia is present, the tachycardia will stop when the product of the mean conduction velocity of the circulating wave and the mean refractory period of the different components of the tachycardia pathway exceeds the length of the tachycardia circuit. Most drugs, however, have a twofold action: on the one hand beneficial (like prolongation of the length of the refractory period of components of the tachycardia circuit); and on the other hand unfavorable (by slowing conduction of the circulatory wave). The net effect of the drug will depend upon the interplay of these changes in relation to the size of the tachycardia circuit.

2) Dissimilar effects of drugs in the A-V and V-A direction

   The effect of a drug on the properties of the accessory pathway in the A-V direction may be quite different from that in the V-A direction.

   The disappearance of the signs of pre-excitation during sinus rhythm following drug administration does not guarantee that conduction over the accessory pathway is no longer possible in a ventriculo-atrial direction and that the patient is cured of his circus movement tachycardia.

3) Effect following acute versus chronic drug administration

   During the study of the effect of drugs in patients with the WPW syndrome, the drug is usually given intravenously or intraatrially over a short period of time. This may result in pharmacodynamics different from those following chronic oral drug administration. This can be the reason for failure of therapy when the drug, which was found to be highly effective when given intravenously, is given orally.

During studies following rapid intravenous administration it also became apparent that the effect of several drugs was shorter than previously assumed. This suggests that failure of oral drug administration may be caused by a dosage schedule that is too widely spread, and suggests the use of long-acting drug preparations when available.

Treatment of Arrhythmias in the WPW Syndrome

1) Drug treatment should only be given when the arrhythmia interferes with the physical and/or psychological well being of the patient.

2) Contributing factors like valvular heart disease, coronary heart disease or sick sinus syndrome should be identified, and when possible, corrected.

3) For prevention of the tachycardia initiating premature beat, quinidine, preferably given as a long-acting preparation, is still the drug of choice.

4) Drug treatment during tachycardia should depend upon the site of origin, type of tachycardia and electrophysiologic properties of the structure involved during tachycardia. Lengthening of the refractory period or block in the accessory pathway can usually be accomplished by procaine amide, quinidine, disopyramide, amiodarone or ajmaiine. Tachycardias based upon a circus movement incorporating the accessory pathway can frequently be controlled by administration of these drugs. When possible, long-acting agents should be given to minimize changes in drug levels. When combinations of drugs must be used, a drug should preferably be given which prevents ectopic activity and lengthens the refractory period of the accessory pathway, like quinidine, plus an agent which lengthens the refractory period of the A-V node like a beta-blocking agent. If, during atrial fibrillation or flutter, a short refractory period of the accessory pathway is present, acute control of the ventricular rate can usually be accomplished by intravenous procaine amide or ajmaline.

Selected References

1. Wellens, H.J.J.: Contribution of Cardiac Pacing to Our Understanding of the Wolff-Parkinson-White Syndrome. Brit. Heart J., 37:229, 1975.

2. Wellens, H.J.J.: Effect of Drugs on Wolff-Parkinson-White Syndrome and Its Therapy. In: His Bundle Electrocardiography and Clinical Electrophysiology. Ed. by Narula, O., F.A. Davis, Philadelphia, 1975.

TABLE I - TYPES OF PRE-EXCITATION

Name	Other Name(s)	Anatomy		ECG
1. Accessory atrio-ventricular pathway	Kent bundle WPW syndrome	Direct connection between atrium and ventricle	KENT	Delta wave short P-delta interval increased QRS width
2. Nodo-ventricular accessory connection	Mahaim fiber	Fiber connecting A-V node with ventricular myocardium	MAHAIM	Small delta wave P-delta interval longer than WPW QRS width less than WPW
3. Fasciculo-ventricular accessory conduction	Mahaim fiber	Fiber connecting the penetrating or the branching part of the bundle of His with ventricular myocardium		
4. A-V nodal bypass tract	James fiber LGL syndrome	Pathway connecting atrium with penetrating part of bundle of His or short circuit within the A-V node	JAMES	Short PR interval Normal QRS width

TABLE 2

EFFECT OF DRUGS ON THE REFRACTORY PERIOD AND CONDUCTION VELOCITY OF THE DIFFERENT PARTS OF THE HEART IN PATIENTS WITH THE WPW SYNDROME

Length of the Effective Refractory Period

	Atr.	AV node	His-Purkinje	Ventr.	Acc.P.
Digitalis	±	+	?	±	-
Procaine Amide	+	0	+	+	+
Quinidine	+	±	+	+	+
Ajmaline	+	0	+	+	+
Diphenylhydantoin	±	-	-	±	±
Atropine	0	-	?	0	0
Propranolol	±	+	?	±	0
Lidocaine	±	0	?	+	+
Verapamil	±	+	?	±	±
Amiodarone	+	+	+	+	+
Disopyramide	+	±	0	+	+

+ = lengthened, "-" = shortened, 0 = no change, ± = inconsistent, ? = not known

Conduction velocity

	Atr.	AV node	His-Purkinje	Ventr.	Acc.P.
Digitalis	±	-	?	±	?
Procaine Amide		±	-	-	?
Quinidine	-	±	-	-	?
Ajmaline	-	±	-	-	?
Diphenylhydantoin	±	+	0	+	?
Atropine	0	+	0	0	0
Propranolol	-	-	0	-	?
Lidocaine	-	±	?	±	?
Verapamil	0	-	0	0	?
Amiodarone	-	-	-	-	?
Disopyramide	-	0	0	0	-

+ = increased, "-" = decreased, 0 = no change, ± = inconsistent, ? = not known

SURGICAL AND PACEMAKER THERAPY OF SUPRAVENTRICULAR TACHYARRHYTHMIAS

Andrew G. Wallace, M.D.

Paroxysmal supraventricular arrhythmias include atrial fibrillation, atrial flutter, atrial tachycardia, junctional tachycardia and other disturbances less common than the above. Frequently, such disturbances of rhythm arise because of diffuse involvement of the atrial chambers by processes such as rheumatic carditis and pericardial disease, or they may arise because of atrial distension secondary to processes which primarily involve the ventricles and which lead to congestive heart failure. Examples of the latter would include acute myocardial infarction,ischemic cardiomyopathy and hypertension.

In other instances which occur with significant frequency, these same arrhythmias may be present in the absence of heart failure, associated with localized rather than diffuse atrial disease, or perhaps conditioned by a congenital abnormality such as the Wolff-Parkinson-White Syndrome or selective disorders involving the sinus node region. In the latter instance, it is well established that a feature of sinus node disease is the propensity of such patients to have paroxysmal atrial dysrhythmias such as PAT, flutter or fibrillation.

Fortunately, in most patients, traditional pharmacologic measures are adequate to either prevent the paroxysm of tachycardia or to control the ventricular rate within accepted limits in the event of an atrial dysrhythmia. Occasionally, pharmacologic methods fail, or they may even exaggerate the severity of the arrhythmia, or it may be sufficiently life-threatening to warrant consideration of a more definitive approach to precluding its occurence or controlling the ventricular rate.

Historically, it is of interest to note that removal of thoracic sympathetic ganglia was first reported to be effective in the control of difficult supraventricular arrhythmias as early as 1930. In the 1950's, it became clear that paroxysmal ventricular tachyarrhythmias occurring in patients with AV block could be prevented by accelerating the ventricular rate by pacing, and current experience supports the view that atrial pacing in patients with sinus bradycardia can reduce the frequency of paroxysmal atrial tachyarrhythmias. It was also demonstrated in the 1960's that atrial stimulation could sometimes terminate reentrant atrial tachycardias and that rapid atrial pacing, faster than the inherent atrial tachycardia, could lead to higher degrees of AV block (through concealment), and thus lower the ventricular rate. Finally, it was demonstrated even more recently that electrophysiological techniques could be used to define localized areas of atrial disease, ablation of which abolished arrhythmias, and that accessory pathways responsible for the tachyarrhythmias associated with the Wolff-Parkinson-White Syndrome and its variants could be identified and surgically divided with abolishment of the arrhythmias.

Thus, today, there are several surgical approaches to the treatment of life-threatening or medically resistant supraventricular arrhythmias. These include:

1) Ablation of the focus responsible for the arrhythmia
2) Division of accessory pathways
3) Cardiac sympathectomy
4) Atrial pacing to prevent tachyarrhythmias
5) Atrial pacing to terminate tachyarrhythmias
6) Atrial or ventricular pacing to preclude bradycardia in the bradycardia-tachycardia syndrome (sinus node disease)
7) Division of the His bundle

There is sufficient evidence now to indicate that these approaches have considerable promise in carefully selected patients and that some may be the preferred approach in selected instances. In only a few cases, however, is the available experience sufficiently great to see clearly the ultimate role and utility of such approaches. Our own view, however, is that surgical approaches will become established as an effective and useful therapy for the control of supraventricular tachyarrhythmias, particularly those which are resistant to medical means and which occur in patients with little or no compromise of ventricular function.

Selected References

1. Gallagher, J.J., Gilbert, M., Svenson, R.H., Sealy, W.C., Kassell, J., and Wallace, A.G.: Wolff-Parkinson-White Syndrome: The Problem, Evaluation and Surgical Correction. Circ., 51:83, 1975.

2. Davidson, R.M., Wallace, A.G., Sealy, W.C., and Gordon, M.S.: Electrically Induced Atrial Tachycardia with Block. Circ., 44:1014, 1971.

3. Haft, J.I., Kosowsky, B.D., Lau, S.H., Stein, E., Damato, A.N.: Termination of Atrial Flutter by Rapid Electrical Pacing. Circ., 36:637, 1967.

4. School, S.F., Wallace, A.G., Sealy, W.C.: Protective Influence of Cardiac Denervation Against Arrhythmias of Myocardial Infarction. Cardiovascular Research, 3:241, 1969.

5. Aroesty, J.M., Cohen, S.I., Morkui, E.: Bradycardia Tachycardia Syndrome; Combined Pharmacological and Pacemaker Therapy. Chest, 66:257, 1974.

6. Moss, J., Roberts, J.: Bradycardia-Tachycardia Syndrome. Prog. in Cardiovasc. Dis., 16:459, 1974.

TACHYCARDIA AND BRADYCARDIA DEPENDENT CONDUCTION DISORDERS

Nabil El-Sherif, M.D.

Many cases of atrio-ventricular (AV) and intra-ventricular (IV) conduction disorders are rate dependent, with the conduction disorder usually associated with either acceleration of the heart rate (tachycardia-dependent) or slowing of the rate (bradycardia-dependent). It is of some significance to remember that in tachycardia-dependent conduction disorders, the abnormality appears at "higher" but not necessarily "high" rates. Thus, a bundle branch block pattern that appears when the sinus rate increases from 70-75 beats/min. is tachycardia-dependent, although a sinus rate of 75/min. is not considered a tachycardia by conventional definition. The same thing is true for bradycardia-dependent conduction disorders. Rate dependent IV conduction disorders usually present in the form of a bundle branch block pattern while AV conduction disorders can take the form of first, second or third degree blocks.

Tachycardia-Dependent Conduction Disorders

Tachycardia-dependent AV and IV conduction disorders are considered consistent with known electrophysiological characteristics of the conduction system when they develop at very short cardiac cycles. Thus, a bundle branch block pattern that develops in early coupled supraventricular premature beats and rapid supraventricular tachyarrhythmias is not considered pathological since the short cycle lengths can approach the normal effective refractory period of the bundle branch system. Usually, an aberration of the right bundle branch block pattern is seen in these cases which reflects a longer effective refractory period of the right bundle branch system compared to the left bundle. It is also a physiological observation that A-V nodal conduction delay and block can develop at very short cycle lengths. In contrast to physiological tachycardia-dependent blocks, a pathological tachycardia-dependent conduction disorder is said to be present when the abnormality develops at relatively long cycle lengths or in other words, at relatively slow heart rates (usually between 50-100/min.). In these cases, a pathological prolongation of the effective refractory period of the conduction system is presumed. Probably the most serious clinical consequence of pathological tachycardia-dependent conduction disorders is the so-called tachycardia-dependent paroxysmal A-V block. The latter may be defined as the sudden occurrence of repetitive block of the atrial impulse during 1:1 A-V conduction (or occasionally 2:1 A-V block), resulting in a transient total interruption of A-V conduction. The onset of the arrhythmia is usually associated with a period of ventricular asystole before the return of conduction or the escape of a subsidiary pacemaker. This period of ventricular asystole, often exaggerated by delayed escape rhythms frequently dramatizes the clinical picture of the arrhythmia. Recent experimental and clinical observations have shown that paroxysmal A-V block following acute myocardial infarction is frequently a tachycardia-dependent phenomenon. The lesion is commonly localized in the His-Purkinje system and the paroxysmal A-V block is temporally associated with the occurrence of second degree A-V block with a minimal increase in conduction delay (so called "Mobitz II" block). In patients with acute myocardial infarction, paroxysmal A-V block may occur on acceleration of the sinoatrial rate, either spontaneously or induced by drugs given for varied therapeutic indications (e.g., atropine sulfate or isoprenaline). (See Figure 1). These observations underscore the potential clinical consequences of rapid atrial rates in patients with acute myocardial ischemia and type II A-V block.

Bradycardia-Dependent Conduction Disorders

In the past, bradycardia-dependent conduction disorders were considered a rare finding. Recent experimental and clinical observations have shown, however, that bradycardia-dependent bundle branch block as well as A-V block are not uncommon. Interestingly enough, several examples of rate-dependent bundle branch block revealed the concurrent development of tachycardia-dependent and bradycardia-dependent block with normal intraventricular conduction at intermediate heart rates. This is shown in Figure 2 which illustrates a rate-dependent left bundle branch block. The record reveals that the bundle branch block pattern develops at cycle lengths shorter than 90 msec. (tachycardia-dependent block) or longer than 152 msec. (bradycardia-dependent block) while normal IV conduction is present at intermediate cycle lengths.

As with tachycardia-dependent conduction disorders, bradycardia-dependent paroxysmal A-V block has the most serious clinical consequences. In these cases intermittent complete A-V block develops at critically long R-R cycles either due to sinus slowing or following the compensatory pause of a premature ectopic beat. Normal conduction usually resumes only after a ventricular escape beat when a subsequent P wave falls within the normal conduction range (see Figure 3). It should be emphasized, however, that the majority of clinical examples of paroxysmal A-V block are tachycardia-dependent and not bradycardia-dependent.

Mechanism

The electrophysiological mechanism for tachycardia-dependent conduction disorders developing at very short cycle lengths is an impulse spread through incompletely repolarized fibers, usually during the latter part of phase 3 of the membrane action potential. Pathological tachycardia-dependnet conduction disorders cannot be explained by impulse spread before completion of repolarization, because this would entail the presence of markedly prolonged action potential durations. However, it has been recently shown that depressed muscle and Purkinje cells can exhibit post-repolarization refractoriness which means that the duration of complete recovery of excitability is greater than that of the action potential. These fibers primarily show a time-dependent rather than a voltage-dependent response to cycle length changes. This response, which is somewhat similar to the normal response of some cells in the sinoatrial and atrioventricular nodes, can adequately explain cases of pathological tachycardia-dependent conduction disorders.

On the other hand, bradycardia-dependent conduction disorders were previously often ascribed to a mechanism of enhanced phase 4 depolarization. Recent observations, however, suggest a more complex electrophysiological mechanism for bradycardia-dependent blocks which does not entail an enhanced diastolic depolarization.

In conclusion, one should be aware of the fact that the observation of an IV of AV conduction disorder in a casual ECG record does not necessarily mean the presence of a permanent conduction defect. Slight slowing of the heart rate may result in normal conduction, thus unravelling a tachycardia-dependent conduction disorder. Occasionally, slight acceleration of the rate may normalize conduction, thus revealing the presence of a bradycardia-dependent block. Thus, as a rule, unless the conduction defect is shown to persist at a wide range of heart rates, a rate-dependent disorder cannot be excluded.

Figure 1

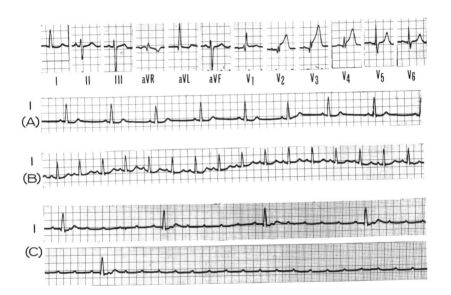

Tachycardia-dependent paroxysmal A-V block following isoprenaline infusion with marked acceleration of the sinus rate. The top record illustrates the patient's 12-lead standard electrocardiogram on admission, showing right bundle branch block, left axis deviation, and acute anteroseptal myocardial infarction. Panel A illustrates the patient's cardiac rhythm on admission and reveals sinus bradycardia at a rate of 48 beats/min. The rhythm strip in panel B was obtained shortly after the start of isoprenaline infusion and shows an increase of the sinus rate to 95 beats/min. with 1:1 A-V conduction. Panel C illustrates the development of sinus tachycardia (130 beats/min.) with a high grade A-V block that terminated in complete A-V block and a prolonged ventricular asystole.

Figure 2

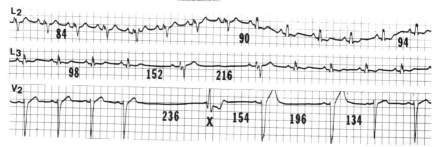

Tachycardia and bradycardia dependent left bundle branch block. "X" represents a ventricular escape beat.

Figure 3

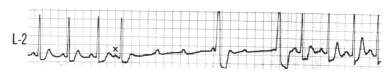

Bradycardia-dependent paroxysmal A-V block following an atrial premature beat (marked "X").

Selected References

1. El-Sherif, N.: Tachycardia and Bradycardia Dependent Bundle Branch Block After Acute Myocardial Ischemia. Brit. Heart J., 36:291, 1974.

2. El-Sherif, N., Scherlag, B.J., Lazzara, R., Hope, R., Williams, D.O., Samet, P.: The Pathophysiology of Tachycardia-Dependent Paroxysmal Atrioventricular Block After Acute Myocardial Ischemia. Experimental and Clinical Observations. Circ., 50:515, 1974.

CURRENT STATUS OF STRESS TESTING AND CARDIAC REHABILITATION

David S. Sheps, M.D.

The resting electrocardiogram is helpful in correlating clinical symptoms and physical findings with underlying coronary artery disease only if the electrocardiogram is positive for the presence of ischemic heart disease. A normal electrocardiogram should not be used as evidence to rule out a cardiac etiology for chest pain. The objectives of exercise testing are:

1) to establish a diagnosis of overt or latent heart disease

2) to evaluate cardiovascular functional capacity, particularly as a means of clearing individuals for strenuous work or exercise programs

3) to evaluate responses to conditioning and/or preventive programs

4) to increase individual motivation for entering and adhering to exercise programs.

Several precautions should be taken before exercise testing. A history should always be taken and a physical examination and resting electrocardiogram should be performed before the test. Contraindications to exercise testing include a recent myocardial infarction (less than 2 months), a recent worsening of angina pectoris, acute non-cardiac illness, and uncontrolled arrhythmia of a severe nature. There are numerous relative contraindications.

FIGURE I

CONTRAINDICATIONS TO EXERCISE TESTING

Cardiovascular	Others
Rapidly progressing angina Impending infarction Massive ventricular aneurysm Dangerous arrhythmia Fixed ventricular rate pacemaker Untreated atrial fibrillation Uncontrolled hypertension Acute myocarditis	Uncontrolled diabetes mellitus, thyrotoxicosis Disabling skeletal-muscle disorders Recent pulmonary embolism Severe pulmonary hypertension Severe electrolyte imbalance Acute infectious disease

The exercise test should always be supervised by a physician and resuscitation equipment should always be at hand. Constant oscilloscopic monitoring of the electrocardiogram during exercise and initial recovery increases the safety of the procedure. The test should be interrupted with the occurence of one of the following signs:

1) Occurence of three or more consecutive premature ventricular beats
2) Onset of an ataxic gait, or
3) Progressive hypotension

The mortality attributed to exercise testing is reported at less than 1 in 10,000 tests. This mortality was not related to the intensity of the exercise test.

Methods of Exercise Testing

Exercise tests are basically divided into single-stage and multi-stage tests. Single stage tests are best typified by the Masters' 2-Step Test, which is well known to all physicians. The exercise consists of walking up and down two steps for one and a half minutes (single test) or three minutes (double test). The major disadvantage of single stage tests is lack of standardization based on myocardial oxygen requirements. The variability of the relative work load imposed on the subject results in a wide range of heart rate responses. For example, the peak heart rate during the double-step test varied between 105 and 192 beats per minute. Therefore, the stress to the myocardium varies depending on the patient's condition and weight. In addition, the double Masters' test provides a lower incidence of positive electrocardiographic findings in patients with documented coronary artery disease. Nevertheless, since it is an easy test to perform, it still is used widely as a screening procedure. The heart rate response, however, should be taken into account in interpreting the electrocardiographic response to this test.

Multi-stage tests are now the method of choice in exercise testing since the intensity of exercise and its endpoint are adjusted to each patient's capacity so that the stress to the myocardium is similar for all subjects. As long as the heart rate is taken into account, the choice of the particular type of exercise is not critical and the bicycle ergometer or the treadmill can be used. The endpoint of the test may be predetermined, i.e., the exercise is stopped when a target heart rate has been reached, or the subject is asked to exercise up to his maximal limits. The target heart rate is usually 80 to 90 per cent of the maximal heart rate. The advantage of maximal exercise testing is that maximal tests provide a higher incidence of positive electrocardiographic findings and the physical work capacity of the subject can be measured.

FIGURE II

TARGET HEART RATE (BEATS/MINUTE) IN MULTISTAGE EXERCISE TESTS

Age Group	Lester et al. (1967, 1968)*	Scandinavian Committee
20-29	175	170
30-39	170	160
40-49	166	150
50-59	162	140
60-69	158	130

* These values correspond to 90% of the predicted maximal heart rate. (After Detry)

The protocol in use in the exercise laboratory at the University of Miami-Jackson Memorial Hospital is Bruce's multi-stage treadmill test which includes seven levels of exercise of increasing severity. Each stage lasts three minutes and the intensity of the exercise is increased every three minutes without interruption of the test by changing both the grade and the speed of the treadmill. With this procedure, it is therefore possible to test both limited patients and trained athletes according to the same protocol in a short time. Figure III is a description of Bruce's treadmill test.

FIGURE III

STAGE	SPEED	GRADE	MINUTES*
Rest	0	0	0
I	1.7 mph	10%	3
II	2.5 mph	12%	6
III	3.4 mph	14%	9
IV	4.2 mph	16%	12
V	5.0 mph	18%	15
VI	5.5 mph	20%	18
VII	6.0 mph	22%	21

* Each stage is 3 minutes long

Interpretation

Many different lead systems are used and there is no question that increasing the number of leads recorded and recording the electrocardiogram during exercise enhances the diagnostic sensitivity of exercise electrocardiography. Criteria for interpretation of exercise electrocardiograms also vary, depending upon the sensitivity and specificity that is desired. Specificity means that the finding is rarely or never demonstrated by normal subjects, while sensitivity refers to the percentage of patients with coronary artery disease that exhibit the phenomenon. The term "ischemic ST depression" refers to any horizontal or downsloping depression of the ST segment. Most authors now require an ischemic ST depression greater than or equal to 1 mm. in order to consider the response abnormal. The overall sensitivity of an ST segment depression greater than or equal to 1 mm. during or after near maximal exercise was 78%. The specificity of this type of test is satisfactory since the percentage of false positive responders was only 11%.

FIGURE IV

TYPES OF ST-T CHANGES IN EXERCISE TESTS

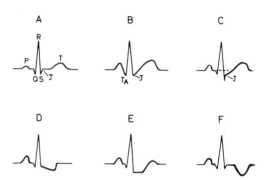

A. Normal electrocardiogram at rest. B. False junctional (J) ST segment depression due to atrial T wave (T_A) C. True junctional ST segment depression. D. Ischemic ST segment depression: sloping down. E. Ischemic ST depression - horizontal. F. Isolated T wave inversion. (After Simpson)

Limitations

Several factors other than the presence of coronary artery disease itself may influence the exercise electrocardiogram. A high percentage of patients with rheumatic heart disease have been reported to have positive exercise tests. These changes were apparently not due to digitalis. Since most of these studies were done in young subjects, the presence of coronary artery disease is unlikely. However, the studies did not include coronary arteriographic data. A possible explanation for these findings is that increased left ventricular work and poor adaptation of cardiac output to exercise caused functional myocardial ischemia without obstructive coronary disease. Hypertension is an important risk factor which is associated with a higher incidence of positive electrocardiographic responses to exercise. This increased incidence of positive responders is even more remarkable when the resting cardiogram is normal. The interpretation of such changes when the cardiogram shows evidence of LV strain is fraught with difficulty since it is not known whether further ST depression occurring on exercise indicates simply an accentuation of the left ventricular strain or the occurrence of myocardial ischemia. Various drugs are known to have an effect on the exertional electrocardiogram. Nitroglycerin decreases heart volume, probably primarily by peripheral venous pooling, both at rest and during exercise. This decreased heart volume during exercise with nitroglycerin certainly contributes to lessening of the depression of the ST segment. In coronary patients, the diagnostic sensitivity of exercise testing will be decreased if the test is performed less than one to two hours after absorption of this drug.

Beta-blocking agents such as propranolol tend to decrease the amount of ST segment depression at the anginal threshold. The mechanism of this action is not completely understood, but nevertheless, it is essential to consider the possible role of this drug in the interpretation of the exertional ECG. Digitalis causes false positive electrocardiographic responses to exercise. These false positive responses can also occur in subjects whose resting electrocardiograms do not show digitalis induced ST segment changes. Therefore, interpretation of the exercise electrocardiogram in a patient taking digitalis is difficult, and ideally, the drug should be stopped before diagnostic exercise testing. Hyperventilation can cause false positive "ischemic" type ST depressions. This has been reported in as many as 15% of patients with normal coronaries and chest pain. In contrast, only 3% of patients with angiographic coronary disease had hyperventilation induced ischemic changes. For this reason, we now routinely include hyperventilation at rest as part of our testing protocol. Physical training has certain predictable effects on the exercise electrocardiogram. At any given level of submaximal exercise, the magnitude of ST segment depression is decreased after physical training. However, the relationship between ST segment depression during exercise and the pressure rate product is unchanged. This suggests that modification of the ECG response to exercise is mainly due to changes in heart rate and blood pressure from physical training rather than to an improved coronary circulation.

Cardiac Rehabilitation

Physical training has been used in the treatment and rehabilitation of coronary patients and its beneficial effects are well known. There are many different types of programs throughout the country, but the basic principles remain the same. For the rehabilitation of the post-myocardial infarction patient the program should be started in the Coronary Care Unit with the prevention of deconditioning and gradual education of the patient throughout his convalescence until the time when he is ready to enter an organized cardiac rehabilitation program for post-myocardial infarction patients. Two months should be allowed after myocardial infarction before the patient is admitted to a regular physical training program. Contraindications to physical training include refractory heart failure, numerous and multifocal premature ventricular beats which increase with exercise, high degree heart block, or a large ventricular aneurysm. The basic objective of a physical training program is to increase the VO_2 max. which is the highest oxygen uptake the individual can obtain during physical work. The intensity of the training program will depend on the individual patient involved taking into account the initial exercise test data which always should be available. The training heart rate should be at least 60% of the submaximal heart rate for that particular patient. If symptoms permit, in patients with exertional angina pectoris, the intensity of the training should be just below the anginal threshold. The patient should be encouraged to use nitroglycerin prophylactically. The program should be progressive and intensity should be frequently adjusted according to the patient's subjective feelings and objective measurements of his physical work capacity. The optimal frequency for such sessions is two to three times a week for sessions lasting 45 to 60 minutes each. Exercise should consist of a warm-up period, a stimulus or training period, and a cool-down period. The warm-up permits gradual circulatory adjustment to exercise. The stimulus period should last 15 to 30 minutes for training effect and exercise should be dynamic. It does not matter what types of exercises are used as long as large muscle groups are utilized.

Some programs use only the bicycle ergometer, while others combine several exercises such as walking, jogging, running, calisthenics, cycling or rowing. Isometric exercises should be avoided because they cause a disproportionate blood pressure elevation. The cooling off period provides a gradual tapering of exercise to avoid sudden decreases in venous return which could cause syncope. Reassessment is generally carried out at 12 weeks after the beginning of an exercise program to determine if a training effect has occured. If physical conditioning has occurred by this time, the patient may then need more strenuous exercise to obtain his target heart rate. If at all possible, it is better to monitor the first training sessions to assure the anticipated physiologic response to the exercise. This may be done by using electrocardiographic methods (telemetry or rhythm strips recorded from defibrillator paddles), or clinically by taking the pulse. After this, the patient should be taught to take his own pulse. Exercises should be pleasurable and should not be inordinately expensive. Competition should be discouraged. Trained personnel and equipment readily available for emergency use are mandatory in this type of program. There have been several reported incidences of exertional ventricular fibrillation occurring in this setting. All of those patients were successfully resuscitated and none went on to experience myocardial infarction. Supervisors should be trained, highly motivated individuals such as physical educators and physical therapists. Education in the physiology of exercise and how it relates to the participants should be an integral part of the program. The exact role of the physician at the sessions depends upon the level of training of ancillary personnel and the extent of personal commitment of the supervising physician. However, it is generally accepted that an effective cardiac rehabilitation program should have a physician present at all sessions. Maximum participant feedback should be encouraged. This can be stimulated through various methods such as an ongoing system of record keeping which the patient fills out himself so that he can see the visual results of his training in terms of changes in heart rate, duration of exercise, etc.

The benefits of a cardiac rehabilitation program are multiple. It is important to communicate with each patient individually and to try to find out what his goals are, since some patients may have unrealistic goals from the outset. However, generally speaking, it is safe to say that a cardiac rehabilitation program will decrease the frequency of anginal attacks with exertion, or at least raise the level of exertion required to precipitate these attacks, and will improve the subject's outlook psychologically. These effects of a chronic exercise program are based on certain observed phenomena occurring after physical conditioning. These include an increase in physical work capacity, a decrease in the blood pressure at rest and comparable levels of work, a decrease in the heart rate a rest and comparable levels of work, a decrease in myocardial oxygen demand (heart rate times blood pressure product at rest and at work), and an altered life style in terms of modification of other risk factors. The main factor influencing the extent of training is the intensity of the effort, with the frequency and the duration exerting lesser effects.

It is important to reemphasize that a rehabilitation program should be an ongoing activity since it is well known that most circulatory parameters return to pre-training levels after a few weeks of detraining. The previously mentioned effects of physical training on well described parameters are well known and widely accepted. However, the mechanism of action of training is not yet well understood. For example, the effect of training on heart volume and myocardial contractility has not been measured. Neither is it known if there is any effect of physical training in coronary patients on collateral circulation or progression of disease, or for that matter, longevity. It is known that the short term prognosis of coronary heart disease is not worsened by training. Some suggest an improvement of this prognosis. Studies to answer this question are difficult to design because one must account for the improvement in other risk factors associated with a training program which usually occurs, such as cessation of smoking, better medical management, etc. Likewise, it is not known whether there is any preventive effect of physical training programs as applied to clinically normal healthy subjects.

In conclusion, much remains to be known about exercise training programs, both in normal people and in coronary heart disease patients. But, at this point in time, it is reasonable to recommend exercise training to those patients who would be receptive to it purely on the basis of an improved outlook on life which almost universally accompanies it.

Selected References

1. Bruce, R.A.: Exercise Testing of Patients with Coronary Heart Disease. Principles and Normal Standards for Evaluation. Ann. Clin. Res., 3:323-332, 1971.

2. Detry, Jean-Marie R.: Exercise Testing and Training in Coronary Heart Disease. William and Wilkins, 1973.

3. Hegge, F.N., Tuna, N., Burchell, H.B.: Coronary Arteriographic Findings in Patients with Axis Shifts or ST-Segment Elevations on Exercise-Stress Testing. Am. Heart Journal, 86:603-615, 1973.

4. Lary, D., Goldschlager, N.: Electrocardiographic Changes During Hyper-Ventilation Resembling Myocardial Ischemia in Patients with Normal Coronary Arteriograms. Am. Heart Journal, 87:383-390, 1974.

5. Rosig, D.R., Reichek, N., Perloff, J.K.: The Exercise Test as a Diagnostic and Therapeutic Aid. Am. Heart Journal, 87:584-596, 1974.

6. Bruce, R.A.: Progress in Exercise Cardiology. Progress in Cardiology, ed. by Yu, D.N., Goodwin, J.F., Lea and Febifer, pp. 113-172, 1974.

7. Zohman, L.R., Cardiac Rehabilitation: Its Role in Evaluation and Management of the Patient with Coronary Heart Disease. Am. Heart Journal, 85:706-710, 1973.

8. Redwood, D.R., Rosing D.R., et al.: Circulation and Symptomatic Effects of Physical Training in Patients with Coronary Artery Disease and Angina Pectoris. N. Engl. J. Med., 286:959-965, 1972.

CORONARY ARTERY DISEASE AND ACUTE MYOCARDIAL INFARCTION

AN OVERVIEW

H. J. C. Swan, M.D.

1. Disease in a major coronary artery which occludes from 60 to 80% of the cross sectional area of that vessel will produce a reduction in blood flow at rest or a serious limitation in the maximal flow possible in the vessel in response to an increased demand for myocardial oxygen supply. Because of the fundamental auto-regulatory function of the distal coronary vascular bed, a marked vaso-dilatation in distal coronary vessels may cause substantive alterations in the distribution of available coronary blood flow, depending upon the presence of multiple lesions in the vascular tree, the severity of the proximal obstruction, the arterial blood pressure and the nature of the collateral blood vessels. The significance of subcritical lesions in remote sections of the proximal arterial tree is that they may affect an area of seriously restricted coronary inflow by modification of collateral blood supply.

2. Cardiac metabolism is essentially aerobic. Anaerobic metabolic function is ineffective, poorly tolerated, and short lived. Since the heart as a pump continues to function on a beat-to-beat cycle, even under-perfused and nonfunctioning segments of myocardium are affected by the function of the adequately perfused fibers.

3. Basic to myocardial dysfunction and myocardial infarction in the presence of coronary artery disease is a discrepancy between the myocardial oxygen demand and the available oxygen supply.

4. Coronary artery disease without myocardial infarction is common. Acute myocardial infarction without coronary artery disease is rare. Coronary artery disease and acute myocardial infarction usually have a cause-and-effect relationship.

5. Acute myocardial infarction is occasioned by: (1) a further acute reduction in coronary inflow to a segment of the myocardium, or (2) myocardial oxygen demand prolonged excessively over the available supply so as to result in non-reversible changes in an area of myocardium.

6. Since coronary artery disease is usually a regional phenomenon in the coronary arteries, its consequences are also regional in the myocardium. However, regional disorders may occur in areas apparently supplied by coronary arteries with lesser degrees of obstructive disorder.

7. Regional coronary artery disease causing a basic imbalance in the relationship of oxygen supply to myocardial fiber oxygen demand is productive first of a depression of myocardial function, second of electrical and metabolic alterations, third of clinical symptoms and fourth of tissue necrosis.

8. Regional disorders of function contribute to ineffective global function and result in an over-all depression of global cardiac pump function disproportionate at times to the degree of regional disorder.

9. A myocardial infarction involving a small area of myocardium and not affecting vital structures (10% of total myocardial mass or less) is usually productive of only a small reduction in over-all cardiac function. On the contrary, a large acute myocardial infarction involving a substantive amount of the myocardium (30% of total myocardium or greater) results in a major depression of over-all global cardiac function.

10. Following myocardial necrosis compensatory mechanisms come into play including alterations in the stiffness of the affected myocardium, the contractile state of the adjacent healthy perfused myocardium, alterations in fluid and electrolyte distributions, and changes in endocrine and autonomic activity. Global myocardial oxygen consumption may be increased while total cardiac work is actually decreased.

11. Rational treatment of acute myocardial infarction includes the definition of the magnitude and significance of pulmonary congestion and edema and the application of methods specifically designed to alter fluid volumes to the problems of low cardiac output and blood flow whose causes may be reversible--hypovolemia, arrhythmias and mechanical defects including mitral regurgitation. Such forms of global depression of cardiac function related as they are to anomalies of regional cardiac behavior are frequently unresponsive to commonly used inotropic agents and are more rationally treated by impedance reduction so as to both improve over-all body perfusion while at the same time preserving or not further jeopardizing ischemic but yet viable myocardium.

12. Once myocardial infarction has occurred, about 20% of patients die suddenly of arrhythmia, about 15-20% die after reaching the hospital, mainly from pump failure, and another 15-20% die within 5 years after hospital discharge, largely from a recurrent infarction or consequences of their first attack. During each of these three critical periods of risk, much has been learned which helps to prognostically stratify within the risk period, and much has been learned about pathogenesis which either forms or could form the basis for new therapeutic approaches which might enhance survival.

Selected Reference

1. Swan, H. J., Forrester, J. S., and Diamond, G., et.al.: Hemodynamic spectrum of myocardial infarction and cardiogenic shock - a conceptual model. Circ. 45:1097, 1972.

PATHOLOGY OF SUDDEN CARDIAC DEATH
AND ACUTE MYOCARDIAL INFARCTION

William C. Roberts, M.D.

A generally agreed upon definition of "sudden cardiac death" is unavailable. Therefore, what constitutes "sudden cardiac death" to one physician may not necessarily do so to another. I define "sudden cardiac death" as that occurring within six hours from onset of symptoms of myocardial ischemia irrespective of whether or not the patient has had previous symptomatic evidence of cardiac disease. Furthermore, histologic evidence of myocardial necrosis is lacking. Obviously, that the sudden death is of cardiac origin must be confirmed by necropsy.

Acute myocardial infarction (AMI) is of two major types: 1) necrosis confined to the inner half of the left ventricular wall (subendocardial), and 2) necrosis involving more than the inner half of the left ventricular wall (transmural).

The degrees of coronary arterial luminal narrowing are similar among patients with fatal ischemic heart disease (IHD) irrespective of whether death occurs suddenly, or after myocardial necrosis, either subendocardial or transmural, has taken place. Certain changes in the coronary arteries are observed routinely at necropsy in fatal IHD:

1) The coronary arteries are diffusely involved by atherosclerotic plaques. Although the lumens of some segments are more severely narrowed than others, all portions of the extramural coronary tree are involved by the atherosclerotic process.

2) In fatal IHD, with rare exception, the lumens of at least two of the three major coronary arteries are > 75% narrowed by old atherosclerotic plaques. The most severe narrowing tends to be in the more proximal portions of the left anterior descending and left circumflex branches; the distal half of the right coronary artery is prone to narrowing that is as severe as that in its proximal portion.

3) The atherosclerotic process is limited to the epicardial coronary arteries, i.e., the major trunks and their near right-angle branches. The intramural (intramyocardial) coronary arteries are spared by the atherosclerotic process.

4) The coronary artery responsible for perfusing the area of myocardial ischemia with oxygen is not necessarily the most severely narrowed of the three major coronary arteries, but its lumen is virtually always > 75% narrowed at some point by atherosclerotic plaques.

5) The coronary arterial luminal narrowing in fatal IHD is produced by complicated atherosclerotic plaques, as opposed to fatty and fibrous plaques. The latter two types of atherosclerotic plaques are world-

wide in distribution, but the complicated plaques, i.e., those containing cholesterol clefts, pultaceous debris, calcium extravasated erythrocytes, etc., are found only in populations which develop symptomatic IHD. The complicated plaques are the ones responsible for severe luminal narrowing. The major component of even the complicated atherosclerotic plaque in fatal IHD is fibrous tissue (collagen) and the lipid component is much less evident. Foam cells actually are relatively infrequent in the coronary arteries in fatal IHD, and the lipid which is present is usually extracellular.

Now to coronary thrombosis in fatal IHD. Some observations:

1) Among patients with fatal IHD, thrombi are infrequent (about 10%) in patients dying suddenly and in those in whom the necrosis is limited to subendocardium.

2) Thrombus is found in a coronary artery in about 55% of patients with fatal transmural acute myocardial infarction.

3) Among patients with transmural myocardial necrosis, the major determinant of the presence or absence of coronary thrombosis appears to be the presence or absence of cardiogenic shock. At necropsy, 70% of patients with fatal AMI with cardiogenic shock have coronary thrombi whereas only about 15% of patients without the power failure syndrome associated with fatal AMI have coronary thrombi.

4) The larger the area of myocardial necrosis, the greater the likelihood of coronary thrombosis. The larger the infarcted area, however, the greater the likelihood of cardiogenic shock. The latter generally indicates that >40% of the left ventricular wall is either necrotic or fibrotic or both, whereas shock is infrequently associated with infarcts or scars involving <40% of the left ventricular wall.

5) When coronary thrombosis is associated with AMI, the thrombus is always located in the artery responsible for perfusing the area of myocardial necrosis. Thus, in anterior wall infarction, a thrombus, if present, will be located in the left anterior descending coronary artery.

6) Thrombi are found in fatal IHD in coronary arteries which already are severely narrowed by old atherosclerotic plaques. At the distal site of attachment of the thrombus, or just distal to this site, the lumen of the coronary artery is nearly always 75% narrowed by old atherosclerotic plaques. Not infrequently, a thrombus may occur in an area between two sites of severe narrowing, similar to a valley between two mountains. If a clot is found in a coronary artery relatively free of old atherosclerotic plaques, embolism rather than thrombosis must be considered.

7) Coronary thrombi in fatal AMI are usually (90%) single, usually (80%) occlusive (as opposed to mural or non-occlusive), short (2 cm long), and located entirely in the major trunks (as opposed to their near right angle branches or intramural coronary arteries). The thrombus,

when only a few hours old, may consist nearly entirely of platelets, but thereafter is composed primarily of fibrin. By definition, the thrombus is adherent to the surface of the arterial wall bordering the lumen.

Since Herrick first used the term "coronary thrombosis" in 1912 to describe the often dramatic clinical event characterized at necropsy by necrosis of portions of left ventricular wall, it has been assumed that the usual cause of AMI is coronary thrombosis. Two factors implicate coronary thrombosis as the precipitating cause of AMI: 1) the occurrence of coronary arterial thrombi in many patients with fatal AMI; and 2) the location of the thrombus in the coronary artery responsible for supplying the area of myocardial necrosis. Five factors, however, tend to indicate that coronary thrombosis is a consequence rather than the precipitating cause of AMI: 1) the very low frequency of thrombi in patients dying suddenly with or without previous evidence of cardiac disease; 2) the increasing frequency of thrombi with increasing intervals between onset of symptoms of AMI and death; 3) the absence of thrombi in fatal transmural AMI nearly as often as they are present; 4) the near absence of thrombi in fatal subendocardial AMI; and 5) the occurrence of thrombi in high percentage only in patients with cardiogenic shock, most of whom have large transmural infarcts.

The key to coronary thrombosis, just like the key to thrombosis occurring anywhere in the body, is slow blood flow, or relative stasis, and sufficient time for the thrombus to form. The absence of these two factors (slow blood flow and time) may explain the absence of coronary thrombosis as the interval from the onset of symptoms of myocardial ischemia to death increases. There is a marked reduction in blood flow in the coronary artery responsible for supplying the area of myocardial infarction. This observation was made in dogs after inducing AMI, and they had normal, i.e., widely patent, vessels. In fatal AMI in humans, the thrombus is always located in an artery already containing considerable atherosclerotic plaques, and therefore, the infarct-induced relative coronary stasis is probably even greater. Cardiogenic shock must further diminish coronary flow.

The type of activity experienced by patients at the time of onset of AMI may reflect slowed blood flow. Nearly 75% of patients with AMI have the onset of chest pain while sleeping, resting, or performing mild activity. Although inactivity may cause slight diminution in coronary blood flow, considerable stasis of blood (infarction-induced plus cardiogenic shock) is usually necessary for a thrombus to form. In contrast to fatal AMI, coronary thrombosis is rarely observed in fatal angina pectoris although the degree of coronary luminal narrowing by atherosclerotic plaques is similar in degree to that observed in AMI. Evidence of thrombus formation is nearly always observed in arteries implanted into the left ventricular myocardium, presumably because of poor blood flow. Thrombus formation does not occur in similar arteries implanted into the left ventricular myocardium but allowed to drain into the right ventricular cavity. Thus, it appears that a period of diminished coronary blood flow is necessary for thrombus to form in a coronary artery. Shock, congestive cardiac failure and inactivity all decrease coronary flow, and with time may allow thrombosis.

Further support for the concept that coronary thrombosis is a consequence rather than a precipitating cause of AMI was supplied recently by Erhardt and associates who observed radioactivity at necropsy in coronary arterial thrombi in patients given radioactive I^{125}-labelled fibrinogen shortly after admission because of AMI. This finding implicates coronary thrombosis as a secondary event occurring some time after the infarction.

In conclusion, there is substantial evidence that acute thrombus formation does not precipitate acute fatal IHD. The major problem is diffuse generalized coronary atherosclerosis with severe (> 75%) luminal narrowing (at least two of the three major coronary arteries).

Despite the above de-emphasis on the role of thrombus in precipitating AMI, I would like to suggest as others have, that thrombosis plays a major role in the organization of the atherosclerotic plaque in the first place. Several observations suggest that atherosclerotic plaques result, at least in part, from the organization of thrombi:

1) The presence of known components of thrombi - namely fibrin and platelets - within atherosclerotic plaques.

2) The occurrence of known components of atherosclerotic plaques - namely foam cells, cholesterol clefts, pultaceous debris, and calcium - in organized hematomas or known thrombi wherever they occur in the body. An example is the left atrial thrombus in the patient with mitral stenosis. Organization of this thrombus may produce typical complicated atherosclerotic plaques.

3) The presence of multiple channels in lumens - a recognized consequence of organization of pulmonary arterial thromboemboli. Multiluminal channels commonly are found in severely atherosclerotic coronary arteries. This observation suggests that thrombi or emboli were at one time present and that they organized. The tissue present between the multiluminal channels is similar to that found in arteries with only one channel. Because the artery with multiple channels has been recognized as the hallmark of an organized thrombus, and because the tissue in both multi and unichanneled arteries is similar, Duguid reasoned that the causative process was similar.

4) The major component of the complicated atherosclerotic plaque, i.e., those capable of causing significant luminal narrowing in the coronary arteries of patients with fatal ischemic heart disease, is fibrous tissue or collagen, not lipid. This is true whether or not hyperlipidemia is present. Foam cells actually are infrequently observed in the coronary arteries in patients with fatal ischemic heart disease. Often the "density" of the fibrous tissue plugging a coronary artery is different in different portions of a plaque, and these subunits may be demarcated by distinct elastic lamellae. These subunits suggest that thrombus is deposited at different times and that the "density" of the resulting fibrous tissue may be determined by the composition of the initial thrombus,i.e., whether platelets or fibrin predominated.

5) Experimentally induced thrombi under proper conditions may be trans-

formed into atherosclerotic plaques closely resembling those observed in human coronary arteries.

The above factors obviously do not prove that thrombosis is the cause of atherosclerosis, but together they strongly suggest that organization of thrombi plays a major role in the development of the complicated atherosclerotic plaque. Indeed, most present serious students of the morphology of the arterial plaque support, in whole or in part, the thrombogenic origin of atherosclerosis. Because the clotting factors in the blood appear to be similar in all population groups and because symptomatic atherosclerosis develops only in those population groups with elevated blood lipids, the latter also play a role in the development of the plaque. Lipids may exert their effect, however, more by their ability to alter the clotting mechanism than by their ability to infiltrate the arterial wall.

Selected References

1. Roberts, W.C.: Coronary arteries in fatal acute myocardial infarction. Circulation 45: 215-230, Jan. 1972.

2. Roberts, W.C.: Relationship between coronary thrombosis and myocardial infarction. Modern Concepts Cardiov. Dis. 41: 7-10, Feb. 1972.

3. Roberts, W.C. and Buja, L.M.: The frequency and significance of coronary arterial thrombi and other observations in fatal acute myocardial infarction. A study of 107 necropsy patients. Amer. J. Med. 52: 425-443, 1972.

4. Roberts, W.C., Ferrans, V.J., Levy, R.I., Fredrickson, D.S.: Cardiovascular pathology in hyperlipoproteinemia. Anatomic observations in 42 necropsy patients with normal or abnormal serum lipoprotein patterns. Amer. J. Cardiol. 31: 557-570, 1973.

5. Roberts, W.C.: Does thrombosis play a major role in the development of the symptom-producing atherosclerotic plaque? Circulation 48: 1161-1166, 1973.

6. Roberts, W.D.: Coronary atherosclerosis and its complications. MEDCOM slide series, 1974.

A CLINICAL VIEW OF CORONARY PATHOLOGY IN MYOCARDIAL INFARCTION

Robert J. Boucek, M.D.

Certain clues revealed by the clinical presentation of patients with myocardial infarction may indicate the probable underlying coronary pathology. Recognition of these clues can help the physician identify those patients at high risk for sudden disaster.

History

An initial clue may come from the character of the chest pain. Dr. Radi Macruz from the University of Sao Paulo, Brazil correlated radiated pain with the location of coronary obstruction (coronary arteriography) in 303 patients. The results are shown in Table 1.

TABLE 1

PAIN DISTRIBUTION AND CORONARY PATHOLOGY IN MYOCARDIAL INFARCTION

CORONARY ARTERY	LOCATION	RADIATION
Anterior Descending	Precordial	Often none Left arm
Right	Precordial	Back Shoulders Bilateral
Anterior Descending and Posterior Circumflex	Precordial	Right and Left Arm Cervical - Back Mandible

Ref: Macruz, R.: Heart Attacks: Pain and Diagnosis. Medical World News, March 22, 1974.

Additional correlations include the observation that patients with chronic angina pectoris (>3 months) generally have long segmental narrowing and obstruction of the right coronary artery in addition to a critical narrowing of a second coronary artery. Nocturnal and rest angina usually indicate triple vessel disease. Non-effort related angina pectoris preceding a myocardial infarction should suggest the possibility of critical narrowing of the coronary ostia (usually the right).

Physical Signs

Clinical signs may be of help in assessing coronary pathology. Abnormal movements of the precordium or the ectopic region are usually found with obstruction of the anterior descending artery. The systolic murmur of papillary muscle dysfunction (occasionally a systolic click) is common. The anterior papillary muscle is suppled by the left coronary and the posterior papillary muscle by both the left and right coronaries.

Electrocardiogram

In general, right coronary artery pathology is revealed by changes in the P-R interval and in leads II, III and AVF. The right coronary artery transports blood to the conduction system proximal to the right and left bundle branches.

Anterior descending coronary artery pathology is revealed by changes in the QRS and the precordial leads V1 through V4. The anterior descending artery via the septal perforating branches transports blood to the right and the superior (anterior) fascicle of the left bundle branches and to the major portion of the ventricular septum. Through the diagonal branches, the anterior descending artery transports blood to the anterior and anterolateral wall, the inferior wall of the left ventricle, and the anterior papillary muscles of both ventricles.

Pathology in the circumflex artery is generally revealed by QRS-T changes in the precordial leads V5 and V6. Left atrial infarctions result from obstruction of a branch artery from the circumflex artery.

Heart Block

The blood supply of the ventricular conduction pathways is shown in Figure 4, page 6. The AV node and the His bundle are in the territory of the right coronary artery. The right bundle branch and the proximal part of the left bundle branch (summit of the ventricular septum) are within the territory of the anterior descending artery (via the first septal perforating artery). The anterior fascicle of the left bundle and the RBB are in the territory of the anterior descending artery. The take-off of the posterior fascicle of the LBB is in the territory of the right and anterior descending arteries. The peripheral branching of the LBB is in the territory of the circumflex artery.

When this vascular arrangement is known, a number of correlations between heart block and likely locations for obstructive coronary disease can be deduced. Briefly, left anterior hemiblocks complicating an anteroseptal myocardial infarction are likely to be due to an obstruction of the anterior descending artery distal to the first long septal perforating artery. Right bundle branch block plus left anterior hemiblock is probably due to obstruction of the anterior descending artery proximal to the first long septal perforating artery. A posterior hemiblock plus RBBB suggest triple vessel obstructive coronary artery disease.

It is commonly appreciated that acute atrioventricular block with inferior infarction is due to right coronary obstruction, is often evanescent and related to ischemia. In contrast, patients with conduction blocks below the bundle of His have thrombotic obstruction of the anterior descending artery, associated with anterior infarction, extensive necrosis, and a poor prognosis. Such patients commonly develop fascicular blocks before proceeding to complete heart block.

Protection against the danger of heart block or asystole in anterior infarction is possible by the insertion of an artificial pacemaker, but sudden death still occurs. Perhaps emergency myocardial revascularization should be considered in patients with anterior wall infarcts complicated by heart block.

Myocardial Failure

Left ventricular failure presenting with atrial arrhythmias, diastolic gallops and possibly reversed splitting of the second heart sound is not uncommon during the initial 3 days following myocardial infarction. It is more common in anterior infarction and aggressive therapy, especially with rapidly acting diuretics, is the best approach to preserve ischemic non-necrotic myocardium. When more severe left ventricular failure occurs, as in patients in their mid-60's (usually males) with a history of previous myocardial infarction(s) presenting as an acute transmural infarction with hypotension and underperfusion of the cerebral, mesenteric, renal or pulmonary circulations, advanced coronary artery atherosclerosis with obstruction in the anterior descending and right coronary arteries is the most likely coronary pathology. Acute obstruction results from a thrombus or intraplaque hemorrhage. Myocardial necrosis is extensive and the prognosis is very poor.

Myocardial Rupture

A critical period following myocardial infarction when myocardial, papillary muscle or septal rupture or thromboembolic complications may occur is from 3 to 9 days. The common clinical setting for rupture of the free wall is a patient older than 65 with a history of hypertension, 75% without previous coronary insufficiency, recurring pain at 3-7 days, and a transmural anterior, anterolateral or posterolateral myocardial infarction. The usual pathology of the coronary arteries is thrombotic occlusion in the proximal region of the anterior descending and less often the circumflex.

The clinical setting for septal perforation differs from free wall rupture by occurring in younger male patients. A sudden circulatory collapse, reappearance of retrosternal pain, and the appearance of a systolic murmur should suggest septal perforation. Obstruction of the right coronary artery is more common with septal perforation than with free wall rupturing.

The major teaching points to be emphasized are:

1. Constant refinement in correlations between clinical presentation and the underlying coronary pathology is the essence of continuing education in the management of patients with myocardial infarction.

2. Clues as to the most likely underlying coronary pathology may come from the character of pain, physical signs, ECG signs of ischemia, and the degree of vascular collapse.

3. Acute heart block provides important clues as to the obstructive site along the coronary artery and represents an ominous complication.

4. Myocardial infarction may extend at 3-6 days when grave complications of myocardial rupture may occur. Potential candidates may be recognized by unique clinical settings.

5. Extensive atherosclerosis and multiple sites of critical coronary narrowing is to be expected in patients with pump failure.

Selected References

1. Hunt, D., et al: Histopathology of heart block complicating acute myocardial infarction: Correlation with the His bundle electrogram: Circulation 48:1252, 1973.

2. Walston, A., et al: Acute coronary occlusion and the power-failure syndrome: Am. Heart J. 79:613, 1970.

3. Friedman, et al: Clinical and electrocardiographic features of cardiac rupture following acute myocardial infarction: Am. J. Med. 50:709, 1971.

4. Campion, B. C., et al: Ventricular septal defect after myocardial infarction: Ann. Int. Med. 70:251, 1969.

ANGINA PECTORIS - CLINICAL PRESENTATION

Robert J. Myerburg, M.D.

The symptom of angina pectoris, according to its classical description, is a form of chest pain having a characteristic quality, location, radiation, mode of onset, and response to either rest or nitroglycerin. The classical description of this symptom complex, as outlined two hundred years ago by Heberden, has not been improved upon by modern clinicians. However, throughout the years, and especially during the past 20 years, it has become increasingly evident that variations in the pattern of the symptom complex may potentially mislead us in our attempts to confirm or rule out the presence of significant coronary atherosclerosis. In addition, symptoms unrelated to cardiovascular disorders may mimic quite closely the quality, location, and radiation of the pain of true angina pectoris. Only a thorough history and physical examination, combined with appropriate use of electrocardiography and exercise tests, will allow us to be reasonably accurate in identifying the presence or absence of angina pectoris clinically.

Substernal squeezing, pressing, or vice-like chest discomfort, radiating into the neck, left shoulder, left arm, and left hand, represents a pain and radiation pattern which is quite typical of angina pectoris. However, the pain of angina may radiate to either shoulder, either arm, or the fingers of either hand; it may radiate to either the anterior or posterior aspects of the neck; it commonly radiates to the interscapular area of the back; and either the lower or (less commonly) the upper jaw may be a site of radiation. In addition, the pain may radiate to the epigastrium or even the oropharynx. Some patients describe "anginal" attacks which are not experienced as pain at all, but rather as episodic shortness of breath on exertion, which has all of the activity-related characteristics of angina pectoris but is described by the patient as dyspnea rather than pain. This form of dyspnea-on-exertion is really an equivalent of angina pectoris, and frequently responds to nitroglycerin.

The physical examination during episodic chest pain may be extremely helpful when the nature of the pain is in question. While many patients are free of abnormal physical findings between attacks of angina pectoris, it is quite common to detect one or more of a number of physical findings during an attack of angina pectoris. These findings may be quite rewarding when there is some doubt as to the diagnosis. The physical findings that commonly accompany an episode of true angina pectoris are tachycardia and hypertension, S_3 and S_4 gallops, apical systolic murmurs related to papillary muscle dysfunction, ischemic bulges on the precordium which are palpated only during the episodic pain, paradoxical splitting of the second heart sound, and pulsus alternans. It is often possible to bring out one or more of these physical findings, short of precipitating an attack of angina pectoris, by stressing the cardiovascular system with the use of handgrip isometric exercises. Should an attack of angina be precipitated, it can usually be rapidly terminated by nitroglycerin.

Selected Reference

Hurst, J. W.: The Heart. Third Edition, McGraw-Hill, 1974.

PROGNOSIS IN ANGINA PECTORIS

Andrew G. Wallace, M.D.

In 1956, Richards, Bland and White published their account of a 25 year followup of 500 patients whom they cared for from the onset of symptoms of angina pectoris until death. Contrary to the opinion which prevailed in the 30's and 40's, their report showed that 80% of their patients survived 5 years and approximately half survived for 10 years. A major point of their study, however, was to call attention to the highly variable prognosis among patients with this diagnosis, some dying within months and others surviving 25 years.

By 1956, it had become clear to White that patients at the highest risk of early death were those with prior myocardial infarction, cardiomegaly by chest X ray, hypertension and resting ECG abnormalities. The Health Insurance Plan of New York refined the predictive value of clinical description of patients with angina, noting that in men under age 55, the annual mortality was 2% per year in the absence of heart failure, hypertension, prior myocardial infarction, or resting ECG abnormality. This annual rate increased to 4% when angina was complicated by hypertension, to 8% with hypertension and ECG abnormalities and to 14% with hypertension, ECG abnormalities and heart failure.

In 1970 Friesinger demonstrated the added prognostic value of coronary anatomy as defined by arteriography: patients with single vessel disease having a 95% five year survival and those with major obstruction of 3 vessels having a 47% five year survival (see Figure 1). Subsequent reports have demonstrated important prognostic information related to the degree of abnormal ventricular function by angiography and the functional state of patients determined by treadmill performance.

Based upon these insights, it now seems certain that the prognosis for 5 year survival can be estimated with great precision in patients with angina. Such estimates can and should provide a logical basis for selecting patients for arteriography, for assessing the need for urgent surgery, and for giving the physician confidence that many patients with angina can be safely treated by medical means, reserving surgical treatment for those with symptoms which fail to respond adequately to medical therapy.

Just as a logic process based on accurate descriptors can be used to accurately assess prognosis without surgery, a similar process can be used to estimate surgical risk, the probability of relief of symptoms after surgery and the likelihood that surgical therapy will prolong life. Surgical risk varies from about 1 to 15% depending primarily on the state of ventricular function and the presence or absence of associated valvular disease. Symptomatic relief averages about 70%, but is greater in patients with positive presurgical exercise tests than in those with negative or indeterminant responses to stress, and also varies with psychological descriptors. Survival appears to be improved in certain subgroups such as significant left main coronary stenosis, and two vessel disease involving the right and anterior descending if ventricular function is good. Survival appears unaltered in other subgroups by surgery and may be worsened by surgical intervention in other subgroups. From these considerations it seem clear that surgical therapy has and will continue to have a role in treatment of patients with angina. The value of surgery in patients with significantly compromised ventricular function is in serious question. The concept that all patients with significant obstructions of one or more coronary arteries need surgery to prolong life is untenable. It follows that medical management has and will continue to have a central role in the management of many patients with angina.

Selected References

1. Reeves, T.J., Oberman, A., et al.: Natural History of Angina Pectoris. Am. J. Cardiol., 33:423, 1974.

2. Friesinger, G.C., Page, E.E., and Ross, R.S.: Prognostic Significance of Coronary Arteriography. Trans. Amer. Assoc. of Physicians, 83:78, 1970

3. Webster, J.S., Moberg, C.V., Rinco, G.: Natural History of Severe Proximal Coronary Artery Disease. Am. J. Cardiol., 23:195, 1974.

4. Sheldon, W.C., Rincon, G., et al.: Surgical Treatment of Coronary Artery Disease: Pure Graft Operations. Prog. in Cardiovas. Dis., 18:237, 1975

5. Ross, R.S.: Surgery in Ischemic Heart Disease. Disease-A-Month, July, 1972.

Figure 1

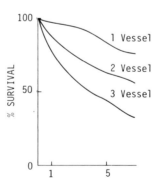

ELAPSED YEARS

The angiographic estimate of the number of diseased vessels has important prognostic significance. (After Bruschke et al., Circ., 47:1147-1153, 1973).

THE INTERMEDIATE CORONARY SYNDROME

Lawrence S. Cohen, M.D.

Combining data from several different series of patients studied angiographically, the average annual mortality for patients with single, double and triple vessel coronary artery disease is 2.2 percent, 6.8 percent and 11.4 percent.

The challenge of this next decade is to define clearly which patients with stable angina are likely to be benefitted by bypass grafting. Certain high risk patients are almost assured of being helped by operation but it is unlikely that all patients with angina pectoris should be considered for surgical therapy.

The management of patients with the intermediate coronary syndrome is also not agreed upon uniformly. There are a variety of names associated with the syndrome, (impending myocardial infarction, progressive coronary insufficiency, unstable angina pectoris, pre-infarction angina, accelerated angina pectoris, status anginosus, and acute coronary insufficiency.)

Because of the variety of names associated with this syndrome it is particularly important to have a standardized definition. The cardinal features of the syndrome are: 1) recurring angina at rest, 2) incomplete relief of pain with nitrites, 3) unstable ECG but without new Q waves, and 4) non-diagnostic enzyme changes.

In determining the best form of therapy, either medical or surgical, it is important to ask what is the natural history. Gazes reported a 20 percent mortality in one year and a 50 percent mortality in ten years. Krauss et al., found that most patients responded to initial medical therapy but 20 percent were dead at the two year period. In the study reported from Johns Hopkins, the operative mortality was 22 percent but two-thirds of the survivors were pain free. In the medically treated group, mortality was lower but the late status of the group was for them to have continued angina pectoris.

It is our current policy to treat patients with the intermediate coronary syndrome initially with medication. Most patients can be stabilized. Then a decision concerning coronary arteriography and operation can be made electively.

Selected References

1. Fischl, S. J., Herman, M. V., Gorlin, R.: The intermediate coronary syndrome. Clinical, angiographic and therapeutic aspects. New Eng. J. Med. 288:1193, 1973.

2. Conti, C. R., Brawley, R. K., Griffith, L., Cohen, L. S., et. al.: Unstable angina pectoris: morbidity and mortality in 57 consecutive patients evaluated angiographically. Amer. J. Cardiol. 32:745, 1973

ACUTE MYOCARDIAL INFARCTION: THE FIRST 24 HOURS

Andrew G. Wallace, M.D.

Most patients who reach the coronary care unit will have chest pain, anxiety and arrhythmias, but they will survive. The first 24 hours on the CCU are used largely to relieve pain and anxiety, to establish the diagnosis of myocardial infarction, and to initiate treatment for arrhythmias as well as efforts which may reduce the likelihood of developing subsequent complications. The pain of acute myocardial infarction in most instances is very intense, contributes to anxiety and may be accompanied by autonomic imbalances which lead either to hypertension and tachycardia on the one hand, or bradycardia with hypotension on the other. Most people stress that the early and rapid relief of pain is vitally important to the management of the patient and is best accomplished with morphine. Morphine should be used cautiously in the patient with bradycardia, but any bradycardia induced by morphine or accentuated by this agent can usually be relieved with small doses of intravenous atropine. Once pain is relieved, anxiety usually diminishes, but if the patient is still overtly anxious despite relief of pain and reassurance, we do not hesitate to give him an agent such as Valium.

The diagnosis of an acute myocardial infarction depends largely on the co-existence of a compatible history, electrocardiographic and serum enzyme changes. Serial electrocardiograms are rarely normal in a patient with an established acute myocardial infarction, but the electrocardiographic changes may be subtle, and in a very significant number of patients Q waves may fail to develop or the QRS complex may be uninterpretable because of prior existing conduction disturbances. Serum enzymes are relied upon very heavily to establish the diagnosis of an acute myocardial infarction. With the standard enzymes available in most hospital laboratories, the enzymes are rarely normal in a patient with acute myocardial infarction, but there is a significant incidence of false-positive results due to heart failure, liver disease, intramuscular injections, etc. The problem of false-positive enzymes has been largely circumvented by the recent development of techniques of analyzing isoenzymes of LDH and CPK. In our experience, these isoenzymes are positive in over 95% of patients with an established acute myocardial infarction, and the incidence of false-positives is less than 2%. There are preliminary data which suggest that if samples are obtained frequently, the CPK curve can be analyzed in such a way as to give some insight into the size of the myocardial infarction. Serial determinations of CPK may not only evaluate infarct size, but may also be used in the future to gauge effects of treatment on reducing the size of the infarction. These are important considerations as infarct size is directly related to the degree of pump failure and mortality in acute myocardial infarction.

Clinical descriptors, obtainable within the first 24-48 hours after the onset of symptoms, allow one to identify patients with an extremely low risk of developing serious complications. These patients are good candidates for a liberal approach to therapy including early ambulation and early discharge from the hospital. The factors which identify these low risk patients include: an age of less than 65, the absence of significant heart failure, the absence of advanced degrees of AV block and pain which responds rapidly to initial therapy and does not recur. When patients remain in such a low risk group for 3-5 days after the onset of symptoms, their subsequent hospital mortality approaches 0% and the occurrence of late complications which require specific therapy is negligible. In such patients we feel that 3 days of electrocardiographic monitoring is adequate. Daily good 6' chest films which fail to show evidence of increasing heart size or pulmonary venous congestion are a good prognostic sign. Hemodynamic monitoring appears to be unnecessary in such patients.

Prophylactic antiarrhythmic agents are effective in reducing the prevalence of ventricular ectopic beats, but there is no evidence that prophylactic antiarrhythmics reduce mortality when compared to the rapid use of similar agents when specific indications arise. There is little doubt that coronary care units have significantly reduced in-hospital mortality (by about one-half) through the early detection and treatment of arrhythmia, and that in this setting at least 50% of the patients who suffer ventricular fibrillation can be successfully resuscitated.*

There is still no evidence that anti-coagulation alters the mortality of the acute myocardial infarction, but there is good evidence that the use of heparin in intravenous infusions reduces the incidence of local phlebitis and that both low dose and standard dose anticoagulation reduce the incidence of thromboembolic complications after acute myocardial infarction.

*
"ARRHYTHMIAS COMPLICATING ACUTE MYOCARDIAL INFARCTION" will be presented in a programmed instruction format in the section on Self Assessment (p.293).

Selected References

1. Ebert, R.: Anticoagulants in Acute Myocardial Infarction. JAMA 225:724, 1973.

2. Wagner, G.S.: Importance of Myocardial Specific enzymes of CPK in Diagnosis of Acute MI. Circ., 47:257, 1973.

BUNDLE BRANCH BLOCK AND MYOCARDIAL INFARCTION

Hein J.J. Wellens, M.D. and K.I. Lie, M.D.

Acquired Bundle Branch Block

Bundle branch block (BBB) as a consequence of myocardial infarction is seen in approximately 10% of patients admitted to the hospital because of acute myocardial infarction. Right bundle branch block (RBBB) is twice as frequent as left bundle branch block (LBBB).

Right Bundle Branch Block

When RBBB develops following acute myocardial infarction, the infarct is nearly always located anteroseptally. Characteristically lead V1 shows a QR pattern.

One quarter of patients with anteroseptal infarction develop RBBB. This is a poor prognostic sign. While anteroseptal infarction without RBBB carries a mortality of 23%, this increases to 74% when RBBB develops. Two-thirds of the patients with acquired RBBB also develop block in either the anterior or posterior fascicle of the left bundle branch. In approximately 40% of patients, the development of RBBB with left anterior hemiblock or left posterior hemiblock is followed by complete infranodal (trifascicular) heart block. As far as the development of complete infranodal block is concerned, the following points are of importance.

1) Complete infranodal block is always preceded by the development of bifascicular block.

2) Patients with RBBB of short duration (less than 6 hours) or delayed onset (more than 24 hours) after infarction do not tend to develop complete infranodal block.

3) In the presence of bifascicular block, a prolonged PR interval (>0.20 sec) carries an 85% risk of subsequent development of complete infranodal block.

4) However, a normal PR interval in the presence of bifascicular block does not exclude the subsequent development of complete infranodal block. Under these circumstances, candidates for the latter can be identified by measuring the HV interval by His bundle studies. If prolonged, there is a 75% chance of development of complete infranodal block.

The high mortality rate in patients with anteroseptal infarction and right bundle branch block is primarily related to the size of the infarction. To protect patients against Adams-Stokes attacks, hopefully thereby saving an occasional patient, prophylactic pacemaker insertion should be carried out in patients with acquired RBBB and a frontal QRS axis of less than -45° (left superior hemiblock) or more than $+90^{\circ}$ (left inferior hemiblock), especially if the PR interval is prolonged. This procedure is probably not necessary if the RBBB develops after 24 hours of infarction or lasts for less than 6 hours.

Left Bundle Branch Block

80% of cases of acquired LBBB following acute myocardial infarction are seen during the phase of bradycardia in patients with high degree intranodal block in association with acute inferior infarction. This rate dependent (Phase 4) LBBB is not associated with a poorer prognosis as compared to patients with high degree intranodal block without LBBB.

20% of cases of acquired LBBB are found in anterior and anteroseptal infarction. This does not seem to result in an increased mortality rate.

Pre-existent Bundle Branch Block

Pre-existent BBB was present in approximately 4% of patients admitted to our CCU because of acute myocardial infarction. Two important differences are found between patients with acquired and pre-existent BBB and acute myocardial infarction.

1) 75% of patients with pre-existent BBB are 70 years of age or older as compared to only 30% of patients with acquired BBB.

2) There is a definite relation between site of infarction and acquired BBB. No such association is found in patients with pre-existent BBB, although the site of infarction cannot be determined in a large number of patients with pre-existent LBBB.

Because of this lack of relation between site of infarction and pre-existent BBB, the development of complete infranodal block following acute myocardial infarction in such patients is very rare. Prophylactic pacemaker insertion therefore does not seem to be indicated in patients with pre-existent BBB. When patients with pre-existent BBB are matched for age and sex with patients without BBB, there is no significant difference in mortality rate.

Differentiation Between Acquired and Pre-existent BBB

If BBB is already present on admission to the hospital, two points are of help in differentiating between acquired and pre-existent BBB.

1) Age. Old age favors pre-existent BBB.

2) QRS configuration in lead V1 if RBBB is present. A QR configuration suggests acquired RBBB. A qR or triphasic QRS pattern supports pre-existent RBBB.

Selected Reference

1. Lie, K.I., Wellens, H.J.J., Schuilenburg, R.M.: Bundle Branch Block and Acute Myocardial Infarction, <u>The Conduction System of the Heart</u>. Ed., Wellens, et. al. Lea and Febiger, Philadelphia, 1976, p. 646.

THE HEMODYNAMICALLY UNSTABLE MYOCARDIAL INFARCTION PATIENT

Alvaro Mayorga-Cortes, M. D.

The most common cause of death in the pre-hospital phase of acute myocardial infarction (AMI) is ventricular fibrillation. After the patient is admitted to an Intensive Care setting, the leading cause of death is pump failure.

Pathophysiology

The mechanisms of cardiac failure in acute myocardial infarction are:

1) Loss of cardiac muscle.
2) Decreased compliance of the left ventricle.
3) Mechanical imbalance due to ventricular dyskinesis.
4) Myocardial metabolic abnormalities.
5) Malfunction of the mitral valve apparatus.

Other precipitating factors which may play a role are hypovolemia, atrial and ventricular arrhythmias, bradyarrhythmias, fever, pericarditis, hypoventilation and electrolyte imbalance.

A cardinal feature of cardiac failure is reduction in forward cardiac output below systemic needs. The insertion of balloon-tipped catheters at the bedside has allowed us to indirectly measure left ventricular end-diastolic pressure (LVEDP) by recording pulmonary capillary wedge pressure (PCW), and also to measure cardiac output by different techniques. The hemodynamic spectrum of the failing infarcted myocardium is characterized by different degrees of decreased cardiac output and stroke volume, elevated LVEDP, arterial desaturation with a wide arteriovenous oxygen difference, functional pulmonary A-V shunting and acidosis with hyperventilation. Systemic vascular resistance is elevated in approximately 40% of the cases and hypovolemia is found in up to 20% of patients on admission.

Diagnosis

A. Moderate to Severe Heart Failure

The incidence and mortality of cardiac failure is shown in a group of patients in Table 1. Clinically, the patient may show different degrees of pulmonary congestion and low cardiac output. Tachycardia, confusion, hypotension, pulmonary rales, sweating, diastolic filling sounds and a palpable dyskinetic ventricle may occur as manifestations of different degrees of heart failure. A chest X ray may show cardiomegaly, pulmonary vascular congestion and alveolar edema, but there may be a significant time lag and be normal in the early stages. Clinical assessment (Table 2) requires rapid estimation of intravascular volume, measurement of urinary output and arterial blood gases. At the bedside a third heart sound and tor therapy and the judicious use of mechanical assist devices may in some cases significantly alter the prognosis. It is also possible that modifications in preload and afterload in the noncomplicated case may reduce the area of infarction with beneficial effects on short and long term prognosis.

It is likely that in the next few years refinement in the techniques that attempt to measure infarct size, i.e., serum MB-CPK, multiple lead chest wall ST segment mapping, and isotopic techniques will allow us to better evaluate the usefulness of these interventions.

Selected References

1. Russel, R.O., et. al.: Left Ventricular Hemodynamics in Anterior and Inferior Myocardial Infarction. Am. J. Cardiol., 32:8, 1973.

2. Chatterjee, K., et al.: Hemodynamic and Metabolic Responses to Vasodilator Therapy in Acute Myocardial Infarction. Circ., 48:1183, 1973.

3. Maroko, P.R., et al.: Modification of Myocardial Infarction Size After Coronary Occlusion. Ann. Int. Med., 79:720, 1973.

TABLE 1

CARDIAC FAILURE IN ACUTE MYOCARDIAL INFARCTION

INCIDENCE AND MORTALITY (100 PATIENTS)

		Incidence	Mortality
I.	NO HEART FAILURE	30%	<5%
II.	MODERATE HEART FAILURE	30%	20%
III.	PULMONARY EDEMA	25%	40%
IV.	SHOCK	15%	90%

TABLE 2

ASSESSMENT OF PUMP FAILURE IN ACUTE MYOCARDIAL INFARCTION

I. <u>CLINICAL</u> - General Appearance, Third Heart Sound, Rales

II. <u>ELECTROCARDIOGRAPHIC</u> - Rate, Dysrhythmia, ST Elevation

III. <u>HEMODYNAMIC</u> - Chest X ray, Urinary Output, Arterial Blood Gases, Ventricular Performance

TABLE 3 - AFTERLOAD REDUCING AGENTS IN ACUTE MI

INDICATIONS:
    SEVERE SYSTEMIC HYPERTENSION
    CARDIAC FAILURE WITH ELEVATED LVEDP
    CARDIOGENIC SHOCK
    ASSOCIATED WITH INTRA-AORTIC BALLOON ASSIST

METHOD:
    CONSTANT HEMODYNAMIC MONITORING
    IV DRIP: START AT 25 MICROGRAMS/MINUTE

MAINTENANCE:
    NORMAL P.C. PRESSURE
    DROP IN MEAN Ao PRESSURE: 20 MM.HG.

CONTRAINDICATIONS:
    HYPOVOLEMIA
    LOW OR NORMAL LVEDP
    SEVERE HYPOTENSION: SBP: <90 MM. HG.

TABLE 4 - MANAGEMENT OF CARDIOGENIC SHOCK SECONDARY TO ACUTE MI

EARLY DIAGNOSIS:
    HEMODYNAMIC MONITORING
    SBP - LESS THAN 85 MM.HG.
        - DROP OF 40 MM.HG. FROM CONTROL
    POOR ORGAN PERFUSION
    ↓

VOLUME EXPANSION: LVEDP AROUND 20 MM.HG.
    ↓

AFTERLOAD REDUCTION
DOPAMINE
INTRAAORTIC BALLOON ASSIST
    GOOD RESPONSE: 3-5 DAYS
    POOR RESPONSE
    ↓

EMERGENCY CORONARY AND LEFT VENTRICULAR ANGIOGRAPHY
SUITABLE ANATOMY: SURGERY

ACUTE PUMP FAILURE--BEDSIDE CORRELATIONS

WITH HEMODYNAMIC MEASUREMENTS

(Including when to use the balloon
flotation--Swan-Ganz--catheter)

H.J.C. Swan, M.D.

1. Hemodynamic measurements: The balloon tipped flow guided catheter has now been demonstrated to be of value in hemodynamic measurements in critically ill patients. Conventionally, the catheter is inserted into the venous system and when its tip lies in the right atrium a small (0.8-1.5 cc.) balloon is inflated. With gentle advancement from the periphery, the flowing blood stream guides the catheter through the right ventricle into the pulmonary artery, where it impacts in a location from which the pulmonary artery wedge pressure is recorded. The balloon flotation catheter can be commonly used at the bedside and does not require fluoroscopy, is remarkably safe for a catheterization procedure, and in the majority of instances, the procedure is accomplished with a minimal delay.

2. Important parameters of physiological functions which are of significance and relevance in patient care decision-making include the level of left ventricular filling pressure, the level of pulmonary artery systolic and diastolic pressure, the cardiac output (by thermo-dilution), the level of pressures on the right side of the heart and other variables. The reproducibility of pressure measurements in the steady state condition is usually within ±2 mm. Hg., and the reproducibility of triplicate cardiac output measurements is ±3.9%.

3. It is possible to measure the absolute level of left ventricular filling pressure as well as of pulmonary venous pressure (essentially equivalent) with accuracies acceptable for diagnostic purposes. Central venous pressure measurements made heretofore relate poorly to levels of left ventricular filling pressure, and decision-making based upon either the absolute value or relative changes in central venous pressures are from time to time significantly misleading.

4. The thermo-dilution method allows for the calculation of the absolute level of cardiac output and stroke volume, and changes in this value occasioned by the natural course of the disease or by therapy. Absolute changes in cardiac output of approximately 0.2 L/min./M^2 are found to be significant.

5. Complications encountered utilizing the balloon flotation catheter system include thrombosis, balloon rupture, arrhythmias (uncommon), catheter knotting, and pulmonary infarction. Rupture of the pulmonary artery by balloon inflation has been reported, and is the only known fatal complication of the use of flotation catheters.

6. The broad correlation of hemodynamic measurements at the bedside with clinical manifestations of acute pump failure is good. High levels (exceeding 18 mm. Hg.) of mean pulmonary artery wedge pressure are seen in patients with clinical and x-ray evidence of pulmonary congestion and edema, a third heart sound and sinus tachycardia. At times, the radiological and physical signs of pulmonary congestion remain after successful lowering of wedge pressure by diuretics or other means. The diagnosis of mitral insufficiency and other important complications of coronary artery disease and acute myocardial infarction is facilitated by the measurements of pressure, blood flow and other variables.

7. Indications for balloon flotation catheterization of the pulmonary artery are present in between 10 and 20 percent of patients with acute myocardial infarction and include patients with complicated myocardial infarction--i.e., multiple infarcts, mitral regurgitation, ruptured ventricular septum, suspected hypovolemia, severe power failure of the heart from other causes, the use of certain interventions including impedance reduction, circulatory assist by balloon or external counterpulsation, and current clinical trials of other innovative interventions including use of propranolol, corticosteroids, glucose-insulin-potassium infusions, etc.

Selected References

1. Swan, H.J., Ganz, W., and Forrester, J., et. al.: Catheterization of the heart in man with use of a flow-directed balloon tipped catheter. NEJM 283:447, 1970.

2. Forrester, J., et. al.: Filling pressures in the right and left sides of the heart in acute myocardial infarction. A preappraisal of central venous pressure monitoring. NEJM 285:190, 1971.

ACUTE PUMP FAILURE--PRACTICAL MANAGEMENT

H.J.C. Swan, M.D.

Progressive steps to interventions of increasing complexity and potency are determined by the initial state of the patient and by favorable or unfavorable alterations occurring in the natural history of the disease state and/or in response to therapy.

1. Initial clinical evaluation of the fundamental cause and nature of acute pump failure includes assessment of the role of rhythm disturbance, pulmonary congestion and edema, or failure of forward cardiac output.

2. Serious alterations in any one of these factors demand immediate clinical intervention directed at its specific correction--cardioversion or Lidocaine for serious arrhythmias, powerful diuretic agents for severe pulmonary congestion or edema and consideration of the etiology of failure of forward cardiac output.

3. For patients with the more serious variants of pump failure not associated with cardiac dysrhythmia, obvious hypovolemia or disorders of cerebral, pulmonary or renal function a balloon flotation catheter should be advanced to record pulmonary arterial wedge pressure and, incidental to its passage to the right ventricle, right atrial mean pressure. When possible, measurement of cardiac output by the thermodilution principle should be obtained.

4. Moderate elevations (18-20 mm. Hg.) of pulmonary capillary wedge pressure but with a cardiac index in excess of 2.5 L/min./M^2 probably requires no treatment or at most one dose of a moderately potent diuretic (Lasix 40-80 mg.). For patients with somewhat higher mean pulmonary capillary wedge pressure or with more serious symptoms, diuretics should be used on one or more occasions. As the mean pulmonary capillary wedge pressure falls to levels of between 14-18 mm. Hg., the symptoms and signs of pulmonary congestion will disappear yet cardiac output will be maintained.

5. For patients with mean pulmonary capillary wedge pressure of less than 14 mm. Hg. no treatment is required unless cardiac index is depressed below 2.4 L/min./M^2. If this is associated with hypotension, then fluid loading should be employed bringing the pulmonary capillary wedge pressure to a value between 14 and 18 mm. Hg. This will occasion a rise in cardiac output and in arterial blood pressure.

6. When cardiac index is reduced substantively to levels below 2 L/min..M^2 and left ventricular filling pressure substantively exceeds 25 mm. Hg.

then the patient may be in the pre-shock level. It is our current practice to employ sodium-nitroprusside as an impedance reduction agent to allow for the more effective emptying of the left ventricle. Sodium-nitroprusside in doses of 16 to 128 Mgm./Min. can be employed under controlled and monitored situations. The first beneficial effect is a reduction of mean pulmonary capillary wedge pressure to values of 15-25 mm. Hg. with improvement of symptomatology. There is usually a small but significant increase in cardiac index which alters favorably over the ensuing hours so that the patient may be weaned from sodium-nitroprusside in 36 to 48 hours under most conditions.

7. In patients with clinical evidence of the shock syndrome or those in whom sodium-nitroprusside or other impedance reduction agents appear to be ineffective, inotropic agents may be used in small doses and with caution--Dopamine and Norepinephrine appear to be the most effective agents in this regard.

8. In patients with profound reduction in arterial blood pressure, yet with optimization of cardiac rhythm and rate, electrolytes, arterial oxygen saturation, pulmonary ventilation and function and peripheral vascular resistance, circulatory assistance by means of an intra-aortic balloon may be effective.

9. In patients who have suffered from severe and profound depression of cardiac function during acute myocardial infarction, careful followup should be instituted. After three months, the patient should be assessed for the feasibility of a definitive study including coronary arteriography and left ventriculography to define residual lesions in the coronary arteries and to determine whether or not operative intervention might improve the mechanical and metabolic functions of the residual healthy myocardium.

Selected References

1. Conn, Howard F., ed.: <u>Current Therapy 1975</u>. W.B. Saunders Company, Philadelphia, 1975.

2. Swan, H.J., and Chaterjee, K.: Vasodilator therapy in acute myocardial infarction. Mod. Conc. Card. Dis. <u>43</u>:119, 1974.

CORONARY ANGIOGRAPHY

Benjamin Befeler, M.D.

Coronary arteriography as a clinical tool has enhanced the interest in coronary artery disease and has provided an objective method to evaluate the natural course of this disease and the effects of different modalities of therapy. Coronary disease represents a monumental epidemiologic problem in the United States. About one-half million persons died of this disease in this country last year, hence the tremendous importance of having a safe and reproducible technique to delineate objectively the anatomy of the coronary vessels in vivo.

The study of the clinical anatomy of the coronary arteries is now commonplace and is widely used in the management of patients with coronary atherosclerosis. Data is now available by which prognosis can also be estimated by angiographic assessment of the location, severity, and extent of atherosclerotic obstruction. The demonstration of normal coronaries or of one vessel disease, with certain exceptions such as the left anterior descending, is associated with an excellent five year survival and dictates medical therapy. On the other hand, the five year survival of patients with severe three vessel disease is such that surgical therapy, when technically feasible, should be undertaken, since overall outcome can now be improved.

Anatomy

Basically there are three coronary arteries. (See Figure 3, p. 5.)

The right coronary artery originates in the right sinus of Valsalva. Then it runs a downward course in the atrio-ventricular groove and onto the inferior surface of the heart. In its proximal third, this vessel gives off several branches. They include the pulmonary conus branch which provides blood supply to the outflow tract of the right ventricle. This is a common collateral pathway to the anterior descending branch of the left coronary artery. When there is proximal obstruction of the right coronary artery, this pathway may become functional. In its mid-third, this vessel gives muscular branches to the right ventricular myocardium. One of these branches is the acute marginal. In the inferior wall, the right coronary artery runs in the atrio-ventricular groove to the crux of the heart where it bends upward, identifying the crux with an inverted U. An important branch at this point is the artery to the AV node. The right coronary artery, when dominant, provides blood supply to the posterior walls of both the left and right ventricles as the posterior descending artery.

The anterior descending runs in the anterior interventricular groove and usually terminates near the apex of the heart. This vessel gives the so-called anterior septal perforating branches, which provide blood supply to the anterior septum. Similar branches, the posterior septal perforators of smaller size, originate in the posterior descending branch which may arise either from the right coronary artery or from the circumflex, depending on which is the dominant vessel. The anterior descending also gives muscular branches both to the right and left ventricle. Among the branches to the left ventricle we find the diagonal branches, sometimes in numbers of two or three. Sometimes the diagonal branches may originate from the proximal circumflex. Collaterals may occur between the branches of the anterior descending and the posterior descending through the septal network.

The circumflex artery runs in the atrio-ventricular groove on the left side as a single vessel for a short distance, and then it bifurcates or trifurcates. When this vessel is anatomically dominant, it runs all the way down to the inferior wall of the heart. It gives several muscular branches to the anterolateral wall of the left ventricle and the major vessel of these branches is the obtuse marginal. After its division, the circumflex sometimes gives off the left atrial circumflex which is a posterolateral branch, providing blood supply to the left atrium. This is an inconstant vessel.

A number of minor coronary abnormalities have become better known with coronary arteriography. For example, several ostia may be present in the right sinus with separate origins of the main right coronary artery and the pulmonary conus branch. Other variants include a single coronary artery originating from the right sinus of Valsalva, and the circumflex branch originating from the right coronary ostium through a separate orifice in the right sinus of Valsalva and running around the conus of the left side. Occasionally one coronary artery originates from the pulmonary artery and this gives origin to a specific clinical picture with an arterio-venous fistula physiology.

It has been established arbitrarily that the dominant coronary is the vessel which goes past the crux of the heart. In humans, in approximately 60% of the cases, the right coronary artery is dominant, and in about 15%, the circumflex is dominant. In the remaining cases, one finds a balanced circulation which means that there is dual blood supply to the inferior wall of the heart.

The combination of coronary arteriography and coronary flow studies with radioactive materials, such as radioactive K, xenon and others, has expanded the possibilities for a more rational approach to surgical therapy. Coronary disease tends to be localized to the proximal segments of the coronary tree (Figure 1), making bypass grafting to intermediate and distal segments possible.

Indications for Procedure.

1) Incapacitating angina pectoris unimproved by medical therapy. These patients are considered for surgical intervention which is usually carried out if high grade proximal coronary obstructions are defined at angiography with good "runoff" beyond the obstructions.

2) Unstable or so-called intermediate anginal syndrome.

3) Angina pectoris in patients with congestive heart failure who are not responding adequately to medical therapy and are considered possible surgical candidates for reconstruction of the left ventricle and/or revascularization. It should be noted, however, that the risk of revascularization surgery is directly related to the degree of pump failure.

4) Post-infarction complications such as symptomatic ventricular aneurysm, perforated septum, gross mitral regurgitation.
5) Angina pectoris in young adults.
6) Atypical chest pain with or without normal resting and exercise electrocardiograms. In this group of patients, the test is performed for diagnostic purpose.
7) Suspected congenital lesions involving the coronary circulation.
8) Asymptomatic individuals with abnormal electrocardiograms. In this category we include persons who may be disqualified from insurance or from their occupations, e.g., airplane pilots.
9) Patients considered for valvular surgery with or without manifestations of coronary artery disease. The additional risk of coronary bypass surgery in patients needing valve replacement is generally small.
10) As a means of evaluating the results of surgical intervention.

Grading of Lesions

0) No arteriographic abnormalities noted.
1) Trivial irregularities in luminal diameter.
2) Localized narrowing estimated to be greater than 50%, but less than 90% of the luminal cross sectional area of a vessel.
3) Multiple narrowing in the same vessel estimated to be greater than 50% and less than 90%
4) Narrowing estimated to be greater than 90% of the luminal cross section area.
5) Total obstruction of a vessel without any filling of the distal segments from the proximal portion.

This scoring system is applied individually to each of the three main branches of the coronary system.

Hazards and Usefulness of the Technique

The hazards of angiographic evaluation relate primarily to the patient population and the experience of the angiographer. A mortality figure of 0.5% and a complication rate of 3 to 5%, related to acute myocardial infarction, systemic thromboembolism and peripheral arterial damage which is usually correctable, are to be anticipated. It also seems clear that angiographic assessment may underestimate, just as postmortem examination may overestimate, the extent of coronary disease. Certain areas within the coronary tree are less well evaluated. The inherent variability of coronary branch distributions may make it impossible to identify a vessel which has been occluded at its point of origin, but this must be uncommon.

This technique has increased our knowledge of coronary artery disease and has allowed us to establish clinical, pathologic and electrocardiographic correlations. It has also been an excellent tool for the selection of candidates for myocardial revascularization and has provided a major objective means of following these patients after surgery.(Figure 2)

Selected References

1. Wells, D.E., Befeler, B., Winkler, J.B., et al.: A Simplified Method for Left Heart Catheterization Including Coronary Arteriography. Chest, 63:959-962, 1973.

2. Proudfit, W.L., et al.: Selective Cinecoronary Arteriography - Correlation of the Clinical Findings in 1000 Patients. Circ., 33:901, 1966.

Figure 1

This illustration shows the distribution of significant coronary obstructive lesions. Since they are predominantly proximal, bypass grafting to more distal segments is readily accomplished.

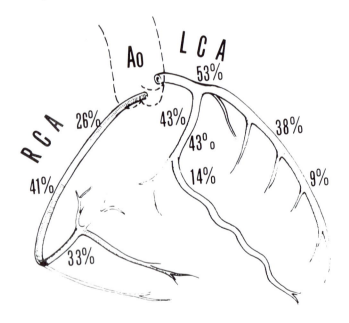

FIGURE 2 - CORONARY ANGIOGRAPHY AND LEFT VENTRICULOGRAPHY AS A PRELUDE TO SURGERY

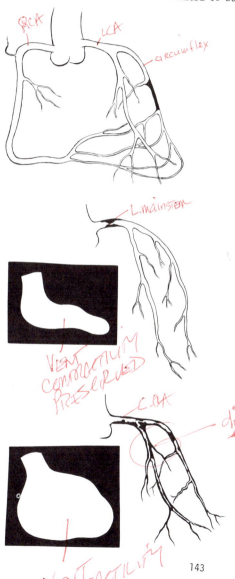

The circumflex is totally occluded. The right coronary supplies excellent collaterals to the distal circumflex. Under these circumstances there is no need for surgery.

The left main stem coronary artery is severely stenosed. Ventricular contractility is preserved (inset). Bypass surgery is indicated and an excellent result is likely.

The left coronary artery shows diffuse involvement. Ventricular contractility is poor (inset). Operation is not indicated as the risk is high and the expected results poor.

SURGERY FOR CORONARY ARTERY DISEASE

Gerard A. Kaiser, M.D.

At the present time we at the University of Miami believe that patients with ischemic coronary artery disease are candidates for coronary artery bypass surgery when their symptoms place them in one of the following groups:

First, the main group of patients are those with chronic unremitting angina who have not responded to medical therapy (including long-acting nitrites and propranolol), and who by coronary angiography are shown to have significant lesions (greater than 75%) in the proximal portion of at least 2 major coronary arteries with good distal runoff and good left ventricular function. Furthermore, a successful bypass procedure requires a distal coronary vessel larger than 1.5 mm. in diameter. There have been 240 patients in this group, 200 males and 40 females. It should be noted that as a group, the female patients did less well than the males, sustaining a higher rate of mortality and a lower rate of symptomatic relief.

The second group of patients are those with unstable angina, often referred to as the "intermediate coronary syndrome" or "preinfarction angina." These patients have persistent pain or a sudden change in the frequency or severity of their symptoms with the development of pain at rest in association with transient electrocardiographic changes, primarily ST-T wave abnormalities without associated enzyme elevation. In this group during the past three years, we have 60 selected patients who have received a saphenous vein bypass graft as an emergency procedure when coronary angiography has indicated that they have significant lesions with good distal vessels for bypass. There have been no fatalities in this group of patients and in our long-term followup, studies have shown a graft patency rate of 98%, which exceeds that of the patients with chronic stable angina (87%). In addition, this group of patients has shown marked improvement in their cardiac function which is even greater than those patients operated on in Group I.

There is a small subgroup of patients in this category who have been operated on for true infarction which is less than 6 hours old. They were thought to have unstable angina, but in retrospect, their enzymes were elevated prior to surgery. Seven patients in this category have been operated upon without a fatality. All developed infarctions which appeared to be smaller and less severe than a comparable group of patients who were treated medically. In the latter group, there were two patients in cardiogenic shock and two other patients who succumbed in the early post-infarction period. It is interesting to note that in the patients with chronic stable angina, the infarction rate following surgery has been 6%, whereas in patients with unstable angina, the infarction rate is 15% However, the mortality rate in patients with unstable angina has been better than the 4% rate noted in the patients operated upon with chronic stable angina as their symptom.

The third group of patients are those who are symptomatic and who have angiographically demonstrated main left coronary lesions or lesions of the left anterior descending proximal to the first septal perforator. These patients have the only anatomic lesions which we believe require bypass surgery in the presence of minimal symptoms.

The fourth group of patients are those with coronary artery disease who have one of the complications of ischemic heart disease, that is, a left ventricular aneurysm or papillary muscle rupture or dysfunction. In this group, it is now our feeling that patients should have a combined operation when anatomic lesions in the coronary arteries allow for bypass, that is, left ventricular aneurysm resection and/or mitral valve replacement combined with bypass surgery. Although the risks for this surgery are greater (10-15%) than for uncomplicated bypass procedures, we believe that the increased risk is justified because of the poor prognosis if revascularization is not done when indicated by the anatomic nature of the coronary arteries.

In summary, we believe that coronary artery bypass surgery using either the saphenous vein or internal mammary artery is a reliable operation which can be performed at low risk (4%) with the expectations of marked relief of the symptoms of angina (90%), improvement in cardiac function (65%), and a high patency rate (87%). The operation is less successful when the prime symptom is that of congestive heart failure. In this latter group of patients, the operative risk is higher and the long-term improvement in symptoms is much less satisfactory.

The early followup (2-5 years) on patients receiving myocardial revascularization indicates that the late infarction rate and the long-term mortality rate following successful bypass surgery is definitely lower than would be expected in a comparable group of patients who have not had bypass surgery. This difference is most notable in patients requiring double and triple coronary artery bypass procedures for multiple vessel occlusive disease. It therefore appears that not only is the quality of life markedly improved in the patients treated surgically, but the data now accumulating supports the view that there is also objective improvement.

Selected References

1. Kaiser, G. A., Ghahramani, A., Bolooki, H., Vargas, A., Thurer, R., Williams, H., Myerburg, R. J.: Role of Coronary Artery Surgery in Patients Surviving Unexpected Cardiac Arrest. Surg., 78:749-754, 1975.

2. Bolooki, H., Vargas, A., Green, R., Kaiser, G. A., Ghahramani, A.: Results of Direct Coronary Artery Surgery in Women. Jr. of Thor. and Cardiovasc. Surg., 69:271-277, 1975.

3. Bolooki, H., Sommer, L., Kaiser, G. A., Vargas, A., Ghahramani, A.: Long-Term Followup in Patients Receiving Emergency Revascularization for Intermediate Coronary Syndrome. Jr. of Thor. and Cardiovasc. Surg., 68:90-100, 1974.

4. Kaiser, G. A., Thurer, R. J., Vargas, A., Williams, W., Ghahramani, A., Bolooki, H.: Indications for Surgical Management of Coronary Artery Disease. Comprehensive Therapy, 1:20-25, November, 1975.

PRACTICAL THERAPY

DIGITALIS AND DIURETICS - PRACTICAL USE

Robert A. O'Rourke, M.D.

The cardiac effects of all digitalis glycosides are alike, and result from augmenting contractility and irritability, and from slowing heart rate and atrio-ventricular conduction. In addition, the digitalis preparations potentiate the vagal effect on the heart. However, the most important effect of digitalis on cardiac muscle is to increase its contractility.

It has been recently shown that digoxin, given as a daily dose without an initial loading dose, can accumulate until a steady state is reached in five to seven days. It is now apparent that this pattern of glycoside accumulation is due to apparent drug elimination characterized by excretion of a per cent of the daily amount of the body stores of cardiac glycosides rather than by excretion of a constant amount each day. Occasionally, a much larger dose of digitalis is required to control arrhythmias than to maintain left ventricular compensation. Under these circumstances it is important to know that the peak action of the drug is reached in 4 to 6 hours. Administration of digoxin in individual doses twice a day may avoid serum concentrations frequently associated with toxicity, while maintaining a more uniform concentration.

The major determinant of the maintenance dose of digoxin is renal function, and the renal clearance of digoxin is directly related to creatinine clearance. Therefore, the half life of digoxin will be increased when there is a marked decrease in creatinine clearance, and the serum half life of the drug will be longer. Hence, the dose of digoxin should be decreased by approximately 50% when the serum creatinine is in the range of 3-5 mg/100 ml, and by 75% when renal function is almost nil. Lean body weight is also a factor. Large muscular patients need more digoxin, not large obese patients.

The recent development of a radioimmunoassay method for measuring the serum digoxin level has been useful in evaluating the therapeutic effect of a specific digoxin dosage, especially when determined on blood drawn at least 6 to 8 hours after the last dose. It is particularly valuable in assessing patients with possible digitalis toxicity and for evaluating patients in congestive heart failure who fail to take their medications as instructed. However, the serum digoxin level is not a substitute for a complete clinical assessment of the patient, and patients with hypoxemia, hypokalemia and hypomagnesemia may have toxic manifestations of digitalis excess in the absence of an elevated serum digoxin concentration.

Although a host of cardiac rhythm disturbances may be caused by digitalis, virtually all of them can be understood by remembering that digitalis may increase atrioventricular block and also increase automaticity. Hence, first, second, third degree block and atrioventricular dissociation may be signs of digitalis intoxication. Similarly evidence of increased automaticity such as ventricular bigeminy or ventricular tachycardia may be the first sign of digitalis intoxication. Hybrid rhythms such as paroxysmal atrial tachycardia with block are a manifestation of both toxic effects of digitalis preparations.

A variety of diuretic agents are available, and in the patient with mild heart failure, almost all are effective. The vast majority of patients requiring chronic diuretic therapy can be well managed with the thiazide group of drugs and have little to gain from the availability of new and more powerful agents. However, in the more severe forms of heart failure, the selection of diuretics is more difficult, and any existing abnormalities in the serum electrolytes must be taken into account.

The "loop diuretics" such as furosemide and ethacrynic acid are extremely potent diuretic agents and are effective in the treatment of severe congestive heart failure. They are the preferred agents in failure associated with acute myocardial infarction. However, hypovolemia and secondary hyperaldosteronism must be avoided. An excessive reduction of blood volume may actually reduce cardiac output, interfere with renal function, and produce profound weakness and lethargy.

Selected References

1. Mason, D.T.: Digitalis Pharmacology and Therapeutics: Recent Advances. Annals of Internal Medicine, 80:520-530, 1974.

2. Frohlich, M.D.: Use and Abuse of Diuretics. Am. Heart J., 89:1-3, 1975.

3. Marcus, F.I.: Digitalis Pharamcokinetics and Metabolism. Am. J. Med., 58:452-459, 1975.

4. Davies, D.L. and Wilson, G.M.: Diuretics: Mechanism of Action and Clinical Application. Drugs, 9:178-226, 1975.

5. Rahimtoola, S.H. and Gunnar, R.M.: Digitalis in Acute Myocardial Infarction: Help or Hazard? Annals of Internal Medicine, 82:234-240, 1975.

ARRHYTHMIAS - PRACTICAL TREATMENT

James A. Ronan, Jr., M.D.

PREMATURE CONTRACTIONS

1. Atrial Prematures: These are seldom treated. However, when they are frequent in the setting of acute infarction, they may precede atrial fibrillation, and digoxin may be indicated.

2. Junctional Prematures: This is also a benign arrhythmia. However, they may reflect digitalis toxicity and withholding the drug is the treatment.

3. Ventricular Prematures: All PVC's do not need to be treated. Multifocal VPC's or PVC's in the setting of an acute myocardial infarction (AMI) need therapy because of the potential for developing ventricular fibrillation. In the setting of an AMI, the treatment of choice is Lidocaine, which is given intravenously. Lidocaine has a half-life of 1.5 hours, hence the time to achieve 90% steady-state concentration during a constant rate infusion is 4 to 6 hours. For this reason, it is important that an initial I.V. bolus be given. The dosage is 1 mg./kg. followed by an intravenous drip of 2 to 4 mg. per minute. If arrhythmias recur, a supplemental bolus of 25 to 50 mg. should be given every 30-45 minutes rather than increase the drip rate until steady-state is reached.

   When oral therapy is indicated, Quinidine Sulfate may be given at a dose of 200 to 300 mg. every six hours. Procaine Amide should be given at three hour intervals (because of its short half-life), a dosage schedule not well tolerated for chronic therapy. Make sure that PVC's are not related to digitalis excess, as the most important therapeutic intervention in this situation is to discontinue the cardiac glycoside.

BRADYCARDIAS

1. Sinus Bradycardia: This rhythm usually requires no treatment unless a reduction in cardiac output or frequent premature ventricular beats result. When sinus bradycardia causes serious consequences of reduced cardiac output (syncope, lightheadedness, confusion, oliguria, hypotension), atropine (IV dose 0.5 to 1.5 mgm) may be of temporary value. Caution should be used in acute myocardial infarction because of the myocardial ischemia which may be produced if sinus tachycardia occurs: occasionally supraventricular tachycardia has resulted and this in turn can cause A-V block. Pacemaker therapy is occasionally necessary for symptomatic sinus bradycardia.

2. **Escape Rhythms:** When the sinus rate slows to such an extent that a lower pacemaker (AV junctional or ventricular) takes over the heart rhythm, it is called an "escape" rhythm. The basic fault is not in the lower, but the upper pacemaker. The ventricular rate is usually 35 to 50 per minute and there is a loss of the mechanical effect of atrial contraction. Treatment is aimed at speeding the supraventricular pacemaker, usually with atropine, elevating the legs or light physical exercise. A pacemaker may be necessary.

3. **Heart Block:** Chronic complete heart block should be treated with a permanent artificial pacemaker. In acute myocardial infarction, complete heart block with a narrow QRS complex, usually seen in inferior wall myocardial infarction, is best treated with a temporary pacemaker if facilities are available and the personnel are experienced with pacemakers and their complications. If those two requirements are not met, the patient can be carefully observed in the Coronary Care Unit and atropine or a slow Isuprel infusion begun. This form of complete heart block is usually transient and clears in one to seven days. In acute infarction, if the complete heart block presents with a wide QRS complex, it is usually due to bilateral bundle branch block. A temporary pacemaker should be placed immediately; there is some evidence that a permanent pacemaker may prevent sudden death in the long term followup.

TACHYCARDIAS

1. **Sinus Tachycardia:** In the healthy person this is not usually detrimental and rates do not usually exceed 140 at rest. However, in the cardiac patient, the tachycardia is usually a reflection of underlying heart failure and must be treated accordingly.

2. **Paroxysmal Atrial Tachycardia:** PAT is one of the reciprocating tachycardias. The goal of treatment is to slow conduction in the A-V junction and thereby break the re-entry cycle. This is accomplished by drugs or maneuvers which increase parasympathetic nerve stimulation to the A-V node. Carotid sinus pressure, the Valsalva maneuver and vasopressors all act reflexively through the carotid baroceptors to slow A-V conduction. Digitalis slows A-V conduction both directly and indirectly through the parasympathetic nervous system. Propranolol in doses of 1 to 2 mg. intravenously is occasionally successful. Electrical cardioversion is rarely needed.

3. **Paroxysmal Atrial Tachycardia with Block (Ectopic Atrial Tachycardia):** This is often a digitalis induced arrhythmia where an irritable atrial focus discharges repetitively as in flutter. Carotid massage will therefore slow the ventricular response, but not abolish the arrhythmia. Withholding digitalis and, if the ventricular response is rapid, I.V. KCl. is the treatment. In those cases not due to digitalis, digoxin will effectively enhance the block at the A-V node when the ventricular response is rapid, and hence slow the rate.

Handwritten annotations at top:
Quinidine: may ↑ AV conduction
thus may give Dig first.
M.A.T.
↑100
varying PR
P wave varying morph.

4. Multifocal Atrial Tachycardia: This rhythm has a rate exceeding 100 per minute, has varying PR intervals, and varying P wave contours. It is commonly seen in chronic lung disease and with digitalis excess. The treatment should be aimed at the underlying disorder. Quinidine and Pronestyl are often helpful.

5. Atrial Flutter: With acute onset of atrial flutter, the atrial rate is usually 300 and the ventricular rate 150 (2:1 flutter). Digitalis may increase the AV block (3:1, 4:1, etc.) and occasionally breaks the flutter. Quinidine may convert to normal sinus rhythm, but should be used only after digitalis has been given in order to avoid the rapid AV conduction which may be produced by quinidine. Electrical cardioversion is particularly effective in this rhythm and may be successful with low energies (10 to 100 Watt-seconds).

6. Atrial Fibrillation: There are two approaches to the treatment of atrial fibrillation:

    1) Allow the atrial fibrillation to persist, but slow the ventricular rate to 60-90/minute
    2) Revert the rhythm to a normal sinus mechanism.

    In general, controlling the ventricular rate and allowing the subject to remain in atrial fibrillation is the treatment of choice if:

    1) There is at least moderate atrial enlargement
    2) The atrial fibrillation has been chronic or recurrent despite drug treatment
    3) The patient is elderly
    4) The underlying cuase of the atrial fibrillation has not been adequately treated (hyperthyroidism, acute heart failure following myocardial infarction)

    Reversion to normal sinus rhythm is usually attempted if none of the above are present or if severe and life-threatening cardiac failure has resulted directly because of the atrial fibrillation. Digitalis slows the ventricular rate through its action on the A-V junction. In many cases, particularly those with paroxysmal atrial fibrillation and no significant cardiac disease, digitalis produces reversion to sinus rhythm. Synchronized electrical (D.C.) cardioversion is the treatment of choice in those who do not respond to digitalis, in emergency situations, or in W.P.W. syndrome. Gradually increasing doses of quinidine are seldom used any more because large doses may be required which approach toxic range and because it may take many days for the proper level to be reached. Anticoagulation is advised for three to four weeks prior to cardioversion in those patients with mitral valve obstruction or with severe heart failure.

7. A-V Junctional Tachycardias: A rate of greater than 60 is "tachycardia" for the A-V junction. It is usually seen in digitalis ex-

cess, acute myocardial infarction, postoperative cardiac surgical cases, and with severe myocardiopathies. In digitalis excess, the main therapy is withholding the digitalis. In the others, digitalis may be helpful. In some instances, the tachycardia is a "reciprocating" tachycardia and may be treated like paroxysmal atrial tachycardia.

8. <u>Ventricular Tachycardia</u>: Ventricular tachycardia is frequently a precursor to ventricular fibrillation, especially in the setting of acute myocardial infarction. Lidocaine in doses of 50 to 100 mg. repeated every few minutes as needed up to a dose of 400 mg. is usually successful in terminating ventricular tachycardia. Electrical conversion at low energies (10 to 100 Watt-seconds) may be used. Procaine amide and quinidine have largely been replaced by the above approach.

Selected References

1. Lown, B., Klein, M.D., and Hershberg, P.I.: Coronary and Precoronary Care. American Journal of Medicine, 46:705, 1969.

2. DeSanctis, R.W., Block, P., and Hutter, A.M., Jr.: Tachyarrhythmias in Myocardial Infarction. Circulation, 45:681, 1972.

2. Gettes, L.S.: The Electrophysiologic Effects of Antiarrhythmic Drugs. Am. J. Cardiol., 28:526, 1971.

MEDICAL TREATMENT OF ANGINA PECTORIS

Robert A. O'Rourke, M.D.

Many patients with the symptom of angina pectoris can be managed with medical therapy. In fact, according to the present state of knowledge of the surgical approaches to the management of angina pectoris, most indications for surgery presuppose a prior trial of medical therapy. Before the institution of a full medical regimen, however, one must be certain of the clinical diagnosis. A thorough history and physical examination, combined with electrocardiography and exercise testing, will permit reasonably accurate identification of most patients.

The clinical types of angina may be described in relationship to the following initiating factors:

1. Effort
   - predictable pain with effort
   - unpredictable pain requiring other factors to be present in order to expose angina of effort, i.e., food or tension
2. Second wind phenomenon
   - angina occurring with the first effort in the morning. Later the same degree of exercise does not produce angina.
3. Tachycardia
   - increases oxygen requirements
   - decreases coronary filling
4. Spontaneous angina
   - sympathetic overactivity associated with an increased heart rate and increased blood pressure; may be pre-infarction state
5. Emotion
   - autonomic discharge provoked by fear, anger or anxiety
6. Thermal - cold
   - reflex vasoconstriction of peripheral and coronary arteries
7. Nocturnal
   - sympathetic discharge (dreams)
   - left ventricular failure - a variant of nocturnal cardiac dyspnea
   - decreased perfusion pressure associated with drop in blood pressure
8. Postprandial - (possible causes)
   - GI "steal"
   - GI disease

Angina pectoris occurs when the myocardial oxygen demand exceeds the capacity of the diseased coronary vessels to deliver oxygen. Accordingly, an effective therapeutic approach to angina pectoris depends on a favorable alteration of this balance by augmenting the capacity of the coronary arteries to deliver blood to the ischemic regions of the myocardium or by reducing the myocardial oxygen demand. In discussing the treatment of angina, it is necessary to consider the major determinants of myocardial oxygen consumption which are:

MYOCARDIAL O₂ CONSUMPTION DETERMINANTS

1) Systolic wall stress (related to ventricular systolic pressure, ventricular size and wall thickness).
2) Heart rate
3) Contractile state of the myocardium.

An increase in systolic blood pressure, heart rate or contractility is associated with an increase in the myocardial oxygen demand and frequently results in the onset of chest pain in patients with occlusive coronary artery disease. Therefore, medical therapy designed to reduce or eliminate exacerbating factors such as systemic hypertension, hyperthyroidism, anemia, congestive heart failure and tachyarrhythmias may reduce the frequency of angina in certain patients despite the fact that the treatment is not specific for angina pectoris.

Specific medications utilized for the prevention or treatment of angina pectoris appear to act primarily by decreasing the myocardial oxygen demand at any given workload rather than by increasing coronary blood flow to ischemic myocardium.

Vasodilators

Sublingual or chewable nitrites (nitroglycerin and isosorbide dinitrate) cause systemic arterial and venous dilatation. The result is a moderate decrease in the systolic arterial blood pressure, a measureable reduction in the left ventricular diameter and a definite decrease in the myocardial oxygen demand despite a slight increase in heart rate and contractility. Whether or not the nitrites also increase collateral coronary arterial blood flow to areas of ischemic myocardium remains unresolved.

Oral nitrites, in the doses usually prescribed, are of no proven efficacy in the treatment of angina pectoris. These compounds are broken down into relatively inactive metabolites during one passage through the liver and usually do not produce the same hemodynamic effects on blood pressure and heart size as when they are taken sublingually. However, there is some new research evidence suggesting that the oral nitrates may produce significant hemodynamic and antianginal effects when given in higher doses than those usually prescribed.

Beta Blockers

Beta blocking agents such as propranolol (Inderal) reduce the myocardial oxygen demand by diminishing systolic blood pressure, heart rate and myocardial contractility at rest and during exercise. Since this drug has a half-life of 2.5 to three hours, propranolol should be given four times a day. The usual therapeutic dose required to decrease the frequency of angina significantly (as compared to a placebo) is 80 to 400 mg a day in four divided doses. This drug should be administered carefully to patients with evidence of reduced left ventricular performance and should not be given alone (without simultaneous digitalis) to patients with signs and symptoms of congestive heart failure. In patients with angina pectoris without congestive heart failure, the dose should be increased until there is a decrease in the resting heart rate by at least 10% and a decrement in the heart rate-systolic blood pressure product (HR x SBP) at any given workload as compared to pre-therapy values.

Selected References

1. Lesch, M. and Gorlin, R.: Pharmacologic Therapy of Angina Pectoris, Mod. Conc. of Cardiovas. Dis., 42:5-10, 1973.

Figure for following article:

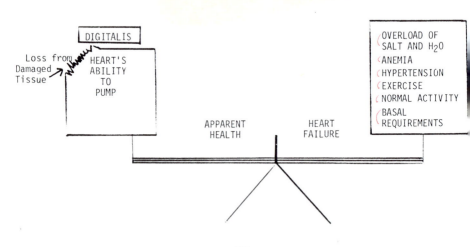

CARDIAC FAILURE - PRACTICAL TREATMENT

Gordon A. Ewy, M. D.

Introduction

Cardiac failure occurs when the heart cannot meet the demands of the body for cardiac output. The spectrum of pump failure is broad, ranging from the patient with symptoms only on severe or prolonged exertion to the patient in cardiogenic shock at rest. A moderate amount of ventricular dysfunction may not be clinically apparent to a patient whose activity is restricted because of another medical disability, whereas a mild degree of impairment results in symptoms and signs of failure when the activity level and the salt and water intake are great.

Ventricular dysfunction can be a segmental problem as is seen in the ventricles of patients with coronary artery disease, or it may be a diffuse defect as is seen in heart muscle failure from a cardiomyopathy (primary myocardial disease), hypertensive, valvular or congenital heart disease. Failing myocardium is characterized by an abnormal ventricular function curve (Fig.5,p.6). Thus, for any given filling pressure, the amount of force generated, and therefore stroke work is decreased in the failing myocardium.

Chronic Congestive Heart Failure (See Figure on previous page)

Chronic congestive failure may result in excessive salt and water retention producing a rise in venous pressure and accumulation of edema fluid.

The goal of therapy in congestive heart failure (CHF) is to effect a more favorable balance between the body needs and hearts ability to supply those needs. Decreasing the body's need is accomplished by decreasing the activity of the patient and limiting excessive salt intake. Complete bed rest may be necessary. In chronic CHF, an important therapeutic maneuver is to have the patient take afternoon naps in addition to limiting strenuous activity. All too often the patient thinks if he has a "bad heart" it can be improved by exercise. In patients with chronic CHF, this concept needs to be changed.

One of the most common predisposing factors to congestive heart failure is hypertension. Once CHF occurs, control of blood pressure is essential to decrease the work load on the heart.

The symptoms of CHF are congestive symptoms and/or symptoms of inadequate cardiac output. Congestion produces symptoms which include dyspnea, edema, nocturia, nausea and anorexia: the major effect of diuretics is to decrease congestion.

Initial diuretic therapy is usually Hydrochlorothiazide 50 mgm daily or b.i.d. Potassium replacement therapy must be given in patients who are receiving diuretics for therapy of CHF. Stronger diuretics, Furosemide (40 mgm tablets), may be necessary. In severe refractory failure, combinations of two or more diuretics may be necessary.

In some patients failure cannot be controlled because of increased work imposed by structural defects such as ventricular aneurysm, valvular obstruction or insufficiency, or congenital defects. These patients need to be evaluated for the possibility of surgical correction.

The other arm of our balance is the heart's ability to pump. We have very few agents that help the heart to function better. Digitalis is the only practical long term inotropic agent. Digitalis excess on the other hand can result in severe dysrhythmias and death. Because of this fact, it must be given with care.

Knowledge of several aspects of digitalis therapy is necessary:

1) Loading dose not always necessary.
2) Size of loading dose should be only three times maintainence dosage.
3) Decrease dose with decreased renal function.
4) Decrease dose with age and decreased body weight.
5) Know what to expect and what not to expect from digitalis therapy.
   The physician often expects too much from digitalis. It is important to remember that at best, digitalis improves the ventricular function curves only moderately and does not return it anywhere near normal in patients with advanced heart failure. It will not consistently return the heart rate to normal in patients with advanced failure. If the stroke volume is decreased because of pump failure, the only way the patient keeps cardiac output up is with a rapid heart rate.
6) Beware of symptoms of signs of digitalis excess.
   Most physicians are aware of the gastrointestinal side effects. Recent publications point to the frequency of central nervous system side effects such as acute fatigue, confusion, and even psychosis. The most frequent arrhythmias from digitalis are premature ventricular beats, second and third degree heart block, AV junctional tachycardia and AV junctional escaped beats. The most serious arrhythmias are atrial tachycardia with block, ventricular tachycardia and bidirectional ventricular tachycardia.
7) Know value of blood determinations.
   Therapeutic range of digoxin is 1 to 2 nanograms/ml. The sample must be drawn at least four to six hours after the last dose. Samples taken before this time are falsely elevated. In the steady state, the serum level can be doubled or halved by doubling or halving the maintenance dose of digoxin.
8) Know how to treat digitalis excess.
   Patients with suspected digitalis should be monitored. Digitalis stopped, diuretics held, electrolytes and renal function evaluated, and patient evaluated. Specific therapy is detailed in reference (1).

Acute Pulmonary Edema

Pulmonary edema results when the pulmonary venous pressure becomes greater than the oncotic pressure - the result is extravasation of fluid into the pulmonary extravascular spaces.

The prime objective in treating pulmonary edema is to reduce this elevated pulmonary venous pressure. Therapy, therefore, depends upon an accurate assessment of the underlying cause. In a patient with mitral stenosis and recent onset atrial fibrillation with rapid ventricular response, (the rapid heart rate shortens diastole to such an extent that the left atrium does not have time to empty via the stenotic mitral valve) the prime objective is to slow the heart rate, allowing more diastolic time for left atrial emptying during diastole. The therapy of choice depends on the clinical status of the patient. If the patient is in an extreme state, the only logical course of action is emergency cardioversion. In less urgent situations, the measures outlined below to quickly reduce venous return should be followed by therapy to decrease the ventricular response to atrial fibrillation by intravenous digitalis: Quabain (full digitalizing dose is 0.75 mgm. Maximal effect is 20 minutes. Initial dose should be 0.2 mgm I.V. followed by 0.1 mgm at 20 minute intervals until desired effect or until digitalizing dose reached) or digoxin (full digitalizing dose 0.75 to 1.5 mgm depending upon patient's lean body mass. Maximal effect is four hours. Initial dose should be 0.5 mgm with 0.25 mgm every four hours until desired response). These patients should be under continuous electrocardiographic monitoring. One also may have to alter the dose if factors that predispose to digitalis sensitivity (such as hypokalemia) are present.

However, the majority of patients in acute pulmonary edema will have left ventricular pump failure. In this situation, one would think acute intravenous digitalization would be the therapy of choice; however, IT IS NOT. Acute intravenous digitalis increases peripheral vascular resistance before it has its inotropic effect and therefore only adds to the overburdened failing left ventricle. The therapy of choice is:

ACUTE DECREASE VENOUS RETURN by the following maneuvers:

1) Sitting the patient upright.
2) Placing his legs over the side of bed in a dependent position.
3) Rotating tourniquets.
4) Oxygen therapy. (Low flow if patient has chronic lung disease)

.... THINK ....

5) Intravenous morphine (Vasodilates, tranquilizes, decreases ventilation)
6) Intravenous Furosemide. (It is interesting that this diuretic lowers pulmonary venous pressure long before its diuretic action).
7) Other maneuvers. (Such as cardioversion or digitalization - see above)
8) Phlebotomy.

The dashed lines between items 1 to 4 and 5 to 8 remind us to stop and think before proceeding. Items 1 to 4 are almost automatic. Intravenous morphine is very helpful, but if the patient has severe dyspnea secondary to chronic obstructive lung disease and not pulmonary edema, morphine could suppress the hypoxia drive with catastrophic results.

Likewise, if the patient's pulmonary edema is secondary to dysrhythmic disorders from digitalis intoxication, digitalis or diuretics would be contraindicated. In the absence of these conditions, Morphine and Lasix are effective additions to the non-invasive maneuvers which decrease venous return. The diuretic response to Lasix will occur within 60 minutes. If there is no response, the dose is doubled.

CARDIOGENIC SHOCK

By definition, cardiogenic shock is inadequate cardiac output with adequate filling pressure. Cardiogenic shock in acute myocardial infarction occurs when greater than 40% of the left ventricular mass is damaged. It is clinically manifested by symptoms and signs of inadequate organ perfusion, i.e. cold clammy skin, inadequate urine output, mental confusion and restlessness.

Experimental observations by Moroko and associates indicate that not all of the damaged or dysfunctioning muscle is irreversibily damaged. A sizeable portion is ischemic; whether this ischemic portion recovers or progresses to necrosis depends upon the critical balance between supply and demand. In acute infarction, the supply is compromised and therefore the greatest chance for recovery of the ischemic myocardium is to reduce myocardial demand. Factors which improve muscle survival are:

1) Decreasing heart rate, i.e. emergency cardioversion if atrial fibrillation; cautious use of beta blockers to slow heart rate in sinus rhythm. Care must be taken if patient is in heart failure.
2) Maintaining adequate coronary perfusion pressure; don't let systolic arterial pressure get below 90)
3) Oxygen therapy.
4) Balloon pumping.
5) Maintain optional filling pressure; some patients can be hypovolemic secondary to diuretic therapy and actually need more volume. Others with elevated pressure need decrease in either afterload (if hypertensive) or preload.

These patients need hemodynamic monitoring with a Swan Ganz catheter and an intra-arterial pressure monitor and therefore need to be transferred from the emergency room environment to a special intensive care area as soon as they are stabilized. The details of the management of such critically ill and hemodynamically unstable patients has been discussed elsewhere.

Selected Reference

1. Ewy, G.A., Marcus, F.I., Fillmore, S.J., Matthews, N.P.: Digitalis Intoxication - Diagnosis, Management and Prevention, Cardiovascular Drug Therapy, 153-174, 1974.

CARDIOPULMONARY RESUSCITATION

Ralph Lazzara, M.D.

Every day nearly 1,000 Americans who suffer a heart attack die before they reach the hospital. Thus, the problem of prehospital sudden death is one of major proportion and represents a major challenge to the medical profession. The patients at highest risk appear to be those with a known history of coronary artery disease, particularly if it is of recent onset; an age of greater than 45; other accompanying cardiovascular diseases such as hypertension; and frequent ectopic beats, particularly if they are multifocal and non-parasystolic in nature. The pattern of pain of unstable angina at rest is particularly significant.

Whatever the factors which might identify those patients at high risk, statistical studies performed in Seattle, Washington and in Miami, Florida reflect that from 15 to 25 per cent of victims of sudden ventricular fibrillation who receive effective cardiopulmonary resuscitation with on-site defibrillation and adjunctive care by well-trained emergency paramedics, where the resuscitated patient is delivered to a hospital with an effective emergency department staff and coronary care unit, will survive to return to a useful life-style.

For instructional purposes, the American Heart Association standards for cardiopulmonary resuscitation have been divided into: 1) Basic Life Support, and 2) Advanced Life Support. Basic Life Support, which is being taught to the lay public, paramedics, and nursing personnel, as well as to physicians, consists primarily of the well-known ABC's of cardiopulmonary resuscitation: A) Airway Management; B) Breathing or Artificial Ventilation; and C) Circulation or External Cardiac Compression. These techniques are outlined in Figure 1 for one and two rescuer resuscitation.

Establishment of adequate advanced life support requires first the insertion of a device to stabilize the airway, either an endotracheal tube or an esophageal airway. Ventilation is then provided using a bag-type ventilator or a respirator of the volume cycled or manually triggered type. The use of 100% oxygen is required since hypoxia is the primary cellular deficiency which must be corrected. A central venous catheter must be placed using either a subclavian vein, an external jugular vein, or an internal jugular vein in order to provide a route for fluid and drug administration.

In patients with a witnessed arrest or in a monitored environment, a single precordial thump may generate a small electrical stimulus in a heart that is reactive. If the heart does not respond, external massage is instituted.

When satisfactory pumping and ventilation are restored and an intravenous line inserted, attention is directed toward the cardiac rhythm. Generally, the rhythm will be ventricular fibrillation, asystole, or ventricular tachycardia. Electrical defibrillation with 200 Joules as an average shock is indicated for ventricular fibrillation or ventricular tachycardia. Lesser shocks should be employed if there is suspicion of digitalis intoxication. Larger shocks may be associated with cardiac damage. Possible causes or contributing factors to these arrhythmias should be sought in the form of drug intoxication (i.e., digitalis, quinidine, electrolyte disturbances, acid-base, or blood gas disturbances). The successful conversion of the arrhythmia may be facilitated by the correction of such disturbances or the use of antiarrhythmic agents such as lidocaine in a dose of 50 to 100 mgm. IV as a bolus. Cardiac asystole is most difficult to deal with because it is commonly the end result of what was initially ventricular fibrillation after prolonged arrest. A high percentage of patients with cardiac asystole are not resuscitatable or have permanent brain damage.

The essential drugs in advanced life support in addition to Lidocaine include the following: Sodium bicarbonate, epinephrine, atropine sulfate and calcium chloride.

Sodium bicarbonate is necessary to treat metabolic acidosis. An initial dose is administered intravenously in a dose of 1 meq/kg by bolus injection. Arterial blood gases should be monitored to determine the degree of acidosis and the need for subsequent sodium bicarbonate therapy.

Epinephrine is useful primarily in asystole to restore electrical activity and in cases of fine ventricular fibrillation to enhance the myocardial electrical potential. Epinephrine is administered in a dose of 5 to 10 ml. of a 1:10,000 solution intravenously. It is rarely necessary to administer catecholamines or other medications intracardiac, since with adequate cardiac massage, intravenous administration should result in delivery of the drugs to the coronary arteries.

Atropine sulfate is used to enhance atrio-ventricular conduction and accelerate the cardiac rate in cases of sinus bradycardia by reducing the vagal tone. The initial dose of atropine sulfate should be 0.5 mg. or less, administered intravenously as a bolus.

Calcium chloride is an inotropic and chronotropic drug which increases myocardial contractility and ventricular excitability. Therefore, calcium chloride is useful in treating electromechanical dissociation and in restoring an electrical rhythm in instances of asystole or fine ventricular fibrillation. The dose of calcium chloride is 2.5 ml. to 5 ml.

Finally, the insertion of temporary transvenous or transthoracic pacer wires may be attempted to induce electrical activity in cardiac asystole or severe bradycardia.

If resuscitation is successful, attention is directed to post arrest complications and the prevention of recurrent cardiac arrest. The most frequent complications are cerebral edema, neurological damage, aspiration pneumonia, and additional cardiac damage resulting in myocardial infarction, hypotension, or cardiac failure. Fractured ribs and gastric distention are common but rarely serious. Ruptured viscus is rare. The duration of time that resuscitation should be continued is difficult to define. Resuscitations that require more than one hour are rarely successful in restoring a functional patient. Prevention of recurrent cardiac arrests involves a thorough clinical evaluation of the circumstances of the previous arrest, assessment of the complications of the arrest, and the use of appropriate measures which may include antiarrhythmic agents or a correction of various clinical disturbances.

SELECTED REFERENCES

1. Stephenson, H.E., Jr., Cardiac Arrest and Resuscitation. C.V. Mosby Company, St. Louis, Mo., 1974

2. Journal of the American Medical Association, February 18, 1974, Volume 227, No. 7 (Supplement).

3. Findeiss, J. C., M.D., ed., Emergency Medical Care, Symposia Specialists, Miami, Florida, 1975.

FIGURE I - The ABC's of Basic Life Support

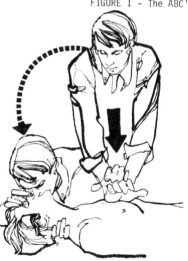
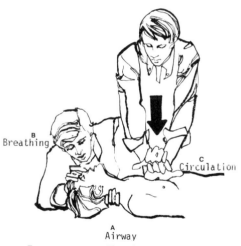

One rescuer cardiopulmonary resuscitation
 -- 15 chest compressions
    (rate of 80/minute)
 -- 2 quick lung inflations

(As per Reference #2 above)

Two rescuer cardiopulmonary resuscitation
 -- 5 chest compressions
    - Rate of 60/minute
    - No pause for ventilation
 -- 1 lung inflation
    - After each 5 compressions
    - Interposed between compressions

HYPERTENSION

PATHOLOGY OF HYPERTENSION

William C. Roberts, M.D.

Other than age and sex, systemic hypertension, hyperlipidema and smoking are the three major factors which increase the risk of development of symptomatic cardiovascular disease. Of the three, two are correctable: smoking, by abstinence; and hypertension, by certain drugs. It is uncertain as yet whether or not reduction in the levels of serum lipids will decrease the frequency of symptomatic cardiovascular disease. Among patients with symptomatic cardiovascular disease, however, hypertension is more common than hyperlipidemia. Because it is more common and because it is correctable by therapy, hypertension deserves far more emphasis than it has received in the past.

To emphasize the devastating effect of hypertension on our society, the frequency of hypertension in the more common cardiovascular disorders is listed in the accompanying table. At least 50% of patients with the listed complications have had hypertension at one time and at least 70% of them have cardiomegaly at necropsy. It is probable that cardiomegaly in most of the patients is caused by hypertension, and that cardiomegaly is a good marker of previous hypertension. It might be better to approach hypertension by asking if the blood pressures were never over 140/90 mm. Hg, how much cardiovascular disease would be eliminated? Complications of atherosclerosis would at least be delayed and dissecting aortic aneurysm and rupture of intracerebral aneurysm would be virtually eliminated.

THE FREQUENCIES OF SYSTEMIC HYPERTENSION AND CARDIOMEGALY IN VARIOUS CARDIOVASCULAR CONDITIONS (THE HYPERTENSIVE DISEASES)

Condition		% with Hypertension*	% with Cardiomegaly or, LVH @ Necropsy†
I.	Sudden death	50	70
II.	Angina pectoris	50	75
III.	Acute myocardial infarction‡	50	75
IV.	Complications of acute myocardial infarction		
	A. Rupture of left ventricular free wall	70	85
	B. Rupture of ventricular septum	70	85
	C. Rupture of papillary muscle	70	85
	D. Left ventricular aneurysm (healed)	70	80
V.	Aneurysm of aorta		
	A. Fusiform, sacular or cylindric	60	80
	B. Dissecting	80	95
VI.	Atherothrombotic obstruction of abdominal aorta or of its branches	70	?
VII.	Cerebrovascular accident (stroke)		
	A. Atherothrombotic cerebral infarction	50	70
	B. Intracerebral hemorrhage	> 90	> 90
	C. Lacunar softenings	> 90	> 95
	D. Charcot-Bouchard aneurysm	> 90	> 95
VIII.	Renal failure	> 90	> 90
IX.	Miscellaneous		
	A. Calcific aortic valve disease of the elderly	50	70
	B. Calcification of the mitral anulus	40	60

* Blood pressure = systolic > 140 or diastolic > 90 mm. Hg. Limited to persons < age 66 years.
† Heart weight = women > 350 and men > 400 gms.
‡ Transmural type. Nearly all patients with fatal subendocardial necrosis have cardiomegaly.

PHYSICAL EXAMINATION IN PATIENTS WITH HYPERTENSION

Michael S. Gordon, M.D.

The physical findings in hypertension can be divided into those which reflect a cause of hypertension, and those which are an effect of hypertension.

I. Findings which suggest a secondary cause of hypertension
   A. The most important clues to a secondary cause are:
      1. Diminished or delayed femoral pulses in coarctation.
      2. Flank bruit in renovascular hypertension. This bruit is most often high pitched, heard best with the diaphragm and is systolic-diastolic or continuous. It is present in 60% of patients with renovascular hypertension and only 5% of essential hypertensives. When listening over the anterior abdomen remember there are other causes of abdominal bruits.
      3. Postural hypotension in pheochromocytoma and primary aldosteronism.
   B. The general appearance may give a significant clue:
      1. There are "no fat pheos". They are hypermetabolic with diaphoresis and tremor.
      2. Look for skin, fat, and face changes in Cushing's disease.
      3. Black patients rarely have renovascular hypertension (but frequently have malignant hypertension)
      4. Age alone may be a clue:
         a. The sudden onset of hypertension in a young patient suggests renal parenchymal disease, e.g., acute glomerulonephritis.
         b. Renovascular disease usually occurs at less than 20 or greater than 50 years, while essential hypertension has its onset in the years between.
   C. Severe retinopathy is consistent with pheochromocytoma, while mild changes are consistent with primary aldosteronism.
   D. Less common findings:
      1. Evidence of peripheral emboli suggests a renovascular etiology.
      2. Polycystic kidneys may be palpated.
      3. Muscle weakness may be demonstrated in primary aldosteronism with hypokalemia.
   E. Finally, certain etiologies associated with high cardiac output and systolic hypertension may be readily recognized on physical examination, including anemia, thyrotoxicosis, hyperdynamic heart syndrome, A-V fistula and aortic regurgitation.

II. Findings which are an effect of hypertension
   A. Funduscopic findings range from early spasm with decrease in retinal artery caliber to exudates and hemorrhages and finally papilledema. The Keith-Wagener classification includes a second

stage before exudates and hemorrhages occur, which is characterized by increased tortuosity and A-V nicking. These latter findings are likely sclerotic changes and not related to hypertension per se. However, the K-W classification remains useful from a prognostic standpoint.
B. The cardiac examination in patients with diastolic blood pressures greater than 100 mm. Hg reveals:
1. a palpable or audible pathologic fourth sound (atrial diastolic gallop) in 75%.
2. The majority of these patients also have a sustained but not displaced left ventricular impulse at the apex.
3. A palpable or audible pathologic third sound occurs in about 1/3 of such patients and follows the development of the S_4.
4. The aortic second sound is enhanced in 80%.
5. A hemodynamically insignificant short, early, crescendo-decrescendo murmur at the upper right sternal edge reflecting turbulence across the aortic valve is heard in 70%.
6. Hemodynamically insignificant aortic regurgitation is heard in 10%. (If in an acute setting, think of dissection.)
7. Later, with overt failure and cardiac dilatation (not just hypertrophy) the murmur of mild papillary muscle dysfunction may appear.
C. Finally, bruits over the carotid and peripheral vessels may be heard.

Selected References

1. Page, I. H., et. al.: Hypertension, a mosaic in medicine. Medcom, Inc., 1971.

2. Kaufman, J. J., et al.: Hypertension - primary and secondary. Ann. Int. Med. 75:761, 1971

3. Fraley, E. E., and Feldman, B. H.: Renal hypertension - current concepts. NEJM. 287:550, 1972.

4. Barlow and Kincaid-Smith: The auscultatory findings in hypertension. Brit. Ht. J. 22:505, 1960.

WORK-UP OF THE NEWLY DISCOVERED HYPERTENSIVE PATIENT

Eliseo Perez-Stable, M.D.

The evaluation of the newly discovered hypertensive patient is a frequent and important clinical problem for the practicing physician. It has been estimated that there are approximately 23 million persons in the United States who can be defined as hypertensives by the criterion of blood pressure above 160/95 mm. Hg. A major health education campaign is under way to detect the more than half of these hypertensive persons who are unaware of their condition. As a result of this campaign it is expected that an increasing number of patients will arrive at primary care centers with recently discovered hypertension.

Hypertension has emerged as the most important of the chronic cardiovascular disorders of man, because it is the one common cardiovascular disease in which treatment has been demonstrated to be effective. Consequently, the main goal of the work-up should be to help the physician in selecting the best therapeutic modality to lower the elevated arterial pressure of his patient.

Approaches to Work-up

There are many different approaches to what constitutes an adequate work-up of a hypertensive patient. It is known that 90 per cent or more of patients have essential hypertension. The physician may limit his work-up to a minimum, running the risk of missing curable forms of hypertension or he may decide to subject all his patients to a complete and expensive work-up. The latter has occurred more frequently.

Purpose of Work-up

A simpler approach which could be used in every uncomplicated hypertensive patient would only include: history and physical examination, CBC, urinalysis, serum potassium, BUN or serum creatinine, blood glucose, serum uric acid and an electrocardiogram. The purposes of this work-up are: 1) Determine the type of hypertension. 2) Identify any coexisting condition which may alter the therapeutic approach. 3) Search for curable forms of hypertension.

1. Determine the type of hypertension -- A history and physical examination is all that is needed to determine the type of hypertension. In patients with malignant or accelerated hypertension, hospitalization and immediate lowering of the blood pressure is mandatory. In less severe forms of the disease it is advisable to withhold therapy until three blood pressure readings during separate outpatient visits are completed. In general, the higher the pressure, the worse the prognosis. Controlled studies have demonstrated that the risk of morbidity and mortality is much higher than was previously suspected for relatively lower blood pressures. These data permit redefinition of clinical severity as seen in Table 2. Patients who are young and/or black carry an even higher risk at any given elevated blood pressure. If the hypertension is labile, the electrocardiographic finding of left ventricular enlargement or complete left bundle branch block would be a strong indication for drug treatment.

The two main mechanisms regulating blood pressure are the peripheral resistance and the cardiac output. Variations in pressure represent primarily variations in the product of cardiac output and peripheral resistance (BP = C.O. X PR). In recent years it has been shown that in labile and early hypertension, the cardiac output is frequently elevated and the peripheral resistance normal. This hemodynamic situation is common in young hypertensives and the arterial pressure may be normalized with the use of drugs which decrease the cardiac output. However, in most cases of uncomplicated fixed hypertension after the age of 40, the cardiac output is normal and the peripheral resistance increased. In these instances, drug therapy should be directed toward arteriolar dilation.

More recently it has been suggested that patients with essential hypertension do not fall into a homogenous group and that they can be separated into three subgroups according to the activation of the reninangiotensin-aldosterone system: low renin (25%); normal renin (60%) and high renin (15%). This hormonal profile may allow the physician to individualize drug treatment. In the high renin subgroup, the hypertension is vasoconstrictor medicated and these patients will respond to the administration of renin-suppressing agents. In the low renin group the elevated blood pressure is volume-dependent and normalization of the arterial pressure may only require the use of diuretics. However, there are some theoretical objections and many practical difficulties in categorizing hypertensive patients in this manner. We consider that at the present time this categorization is impractical as a routine procedure and should be reserved for special situations or as a research tool.

2. <u>Identify any coexisting condition which may alter the therapeutic approach</u> -- This is an important aspect of the evaluation of the hypertensive patient which frequently does not receive adequate consideration. In advanced age or in the presence of extensive arterial disease it may not be rewarding to look for diagnoses for which therapy is not indicated.

The presence of azotemia is no contraindication to lower the blood pressure. Drug-induced reduction of hypertension is important in patients with renal failure. With hemodialysis or transplantation now available to treat uremia, complications of hypertension have become the most common cause of death in end-stage renal failure. Cerebrovascular disease, manifested by transient ischemic attacks (TIA), a previous stroke and occlusive disease of the extracranial arteries, are not contraindications for antihypertensive drug therapy, although the physician has to proceed cautiously and must avoid sudden or drastic reductions of arterial pressure which may compromise cerebral perfusion. The presence of angina pectoris, heart failure or left ventricular enlargement are signs of poor prognosis, but certainly strong indications to reduce the blood pressure.

3. Search for curable forms of hypertension-- The more common causes of curable forms of hypertension are: Coarctation of the aorta; Cushing's syndrome; the use of birth control pills; primary aldosteronism, pheochromocytoma and renovascular hypertension. The frequency of these curable forms is unknown, but probably much less than the 10 per cent figure frequently quoted.

The diagnoses of hypertension due to coarctation of the aorta, Cushing's syndrome and use of birth control pills are suspected by history and physical examination.

Estimates of hypertension due to oral contraceptive drugs range from 0 to 20%. Regardless of the actual incidence, it is clear that only a small number of women develop significant hypertension despite the fact that most have increased levels of renin substrate and high plasma renin activity. Women using oral contraceptives should have their blood pressure determined every six months. If hypertension is detected, the "pill" should be stopped. Although the plasma renin activity and renin substrate level may fall quickly, it may require two to six months for the blood pressure to return to normal.

Pheochromocytoma is a rare cause of episodic or fixed hypertension which almost never occurs in the absence of headaches, palpitations, excessive perspiration, anxiety and weight loss. In the presence of these manifestations the diagnosis is established by demonstration of significantly increased catecholamine production and not by pharmacologic testing. The routine use of urinary VMA determinations in the evaluation of every hypertensive patient is not justified. Pheochromocytomas are so uncommon that only a few medical centers have much experience in their management. Successful treatment requires careful orchestration of the efforts of endocrinologists, anesthesiologists, the surgical team and internist.

The screening test for diagnosing primary aldosteronism is the serum potassium. Normokalemic primary aldosteronism is an uncommon form of a rare cause of curable hypertension. Its existence as a valid entity has been questioned by some investigators. The diagnosis of primary aldosteronism is suspected when serum potassium is less than 3.5 mEq/L and urinary potassium is more than 30 mEq/24 hours in the absence of diuretic therapy. The diagnosis is established by the demonstration of excessive aldosterone production in the presence of suppressed plasma renin activity. The differentiation between an adenoma or hyperplasia of the adrenal cortex as the cause of the aldosteronism is difficult and usually only possible in specialized medical centers. We recommend the referral of suspected patients to a medical center with facilities to diagnose this condition.

The most common cause of curable hypertension is renovascular hypertension, that is, high blood pressure secondary to stenotic lesions of one or both main renal arteries or their branches. The incidence of renovascular hypertension is unknown, but certainly is less than the reported figures of 10 to 30 per cent. It has been estimated by most investigators to be 5 per cent of the entire hypertensive population. We believe this to be a gross exaggeration. We estimate its incidence to be 5 to 10 per cent of patients over 40 years of age with diastolics of 120 mm. Hg. or higher and also 5 to 10 per cent of younger patients with diastolics over 110 mm. Hg. Of the 23 million hypertensives only 15 per cent have these levels of arterial pressure and hence, we consider its frequency to be probably around 1 to 2 per cent of the entire hypertensive population.

The most common lesions responsible for renal arterial stenosis are fibromuscular dysplasia and arteriosclerosis. Fibromuscular dysplasia occurs in young patients, predominantly women. Usually the vascular lesion is limited to the renal artery and in more than 2/3 of the cases is unilateral. Arteriosclerotic lesions are seen in older patients, predominantly men, and are frequently bilateral and are associated with other vascular lesions outside the kidney. Both forms are rare in blacks.

Screening for renovascular hypertension starts with the history and physical examination. We should not search for renovascular hypertension in patients for whom surgical treatment is not indicated, even if a hemodynamically significant lesion is found. Such patients include those over 50 years of age with extensive extrarenal arterial occlusive disease, diabetes mellitus, poor surgical risks, or those who respond well to drug therapy. Another important consideration is the severity of the hypertension. Mild elevations of the arterial pressure, which can be easily controlled with simple antihypertensive drugs, do not warrant an expensive and sometimes hazardous investigation. The only important finding on physical examination which suggests renal artery stenosis is the presence of an abdominal high-pitched bruit of systolic-diastolic (continuous) duration which is found in about 50% of cases. A systolic bruit of short or medium duration is not considered of diagnostic significance.

Only after the decision has been made that a search for renovascular hypertension is indicated does one proceed in obtaining an intravenous pyelogram. The use of an IVP as part of the routine work-up of every hypertensive patient should be condemned and is an example of poor medical judgment. A rapid sequence IVP is the most commonly used screening test. The finding of a difference in renal size of more than 1.5 cm., scalloping of the ureters and a delay in the appearance and/or disappearance of the dye in the affected kidney are considered to be positive findings. However, a false negative IVP is found in 10 to 20 per cent of cases with proven renovascular hypertension.

Another approach is to perform an arteriogram in patients in whom we strongly suspect the diagnosis, omitting the IVP. If the arteriogram is negative, the work-up is concluded and we treat the patient with antihypertensive drugs. In the presence of an anatomic lesion it is mandatory to determine its functional significance before recommending a surgical correction or a nephrectomy. The most acceptable method to evaluate the significance of a renal artery lesion is bilateral catheterization of the renal veins to compare the renin activity in renal venous blood from the two kidneys. In instances of segmental arterial occlusion it is necessary to selectively catheterize the primary branches of the renal vein. Only in patients with renal vein renin activity at least 1.5 times greater on the side of the lesion than on the contralateral side should surgery be recommended. Before performing renin studies of this nature, it is essential to induce an acute volume depletion with a weight loss of 3 per cent or more and withhold all medications which affect renin activity for at least a week. The volume depletion can be achieved by subjecting the patient to three days of a sodium intake of 10 mEq, a potassium intake of 90 mEq. and diuretic therapy in amounts equivalent to 100 mg. of hydrochlorothiazide.

Table 1. TYPES OF HYPERTENSION

Potential Hypertension
  Strong genetic history

Labile Hypertension
  Occasional elevation

Borderline Hypertension
  Systolic 140 to 149 mm. Hg.
  Diastolic 90 to 94 mm. Hg.

Mild Hypertension
  Systolic 150 to 159 mm. Hg.
  Diastolic 95 to 104 mm. Hg.

Moderate Hypertension
  Systolic 160 to 179 mm. Hg.
  Diastolic 105 to 114 mm. Hg.

Severe Hypertension
  Systolic 180 mm. Hg. or greater
  Diastolic 115 mm. Hg. or greater

Accelerated Hypertension
  Retinal hemorrhages or exudates

Malignant Hypertension
  Papilledema

Selected References

1. Veterans Administration Cooperative Study Group on Antihypertensive Agents: Effects of Treatment on Morbidity in Hypertension. JAMA 202:1028, 1967, JAMA 213:1143, 1970, Circulation 45:991, 1972.

2. Kaplan, N. M.: Clinical Hypertension. New York, Medcom Press, 1973.

3. Simon, N., Franklin, S. S., Bleifor, K. H., et al: Cooperative Study of Renovascular Hypertension. Clinical Characteristics of renovascular hypertension. 220:1209, 1972.

RADIOLOGIC EVALUATION OF HYPERTENSION

James R. Lepage, M.D.

A classification of secondary causes of hypertension which has been useful to the radiologist includes:

A. Nephropathies
   1. Parenchymal (nephritis, polycystic disease, neoplasias, etc.)
   2. Vascular (stenosis, nephrosclerosis, fistula, embolism)
   3. Obstructive
B. Endocrinopathies
   1. Adrenal
      a. Pheochromocytoma b. Aldosteronism c. Cushing's disease
   2. Thyroid (hyper and hypothyroidism)
   3. Pituitary (Cushing's disease)
   4. Hyperparathyroidism
C. Coarctation of the Aorta

The following types of radiological investigations are useful in patients with systemic arterial hypertension:

A. Conventional chest roentgenograms. Changes in heart size and configuration are of great importance. Left atrial and/or left ventricular enlargement may suggest a source of systemic arterial embolization. The lungs may show evidence of cardiac decompensation and patchy infiltrates may be observed in the uremic lung. Notching of the ribs may be indicative of coarctation of the aorta. Studies of the bony skeleton may reveal signs of osteonephropathy. Radiographic evidence of subperiosteal bone reabsorption suggests hyperparathyroidism.

B. Hypertensive intravenous urogram. Rapid injection of a large volume of contrast media should be followed by coned-down views of the kidneys, exposed one, two, three and five minutes following the injection of the contrast agent. Decreased renal blood flow causes loss of renal mass, reduction in the volume of the glomerular filtrate and consequently of urine volume, enlargement of the contralateral kidney, and paradoxical increase in urine concentration of the affected kidney because of the retained capacity of the tubules for water reabsorption. Rapid sequence intravenous pyelography has been considered 80% accurate in predicting a functional stenosis with about 10% false-positives and 10% false-negatives. Unilateral or bilateral renal disease may be characterized by changes in kidney morphology or function. The urographic signs of renovascular hypertension include:

   1. Delayed appearance time: delayed and/or diminished "early" nephrogram.
   2. Reduction of renal length and parenchymal thickness: homolateral renal atrophy (right kidney 2 cms. smaller than left; left kidney 1.5 cms. smaller than right) with or without contralateral renal hypertrophy.

3. Late hyperconcentration.
4. Ureteral and/or pelvic notching by arterial collaterals.
5. Decreased volume of the pelvocalyceal system ("spidery" calyces).
6. Prolonged nephrogram.
7. Delayed "washout" during diuresis.
8. Focal or diffuse parenchymal atrophy.

C. Angiography. Aortography may be indicated whenever nephrogenic hypertension is suspected clinically, radiographically, isotopically, or by selective renal blood sampling. Diseases involving the orifices of the renal arteries, the main renal artery and/or its branches, the kidney parenchyma, the pelvocalyceal-ureteral system, and the renal veins may be demonstrated by angiography.

Atherosclerosis, dysplasias of the renal artery, aneurysms and arteriovenous fistula, thromboembolic occlusion of the renal arteries, cysts, and tumors are among the lesions discovered by selective renal arteriography.

The finding of a stenotic arterial lesion alone is not enough for the diagnosis of unilateral renovascular hypertension. Fifty to sixty percent of normotensive individuals at autopsy have various degrees of stenosis of the renal arteries. The important point is to prove that the stenosis is functional in the sense of causing ischemia with secondary hyperproduction of renin.

D. Renal vein studies. Selective sampling of renovenous blood is probably the most informative test for unilateral nephrogenic hypertension. The patient should be prepared with a low sodium diet, diuretics and must lie flat for four hours beforehand. Blood sampling should not be limited to the renal veins and should include sampling of blood from the distal and proximal inferior vena cava. Selective renal venography should be done bilaterally upon completion of the renal blood sampling.

The overall operative mortality of 6% for patients with renovascular hypertension indicates the importance of the radiologic diagnosis and dictates great care in patient selection. Surgery is likely best avoided in patients older than 50 with impaired renal function and evidence of generalized atherosclerosis, especially if they have left ventricular failure. In carefully selected and appropriately reconstructed patients the postoperative cured and improved rate approaches 80%.

Some special comments regarding specific secondary causes of hypertension are pertinent to radiologic evaluation. Primary hyperaldosteronism may be caused by unilateral or bilateral tumors (in about 6%). Very rarely are there tumors in heterotopic locations. Several cases of adrenal carcinoma causing primary aldosteronism have been reported. Preoperative diagnosis can be attained in almost every case by appropriate clinical tests, adrenal vein sampling for aldosterone and adrenal venography.

When pheochromocytoma is suspected, arteriography is usually more informative than venography. Precautions with intravenous regitine are mandatory. The test injection should be carefully monitored. A hypertensive crisis may follow the angiographic examination or even the test injection.

The chief causes of secondary hypertension are stenosis of the renal artery, primary hyperaldosteronism and adrenal hypersecretion of 18-hydroxydeoxycorticosterone.

Intravenous urography remains the best screening test. Renal and adrenal arteriography, adrenal venography, and renal venous blood sampling for renin determination are also widely used radiological techniques, whenever nephrogenic or adrenogenic hypertension is suspected. Such exact determination of secondary causes of hypertension is extremely important, as surgical treatment is indicated in the presence of unilateral renal vascular or parenchymal disease in good-risk patients with definite criteria of renal ischemia, primary hyperreninism, pheochromocytoma, and primary aldosteronism.

SELECTED REFERENCES

1. Bookstein, J. J., et al: Radiographic Aspects of Renovascular Hypertension . JAMA 220: 1218-1230, 1972.

2. Epstein, M.: Renovascular Hypertension vs. Renovascular Disease, Hypertension. 1:16-19, 1975.

3. Franklin, S. S., et al: Operative Morbidity and Mortality in Renovascular Disease, JAMA 231:1148-1153, 1975

4. Maronde, R. F.: The Hypertensive Patient, JAMA 233:997-1000, 1975.

PRACTICAL THERAPY OF HYPERTENSION

Eliseo Perez-Stable, M.D.

Chemotherapy is the only practical solution to the hypertension problem. The impact of an extensive work-up of patients for curable hypertension in reducing morbidity and mortality in the hypertensive population has been minimal. Worse than doing too little work-up before starting therapy is to delay antihypertensive chemotherapy until an extensive work-up is completed. A complete history and physical examination, urinalysis, biochemical profile, chest x-ray and an electrocardiogram is all that is needed in most instances.

Prior to beginning a course of life-long treatment, the patient with mildly elevated blood pressure should be seen on at least three separate visits to document fixed hypertension. The effectiveness of treatment has been well demonstrated in patients with diastolic pressure of 105 mm. Hg. or higher. When the diastolic pressure is between 90 and 104 mm. Hg. the beneficial effects of drug therapy are less clear. There are no studies available evaluating antihypertensive chemotherapy in young individuals with slight elevation of the diastolic pressure or in patients with isolated systolic hypertension or labile hypertension.

The goal of therapy is to lower the blood pressure to normal or to the lowest level that the patient will tolerate. Usually a diastolic pressure of 90 mm. Hg. or lower may be achieved without serious side effects. Chemotherapy frequently requires the use of more than one drug. Polypharmacy is scientifically justified and often necessary because frequently a single drug will not reduce blood pressure without also inducing prohibitive untoward effects. Since many drugs produce their hypotensive effect by different mechanisms, they can be combined so that their therapeutic effects are additive. Also, two drugs may be combined in order to counteract their individual side-effects. For example, a direct vasodilator induces a reflex tachycardia which can be suppressed by agents which depress the activity of the adrenergic nervous system.

Antihypertensive drugs can be divided into three groups according to their mechanism of action: 1) Diuretics; 2) Agents which decrease the activity of the adrenergic nervous system; 3) Direct vasodilators.

1. Diuretics. Thiazide derivatives are the most frequently used. Their antihypertensive action is related to a natruretic effect with a consequent fall in body weight, plasma volume and cardiac output. Roughly 1 to 2 liters of extracellular fluid are excreted and this loss is more or less maintained as long as the patient remains under treatment. Several weeks after starting diuretic therapy, the cardiac output tends to return to normal and the peripheral resistance to decrease. The dose of thiazide varies from 25 to 100 mg. daily of hydrochlorothiazide or its equivalent. The use

of "loop" diuretics, such as furosemide or ethacrynic acid does not offer any advantage unless there is such marked reduction of glomerular filtration rate that thiazides are ineffective as diuretics. Loop diuretics and thiazide related drugs have in common the induction of hypokalemia, hyperreninemia and some decrease in carbohydrate tolerance. They have been used in combination with potassium sparing diuretics like spironolactone and triamterene to prevent potassium depletion. Less common side effects of thiazides are related to hypersensitivity reactions and include rash and thrombocytopenic purpura. Diuretic therapy alone controls the hypertension in a great number of patients, but if, after its use, the blood pressure remains elevated then one of the other two types of drugs should be added.

2. Agents which decrease the activity of the adrenergic nervous system. Rauwolfia derivatives, methyldopa, guanethidine and propranolol are the most widely used. Rauwolfia derivatives have their major action peripherally through depletion of norepinephrine stores, but an important component of their action is on the central nervous system. The daily dose of reserpine should never exceed 0.25 mg. and its major unwanted reaction is depression in susceptible individuals. Methyldopa interferes with the conversion of dopa to dopamine by competitive inhibition of the enzyme dopa decarboxylase and results in the formation of alpha methyldopamine and, in turn, alpha methylnorepinephrine. This compound replaces norepinephrine in nerve-ending stores, and is, in turn, only a "weak transmitter" of adrenergic stimuli. Methyldopa also has an effect in the central nervous system. The dose varies between 0.5 to 3.0 gm/day. A serious side effect of methyldopa is hemolytic anemia. Fortunately, it is quite rare, although the induction of a positive direct Coomb's test is fairly common. A type of supersensitization reaction characterized by low-grade fever, elevation of SGOT and jaundice has been described. Sleepiness and dry mouth are common secondary effects. Both rauwolfia derivatives and methyldopa in therapeutic doses decrease the peripheral resistance and do not affect the cardiac output.

Guanethidine is usually reserved for patients with severe forms of hypertension. This agent produces a depletion of the stores of norepinephrine in the nerve ending. Since it does not penetrate the blood-brain barrier and, therefore, has little adrenergic neuronal blocking activity within the central nervous system, depression does not occur. To become effective, guanethidine must utilize the "membrane-pump" of the sympathetic nerve ending to enter the nerve. Tricyclic antidepressants block the entry of guanethidine into the neuron and thus sharply interfere with or reverse the action of the drug. Amphetamine and other drugs can competitively displace guanethidine from the neuron and reverse its antihypertensive effect. The hypotensive effect of guanethidine is mainly due to a decrease in cardiac output, with a minimal effect on the peripheral resistance. Lack of ejaculation and postural hypotension are the two main complications.

When used alone, rauwolfia derivatives, methyldopa and guanethidine tend to increase renal tubular reabsorption of sodium with a resultant expansion of plasma and extracellular volume. In these circumstances the antihypertensive effect is partially neutralized. This phenomenon explains some instances of drug resistance and can easily be overcome by the addition of diruetic drugs.

Propranolol is a beta adrenergic blocking agent not yet approved by the FDA for the treatment of hypertension. Its mechanism of action is complicated. On one hand it blocks beta receptors in the heart and thus reduces the aforementioned cardiac component of elevated blood pressure; it has been recommended for treatment of hypertensive patients with high cardiac output. More recently it has been demonstrated that propranolol is the most potent hyporeninemic agent presently available. By interfering with renin release in the juxtaglomerular apparatus, propranolol reduces plasma renin activity by more than 80%. Its use has been recommended in high-renin forms of hypertensive states. Bronchial asthma and active peripheral arterial occlusive disease are absolute contraindications and congestive heart failure a relative contraindication to the use of propranolol.

3. Direct Vasodilators. Hydralazine is the only one presently available for oral use. It acts directly on arteriolar smooth muscle with a resultant decrease in peripheral resistance. Since the sympathetic system is not directly affected, the decrease in blood pressure stimulates arterial baroreceptors inducing a reflex hyperactivity of the sympathetic system with increase in heart rate, stroke volume and myocardial oxygen requirement. Unfortunately, the hypotensive effect of decreasing peripheral vascular resistance is neutralized in part by the increase in cardiac output. Daily doses over 200 mg. may precipitate a hypersensitivity state resembling disseminated lupus erythematosus. All manifestations of the latter, except the renal lesion may occur. Combined use of propranolol with hydralazine prevents the reflex increase in cardiac output, thus enhancing the antihypertensive action of hydralazine. Minoxidil is an interesting investigational oral drug with a potent direct vasodilator effect. Like other vasodilators, it is most effective when combined with an agent which inhibits the sympathetic response of the heart and with a diuretic to prevent secondary fluid retention. Preliminary studies have shown a dramatic effect of this drug in patients with severe, resistant hypertension. Several patients previously requiring chronic hemodialysis no longer require it, and control of blood pressure without orthostatic hypotension has been most impressive.

Hypertensive Crisis

Hypertensive crisis is a sudden, life threatening elevation of blood pressure usually but not always associated with a diastolic pressure of greater than 130 mm. Hg., a situation in which it is necessary to lower the blood pressure rapidly and effectively.

Hypertensive emergencies may be classified into two groups: (1) Situations demanding immediate reduction in blood pressure (minutes-hours) as in hypertensive encephalopathy, hypertension with aortic dissection, hypertension with cerebral or subarachnoid hemorrhage and severe hypertension with left ventricular failure. (2) Situations that require prompt reduction in blood pressure (hours-days) as in accelerated hypertension (hypertension associated with retinal hemorrhages and exudates), malignant hypertension (hypertension associated with hemorrhages, exudates and papilledema) and severe hypertension associated with rapid deterioration of renal function.

The treatment should be guided to lower the blood pressure as rapidly and as safely as possible. Once this is accomplished the patient should be switched to an effective regimen of oral therapy for continued blood pressure control. The following drugs are useful in treating hypertensive crisis.

Sodium nitroprusside, diazoxide and hydralazine are direct vasodilators. Trimethaphan (Arfonad) is a ganglionic blocking agent. Diazoxide has the advantage of simplicity of administration in a single 300 mg. dose given rapidly intravenously. Nitroprusside is more effective but requires continuous intravenous administration with constant monitoring of the blood pressure.

HEMODYNAMIC EFFECTS OF DRUGS USED TO TREAT HYPERTENSIVE CRISIS

	Heart Rate	Mean Blood Pressure	Cardiac Output	Peripheral Resistance
Sodium Nitroprusside	↑	↓↓	↓	↓
Diazoxide	↑	↓↓	↑	↓↓
Trimethaphan (Arfonad)	↑	↓↓	↓	↓
Hydralazine	↑	↓	↑	↓

SELECTED REFERENCES

1. Veterans Administration Cooperative Study Group on Antihypertensive Agents. JAMA, 202:1028, 1967; JAMA, 213:1143, 1970; Circ., 45:991, 1972.

2. AMA Committee on Hypertension. Drug Treatment of Ambulatory Patients with Hypertension. JAMA, 25:1647, 1973.

3. Bhatia, S.K., Frohlich, E.D.: Hemodynamic Comparison of Agents Useful in Hypertensive Emergencies. Am. Heart J., 85:367, 1973.

ADVANCES IN DIAGNOSIS

THE ECHOCARDIOGRAM IN CARDIAC DIAGNOSIS

Stuart Gottlieb, M.D.

I. Introduction

Medical application of diagnostic ultrasound evolved from technical knowledge related to naval sonar accumulated during World War I and World War II and the use of pulsed ultrasound for the non-destructive testing of metals in the early 1940's. "Ultrasound Cardiography," originally introduced by Edler and Hertz, is finding increasing application as a reliable non-invasive tool which may be taken to the bedside of an acutely ill patient when necessary. The possibility of performing repeated studies offers the opportunity to assess the effects of medical or surgical therapy and to monitor clinical progress over an extended time. Its rapidly rising popularity is largely the result of expanding interest, particularly in the areas of cardiac dynamics and pediatric echocardiography. The echocardiogram recorded simultaneously with other non-invasive physiologic indicators such as the electrocardiogram, phonocardiogram and carotid pulse provides a superlative tool for studying the genesis of cardiac sounds.

Echographic identification of structures depends upon recognition of the movement of a target and its position with relationship to other structures. The identity and anatomical relationship of intracardiac structures have been established by the ultrasonic detection of microbubbles formed following intracardiac injections of various substances.

Diagnosis depends upon an understanding of normal cardiac structural relationships, their patterns of motion, and their dimensions. An increased intensity of the returning echoes reflects the presence of calcification as in calcific mitral stenosis. Echo producing interfaces which are not normally present must also be recognized, and occur, for example, with pericardial effusion and atrial myxoma. Increasingly important in diagnosis is consideration of the inter-relationship between cardiac pressures and compliance upon the one hand, and myocardial and valvular motion on the other.

II. Technique

The patient is positioned comfortably, usually in the supine or semirecumbent position. The left decubitus position is frequently helpful in emphysematous or obese individuals, since the heart is brought nearer to the anterior chest wall and transducer resulting in less attenuation. The lateral displacement of the heart, which occurs in this position, also enlarges the effective examination window. Studies may be monitored in the A-mode or M-mode, but recording is performed in the M-mode (Fig. 1). The sound beam is directed from the third or fourth intercostal space toward the anterior mitral valve leaflet which may be then used as an intracardiac landmark for the identification of other structures.

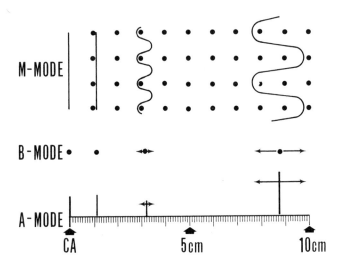

Fig. 1 - Returning echoes are displayed as vertical deflections or spikes along a horizontal baseline (A-mode) which is calibrated in distance from the transducer or crystal artifact (CA). The height or amplitude of the spikes reflects the intensity of the returning signal. While the spikes can be seen to move on the oscilloscope screen (arrows), the motion cannot be recorded in this mode. To record motion, the spikes are just converted into data (B-mode), the brightness of which is proportional to the amplitude of the spikes seen in the A-mode (brightness modulation). These dots are then swept across the oscilloscope screen at a uniform rate of speed, creating a wave form which characterizes the motion of the particular target (M-mode). A grid of dots which establishes distance in the horizontal direction and time in the vertical direction is superimposed on the tracing.

Feigenbaum has suggested that the left heart be systematically considered in four basic positions along its major axis (Figure 2). In position one, the ultrasound beam intersects the anterior and posterior walls of the aortic root including the right and non-coronary aortic cusps, and the posterior wall of the left atrium. As the sound beam is directed inferiorly and slightly laterally (Position 2), continuity between the anterior wall of the aortic root and the interventricular septum can be demonstrated. At the same time, the continuity of the posterior aortic root wall and the anterior mitral leaflet is seen. The lesser diameter of the left ventricular chamber in systole and diastole is measured (Position 3) immediately distal to the mitral leaflets. Here also, measurements of interventricular septal and posterior myocardial thickness can be made. As the ultrasound beam is directed still further laterally and inferiorly toward the apex of the heart (Position 4), the region of the postero-medial papillary muscle is encountered. Attention to technical detail and instrument setting is extremely important and requires considerable experience.

Technical limitations may be encountered in the obese or emphysematous individual or in the presence of surgical or congenital deformity of the chest wall. In such patients, attenuation of the sound beam related to the presence of air or bone interposed between the transducer and the target structure may make acquisition of an adequate study impossible. For most cardiac examinations, this will amount to fewer than 10% of patients.

The tricuspid and pulmonic valves may also be demonstrated. The full diagnostic value of echograms obtained from the latter has yet to be explored.

III. Applications

The following represent the major areas of clinical application of echocardiography. Where not otherwise indicated, the procedure may be regarded as clinically accepted as opposed to being investigational.

1. Mitral Valve
   a. Normal Mitral Valve (Fig. 3)

   Motion of the normal mitral valve produces a characteristic echographic pattern which reflects: (a) compliance of the valve leaflet; (b) the amplitude of leaflet motion (the degree of shortening, if any, of the sub-valvular apparatus); (c) flow across the mitral orifice (and, indirectly, the factors resulting in alteration in flow); (d) the presence of leaflet calcification or thickening. A concise but detailed discussion of the techniques involved in echocardiography and the hemodynamic factors affecting mitral leaflet motion appears in a recent monograph by Feigenbaum.

   b. Mitral Stenosis (Figs. 4 and 5)

   The diagnosis of mitral stenosis may be made with great accuracy even in the absence of characteristic clinical or physical findings. Reduction in diastolic slope (EF) velocity, below 40 mm/sec. (normal 70-140 mm/sec.), with reduction in prominence of the A-wave, a reduced overall amplitude of leaflet motion (normal 24-35 mm.) and abnormal motion of the posterior mitral leaflet also

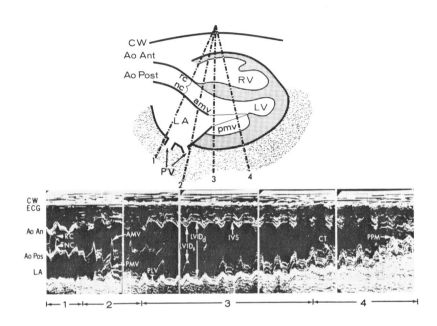

Fig. 2 - At the top is a diagrammatic representation of a sagittal section along the major axis of the left ventricle in the path of the ultrasound beam. The basic four regions are identified. Below, an "M-Mode" scan along the major left ventricular axis is formed by a composite of individual polaroid pictures. See text for explanation. Note the tapering of the left ventricular chamber dimension. Compare this study with Figs. 5 and 6. Ao Ant = anterior aortic root wall; Ao Post = posterior aortic root wall; AMV = anterior mitral valve leaflet; CW = chest wall; CT = chordae tendineae; ECG = electrocardiogram; IVS = interventricular septum; LA = left atrium; LV = left ventricle; RV = right ventricle; $LVID_d$ = left ventricular internal diameter in diastole; $LVID_s$ = left ventricular internal diameter in systole; RC = right coronary aortic cusp; NC = non-coronary aortic cusp; PLV = posterior left ventricle; PMV = posterior mitral valve leaflet; PPM = posteromedial papillary muscle; PV = pulmonary veins.

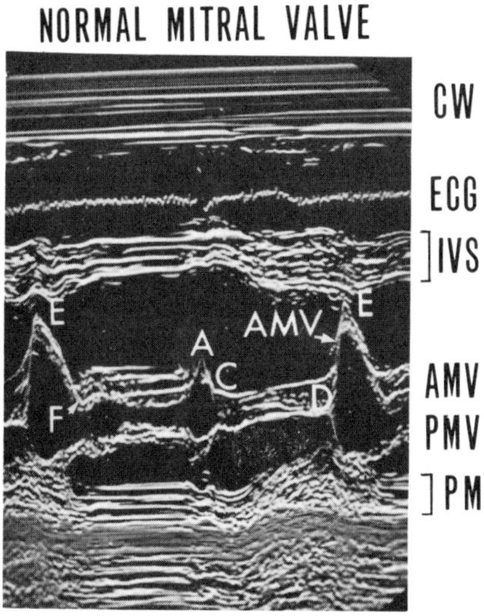

NORMAL MITRAL VALVE

Fig. 3 - Normal Mitral Valve - The anterior mitral leaflet (AMV) and posterior mitral leaflet (PMV) move in opposite directions. The E-F slope reflects flow across the mitral valve orifice during the passive phase of ventricular filling which causes the leaflet to return to a partially closed position. Re-opening occurs as a result of atrial contraction (A). C-D = valve closure during systole; PM = posterior myocardium. Other abbreviations are the same as in Fig. 2.

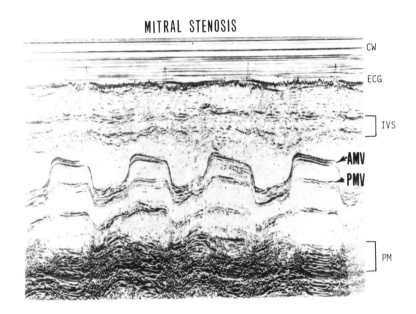

Fig. 4 - Mitral Stenosis - Flattened diastolic slope, reduced amplitude, and abnormal motion of the posterior leaflet (PMV) in the same direction as the anterior mitral leaflet (AMV) are typical of mitral stenosis, as is a reduced or absent A wave.

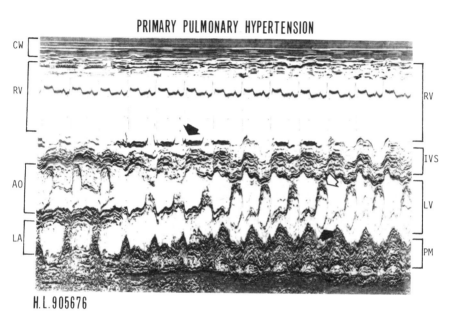

Fig. 5 - Primary Pulmonary Hypertension - The right ventricular dimension (RV) is enlarged and bits of the tricuspid valve are evident (solid arrow, left). Septal motion is abnormal, reflecting volume as well as pressure overload of the right ventricle. The diastolic slope of the anterior mitral valve leaflet closure (open arrow, right) is reduced due to a reduction of flow across the mitral orifice secondary to increased pulmonary vascular resistance. Notice that the posterior mitral valve leaflet (solid arrow, right) continues to move in its normal posterior direction.

allow estimation of the relative severity of mitral stenosis and shortening of the subvalvular apparatus. The presence of calcification is indicated by an increase in the width and brightness of the echoes originating from the mitral leaflet. Subjective estimation of leaflet calcification from the echocardiogram has been found to correlate more closely with surgical and pathologic findings than fluoroscopy or radiographs. Similar patterns of reduced diastolic slope velocity "pseudo-mitral stenosis" are produced in hemodynamic circumstances resulting in reduced flow rates across the mitral orifice. Such situations exist with primary pulmonary hypertension and with increased left ventricular diastolic pressure resulting from left ventricular failure or pressure elevation associated with reduced myocardial compliance, as in aortic stenosis or hypertrophic cardiomyopathy. Under these circumstances, the posterior mitral leaflet continues to move normally in the direction opposite to that of the anterior leaflet. In contrast, in true mitral stenosis the posterior leaflet moves in the same direction as the anterior leaflet. The A-wave is also usually prominent in "pseudo-mitral stenosis" reflecting the increased atrial component (S4).

c. Mitral Regurgitation (Fig. 6)

No consistent characteristic features of mitral regurgitation on a rheumatic or non-rheumatic basis have been identified. Most often, the echocardiogram reflects the volume overload of the left-sided chambers, i.e., dilated ventricle and atrium and increased amplitude of movement of the interventricular septum and posterior myocardium. Frequent findings are those of a high amplitude of leaflet motion and an increased diastolic slope velocity. These findings are not present in some cases of known regurgitant lesions, and their presence is not pathognomonic since, in our experience, they may be seen in other high flow states. An accuracy of about 50-60% may be expected using these criteria for the diagnosis of mitral regurgitation. The anterior and posterior leaflets, normally apposed during systole, have been described to remain partially separated in some patients with mitral regurgitation. The multiplicity of echoes frequently present in these patients, presumably resulting from redundancy of the leaflets and subvalvular apparatus, may make exact systolic identification of the leaflets difficult.

d. Ruptured Chordae Tendineae (Fig. 7)

Markedly increased amplitude and erratic motion of both anterior and posterior mitral leaflets have been described. We have also identified leaflet prolapse into the left atrium due to ruptured chordae tendineae via the suprasternal approach.

e. Mitral Leaflet Prolapse (Fig. 8 and 9)

In patients with the syndrome of systolic click and systolic murmur, an abnormal late or holosystolic posterior motion of

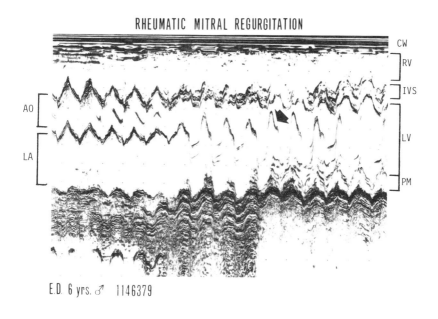

Fig. 6 - Rheumatic Mitral Regurgitation in a 6 year old child. Images of ultrasound beam from the aortic root and left atrium (left) along the major left ventricular axis into the left ventricular cavity (right). The echo findings are non-specific and reflect only a high flow across the mitral valve (high amplitude, rapid opening and diastolic slope velocities of the anterior mitral leaflet) (arrow). There is also evidence of volume overload of the left heart (enlarged left atrium and ventricle with increased movement of the interventricular septum and posterior myocardium).

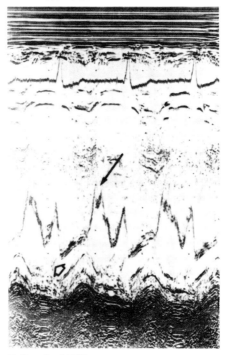

Fig. 7 - Ruptured Chordae Tendineae. A coarse fluttering motion and notching (solid arrow) is seen after initial opening of the anterior mitral leaflet. The posterior leaflet (open arrow) continues to move normally.

MITRAL PROLAPSE

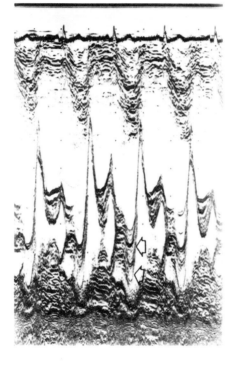

Fig. 8 - Mitral Prolapse - Both anterior (upper arrow) and posterior (lower arrow) mitral leaflets prolapse toward the left atrium during late systole.

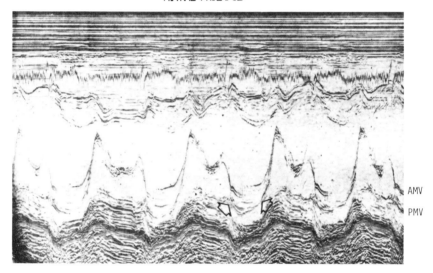

Fig. 9 - Mitral Prolapse - There is holosystolic prolapse of the mitral leaflets toward the left atrium (arrows).

both leaflets toward the atrium is frequently demonstrated. Most often, the abnormal motion involves the posterior leaflet to a greater degree. Occasionally, provocative maneuvers which reduce ventricular volume are necessary to elicit these abnormal findings.

    f. Aortic Regurgitation (Figs. 10 and 11)

Indirect evidence of aortic regurgitation may be obtained from the echographic appearance of mitral leaflet motion. Approximately 40-60% of the patients with chronic aortic regurgitation will demonstrate high frequency oscillatory movement of the anterior mitral leaflet during passive ventricular filling. Premature closure of the mitral valve, as well as increased motion of the interventricular septum and posterior myocardium, have been associated with acute severe aortic regurgitation.

    g. Idiopathic Hypertrophic Subaortic Stenosis (IHSS) or Asymmetric Septal Hypertrophy (ASH) (Fig. 12)

Hypertrophic cardiomyopathy may be demonstrated by echocardiography and the presence or absence of left ventricular outflow tract obstruction determined by assessing mitral leaflet motion. In the presence of ventricular outflow obstruction, a characteristic abnormal systolic anterior motion (SAM) of the anterior mitral leaflet is observed. The gradient across the left ventricular outflow tract appears to correlate quantitatively with the duration and degree of narrowing produced by the abnormal leaflet motion. Attempts to evaluate the effects of medical and surgical therapy for IHSS have been made by assessment of the SAM. The variable and unpredictable nature of outflow tract obstruction makes the use of provocative testing with amyl nitrate, isuprel or valsalva maneuver necessary if no abnormal mitral leaflet motion is noted at rest. Echographically determined inter-ventricular septal thickness to posterior myocardial thickness ratios in excess of 1.3 have been described as a pathognomonic characteristic of hypertrophic cardiomyopathies and are demonstrable even in the absence of resting gradients.

    h. Left Atrial Myxoma (Fig. 13)

Obstruction of the flow of blood across the mitral orifice results in a strikingly diminished diastolic slope velocity of the anterior mitral leaflet resembing mitral stenosis. In addition, multiple echoes originating from the tumor may be seen immediately behind and separate from the anterior mitral leaflet as the mass prolapses from atrium to ventricle during diastole. Differentiation from a thickened leaflet of mitral stenosis is occasionally difficult but can be made by proper variation in gain settings and direct examination of the left atrium.

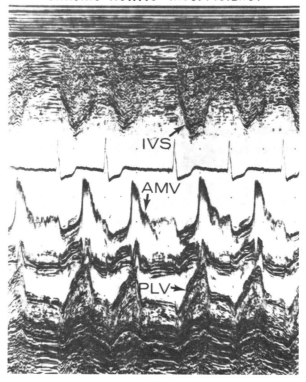

Fig. 10 - Chronic aortic regurgitation - A high frequency oscillatory movement of the anterior mitral leaflet (AMV) is present. The large diameter of the left ventricle and increased motion of both the interventricular septum (IVS) and posterior left ventricle (PLV) reflect diastolic overloading. The time of closure of the mitral valve is normal with respect to the simultaneous ECG.

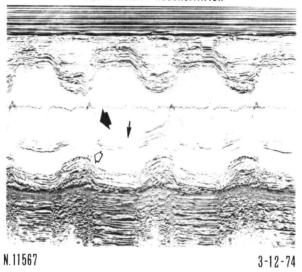

Fig. 11 - Acute aortic regurgitation - Closure of the anterior mitral leaflet (large solid arrow) and the posterior mitral leaflet (open arrow) is approximately 200 msec. before the expected time of closure (vertical solid arrow). This is caused by the volume and pressure overload resulting from severe aortic regurgitation. The volume overload is also reflected by the dilated hyperdynamic left ventricle.

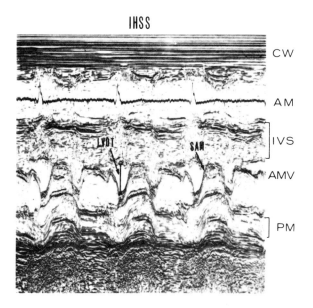

Fig. 12 - Idiopathic hypertrophic subaortic stenosis (IHSS). The left ventricular outflow tract (LVOT) is completely occluded by the abnormal systolic motion (SAM) of the anterior mitral leaflet (AMV). The interventricular septum (IVS) is nearly twice as thick as the posterior myocardium. Such asymmetrical septal hypertrophy (ASH) is characteristically associated with hypertrophic cardiomyopathies.

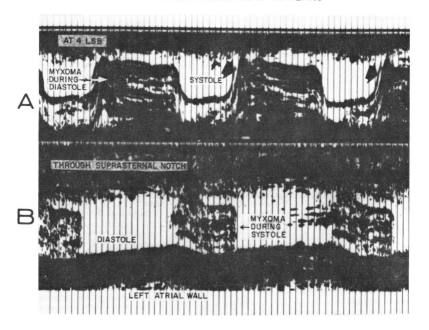

Fig. 13 - Left Atrial Myxoma - A. A dense cluster of echoes which originate from the tumor is present behind the anterior mitral valve leaflet during diastole as the myxoma prolapses from the left atrium into the left ventricle (arrows). B. Direct examination of the left atrium through the suprasternal notch demonstrates the presence of the tumor mass during systole only.

2. Aortic Valve and Aortic Root (Fig. 2)

The box-like configuration produced by motion of the right and non-coronary aortic cusps offers limited information in comparison to that obtainable from the mitral valve. Calcific aortic stenosis results in echoes of increased intensity and reduced amplitude of separation of the aortic valve cusps during systole. Premature motion of the aortic cusps toward closure has been noted in situations of reduced flow across the valve. In obstructive forms of IHSS, the premature closure occurs at mid-systole and coincides with maximum outflow tract obstruction produced by the abnormal motion of the mitral leaflet. Premature aortic cusp closure also may occur with discrete subaortic stenosis. Gradual early leaflet closure occurs with decreased cardiac output. Measurements of the aortic root diameter have been used in the selection of prostheses prior to valve replacement. We have recently diagnosed vegetative involvement of the aortic cusps in two cases of candida endocarditis. Bacterial involvement of the aortic cusps has been described by Feigenbaum and Gottlieb. (Fig. 11)

3. Tricuspid Valve

The pattern of tricuspid valve motion is identical to that of mitral movement in normal subjects. The initial opening movement is frequently identified in the normal patient, but recording of the entire systolic and diastolic trace usually reflects right ventricular enlargement. Tricuspid stenosis and right atrial myxoma produce patterns obstructed flow identical to those seen in the left heart. Tricuspid movement, however, seems more subject to variability in diastolic slope velocities than does the mitral valve, and echographic demonstration of right atrial myxomas is made with greater technical difficulty than those involving the left atrium. In our experience, radioisotope techniques have been of particular help in the study of obstructive lesions proximal to the pulmonic valve.

4. Pulmonic Valve

The pulmonic valve may be demonstrated with some technical difficulty superior and lateral to the aortic valve cusps. No pathognomonic alterations in valve motion have yet been described, but changes in movement have been observed in pulmonary hypertension, pulmonic valvular and subvalvular stenosis.

5. Valvular Prostheses

   a. Mitral

Patterns of poppet motion with various valvular prostheses have been described. Echographically determined measurements of ball diameter and poppet excursion have been compared to similar measurements in the valve prior to implantation with excellent correlation. Opening and closing velocities appear to vary to some extent with patient position, prosthesis type, and poppet composition. While a few cases of prosthetic valve dysfunction have been diagnosed, the general application of echocardiography to evaluation of prosthetic valve function has been limited.

b. Aortic

The position of the aortic valve replacement is unfavorable due to sound attenuation by the sternum and the direction of the long axis of the prosthesis. Experience in this application has been limited and study must still be regarded as investigational.

6. Left Ventricle

a. Pericardial Effusion (Fig. 14)

Diagnosis rests on demonstration of an echo free space separating the posterior and anterior myocardium from their opposing pericardial interfaces. The sensitivity of the echographic technique equals that of carbon dioxide or positive contrast angiography and is slightly greater than that of the radionuclide angiocardiogram or static isotope blood pool imaging. Limited information relative to myocardial dynamics is available by echocardiography in the presence of sizable pericardial effusion since increased translatory motion of the myocardium is usually present. The amount of pericardial fluid present may not be accurately quantitated by this technique though some attempts at gross quantitations have been made. Radioisotope imaging procedures may be indicated when loculated pericardial collections are suspected, as these may not be demonstrated by echocardiography.

b. Posterior Free Wall and Interventricular Septal Motion (Figs. 2, 15)

The pattern and velocity of posterior myocardial motion in the normal individual in the presence of myocardial ischemia, following myocardial infarction, and in response to a number of pharmacologic agents have been described. The technique requires careful standardization since measurements are highly dependent on transducer placement. Similarly, endocardial and epicardial echoes exhibit widely different velocities of motion. In the detection of focal areas of abnormal contractility, the technique is limited by the inaccessability of a large portion of the left ventricle to the ultrasound beam. Moreover, the presence of hypo or frankly dyskinetic segments may actually result in a compensatory increase in heart wall motion in the nondiseased region examined. Subjective impressions of posterior free wall and interventricular septal motion are frequently of value in differentiating congestive cardiomyopathy from focal ischemic disease or infarction. The pattern of diminished motion is usually generalized in the former and localized in the latter.

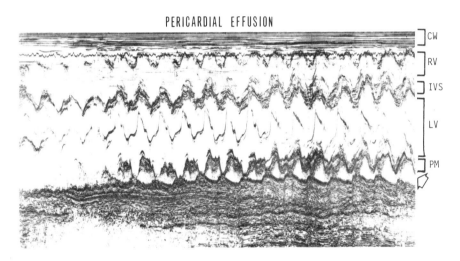

Fig. 14 - Pericardial effusion - Sweep along major axis of the left ventricle demonstrates the presence of pericardial effusion behind the posterior myocardial wall (PM) of the left ventricle (arrow). The amount of fluid increases as the sweep continues inferiorly toward the cardiac apex.

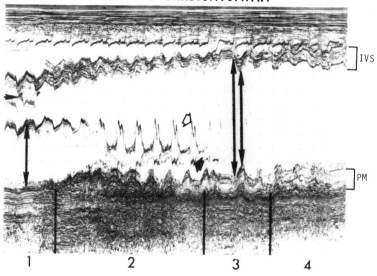

Fig. 15 - Congestive cardiomyopathy - There is generalized decreased motion of both septum and posterior myocardium. The left ventricle is enlarged (arrows, position 3) and there is posterior displacement of the mitral valve echoes from their normal position at the end of the posterior wall of the aortic root. Position 2: solid arrow, posterior mitral leaflet; open arrow, anterior mitral leaflet. In position 1, the right coronary cusp of the aortic valve can be seen (small arrow). Note enlarged left atrium behind the aortic root (large vertical arrow).

c. Posterior Left Ventricular and Interventricular Septal Thickness (Fig. 16)

The thickness of the interventricular septum and free posterior wall of the left ventricle may be determined echographically. Calculations of left ventricular mass have been made by combining the use of these measurements with those of left ventricular chamber dimensions. The same authors indicate that the per cent change in left ventricular wall thickness in systole and in diastole may serve as a useful index of left ventricular function.

While such measurements may be made with a high degree of accuracy, the derived calculations and their application remain largely investigational. As mentioned previously, ratios of interventricular septal thickness to posterior myocardial thickness greater than 1.3 appear to reflect the asymmetrical septal hypertrophy of hypertrophic cardiomyopathy even in the absence of resting gradients across the left ventricular outflow tract.

d. Chamber Dimensions, Functional Measurements (Fig. 16)

Systolic and diastolic chamber diameters may be measured between the endocardial surfaces of the interventricular septum and posterior left ventricular myocardium. The region from which these measurements are made must be carefully standardized if reproducible results are to be obtained during successive examinations.

Through a series of mathematical assumptions and calculations, left ventricular volumes may be calculated along with stroke volume, ejection fractions and cardiac output.

Serial measurements in the same patient appear to be a particularly attractive application of this technique. Chamber dimensions have also been used to calculate the velocity of left ventricular diameter change and circumferential fiber shortening as an index of myocardial contractility. These diameters have also been combined with left ventricular pressures to quantitate compliance, and Popp et al., have applied these techniques to the estimation of valvular regurgitation.

Experience with these applications is limited and, while potentially of considerable pathophysiologic interest, their place in patient management is not yet clearly established. The inability to obtain echograms technically adequate for quantitative assessment in a significant percentage of patients poses a limitation for this method.

CHAMBER DIMENSIONS

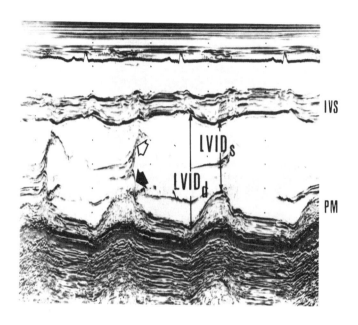

Fig. 16 - Left ventricular wall thickness and internal dimensions in diastole (LVIDd) and in systole (LVIDs), may be measured just inferior to the mitral valve leaflets. Open arrow, anterior mitral valve leaflet; solid arrow, posterior mitral valve leaflet.

7. Right Ventricle (Fig. 17)

The echocardiogram may be used to detect so-called volume overload of the right ventricle. Right ventricular dimensions are increased and there is an abnormal pattern of motion of the interventricular septum. Two types of abnormal septal motion have been described: Type A, in which septum and posterior ventricle move in the same direction; and Type B, which involves flattening of septal motion during systole. These findings may be associated with atrial septal defect, tricuspid regurgitation, anomalous pulmonary venous return, and Ebstein's anomaly, and therefore require careful integration with other clinical and laboratory information.

8. Congenital Heart Disease

   a. Atrial Septal Defect (Fig. 17)

   Patients with hemodynamically significant atrial septal defect display the echographic findings of right ventricular diastolic overload. Uncomplicated pressure overload of the right ventricle, as in pulmonic stenosis, and ventricular septal defects does not produce this echographic pattern. Echographically, ostium primum defects are associated with a left ventricular outflow tract measuring less than 20 mm. and diastolic apposition of the anterior mitral leaflet to the interventricular septum.

   b. Ebstein's Anomaly

   Increased tricuspid valve motion and delayed tricuspid closure, even in the presence of pre-excitation have been described. Some cases have also demonstrated abnormal interventricular septal motion, usually of the type B variety. Failure to demonstrate these findings, however, does not necessarily exclude the diagnosis of Ebstein's Anomaly.

   c. Other Congenital Lesions

   A number of other congenital lesions have been reported to have highly suggestive, if not characteristic, findings. Characteristic echocardiographic patterns have been described in association with valvular dysplasias, hypoplastic right and left heart syndromes and single ventricle. The ease with which the interventricular septum is demonstrated echographically in these cases offers some advantage over contrast angiography. Abnormal echocardiographic findings have also been associated with conditions involving abnormalities of the great vessels, including double outlet right ventricle, complete transposition, and over-riding of the aorta as in Tetralogy of Fallot (Fig. 23).

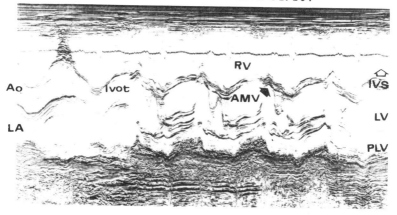

Fig. 17 - Septum primum ASD. Volume overload of the right ventricle has resulted in enlargement of the right ventricular cavity (RV) dimension and paradoxical movement of the interventricular septum (IVS) in which the IVS moves anteriorly in systole (open arrow). Also typical of the echographic findings in this form of endocardial cushion defect is diastolic apposition of the anterior mitral valve leaflet (AMV) to the IVS (solid arrow) and narrowing of the left ventricular outflow tract (LVOT) corresponding to the swan neck deformity seen at angiography. Ao, aorta; LA, left atrium; LV, left ventricle; PLV, posterior left ventricular wall.

The potential use of echocardiography in the selection of cyanotic neonates for catheterization is of obvious importance because of the high mortality associated with catheterization in this group of patients. Thus far, the number of centers in which the study has attained a sufficient degree of diagnostic reliability to obviate catheterization has indeed been limited. Experience with echocardiography in congenital heart disease is still limited but remains one of the most exciting areas of potential application.

Selected References

1. Feigenbaum, H: Clinical Applications of Echocardiography. Prog. in Cardiovas. Dis., 14:531, 1972.

2. Feigenbaum, H.: Echocardiographic Examination of the Left Ventricle. Circ. 51:1, 1975.

3. Gottlieb, S., and Gramiak, R.: Cardiologic Application of Diagnostic Ultrasound. Waverly Press, Inc., Baltimore, 1975.

RADIOISOTOPE CARDIOGRAPHY (CARDIAC SCINTIGRAPHY)

Stuart Gottlieb, M.D.
Nilza Kallos, M.D.

Increasingly aggressive medical and surgical management of patients with coronary artery disease has stimulated interest in non-invasive radioisotopic methods of assessing the myocardium. Cardiac scintigraphic techniques are now available to evaluate:

  I. Myocardial perfusion
 II. Left ventricular wall motion
III. Left ventricular performance

These methods show considerable potential for providing clinically useful data for the management of the acutely ill patient as well as possibly identifying those sub-groups of patients likely to benefit by more invasive studies and surgery.

I. Myocardial Perfusion

Myocardial perfusion may be assessed by performing a myocardial image study. Such studies may be divided into two general categories:

  A. A so-called "hot spot scan" where radionuclide concentrates in the region of acute myocardial ischemia-injury, and
  B. A so-called "cold spot scan," where there is lack of radionuclide concentration in the area of acute myocardial ischemia or of previous myocardial infarction.

A. Myocardial Imaging Using a Hot Spot Scan

The most commonly used agents are: Technetium 99m pyrophosphate, Technetium tetracycline and Technetium glucopheptonate. Again, these radionuclides concentrate in an area of recent myocardial injury. The best results have been obtained with Technetium pyrophosphate. This radionuclide is a bone seeking agent. When there is myocardial death, microscopic crystals of hydroxyapatite, the chief constituent of bone, form within the mitochondria. Since the hydroxyapatite is a crystal containing calcium and phosphate, there will be uptake of the labelled pyrophosphate by the calcium in the crystal, therefore producing a concentration (hot spot) in the region of infarction. This hot spot scan becomes positive 16 to 24 hours after a myocardial infarction and persists for about 10 days to 2 weeks.

The incidence of false positive results is about 10%, and of false negatives, 4%. One importance cause of false positive pyrophosphate scans is a left ventricular aneurysm. The reason for this is unknown. However, a ventricular aneurysm that is positive with a pyrophosphate scan persists as positive indefinitely, while a fresh myocardial infarction will become negative 10 days to 2 weeks after the infarction.

Technetium 99m pyrophosphate is presently being used for the detection of acute myocardial infarction in many laboratories and has been found to have a high degree of accuracy (approximately 90%) in detecting both acute transmural and nontransmural infarcts.

B. Cold Spot Scan

A cold spot scan demonstrates a lack of radionuclides in the area of ischemia-injury or previous infarction. The most commonly used agents for these studies are: Potassium 43, Rubidium 81, Thallium 201 and Cesium 131.

Of these agents, Thallium 201 is the newest and most promising radionuclide for the investigation of myocardial perfusion. The chemical behavior of Thallium is similar to that of potassium and hence it is taken up by normal myocardium. Therefore, if there is an area of ischemia-injury or of fibrosis due to a previous myocardial infarction, the Thallium scan will show this area as a region of less activity when compared to the rest of the myocardium.

In the evaluation of ischemic disease, Thallium 201 appears to be more sensitive than exercise testing, especially for one vessel disease. However, good correlation with coronary angiography is only obtained with Thallium if this substance is injected into the patient at the point of maximal stress during an exercise tolerance test. Thallium studies are also of potential value in selecting patients likely to benefit by coronary artery bypass surgery and in assessing alterations in the coronary circulation and myocardial perfusion following such surgery.

II. Left Ventricular Regional Motion

There are technical limitations to the use of diagnostic ultrasound for the assessment of left ventricular wall motion and left ventricular performance. As a result, several new techniques utilizing commonly available radiopharmaceuticals and nuclear imaging devices have been developed for these purposes and have been found to be accurate, efficient and practical.

An area of abnormal regional left ventricular wall motion can be evaluated best by ECG gated scintiphotos. A gating machine connected with the ECG triggers a gamma scintillation camera in both systole and diastole. This makes it possible to obtain a separate picture of the left ventricular blood pool during both phases of the cardiac cycle. By superimposing these pictures, one can evaluate the left ventricular wall for areas of dyskinesis, hypokinesis or akinesis. Technetium 99 albumin is the isotope commonly used for these studies.

This method permits evaluation of wall motion in areas presently inaccessible to the ultrasound beam, specifically the antero-apical portions. Interventricular septal and posterior myocardial wall movement may be visualized by obtaining these scintigraphic studies in the left anterior oblique projection as well as in the routine right anterior oblique projection.

III. Left Ventricular Performance

By following the passage of a radioactive bolus through the heart chambers and lungs, a gamma camera, with the help of a small computer, can describe flow curves (time-activity curves) of the right ventricle, lung and left ventricle. From these curves, measurements of cardiac output, left ventricular ejection fraction, left ventricular end diastolic volume, pulmonary blood volume and transit times can be obtained.

A 1.2:1 left to right shunt can be detected by this technique by seeing a recirculation peak in the flow curves of the right ventricle or lung, and recent studies suggest that such shunts may be accurately quantitated by this method as well.

We have recently demonstrated the reliability and practicality of measuring left ventricular ejection fraction, cardiac output and pulmonary blood flow at the bedside using an inexpensive probe device (similar to the one used for I^{131} thyroid uptake). The technique is simple, takes 10 to 15 minutes, and requires the intravenous injection of only a small amount of radioactivity. Hence, important data on ventricular performance may be made immediately available in the critically ill patient.

Over the past several years we have shown the immediate clinical utility and practicality of having available diagnostic ultrasound and several types of nuclear imaging and counting devices within a single integrated cardiovascular laboratory since the information they provide is often complimentary. Such a setting optimizes the opportunity to combine the technical expertise of the nuclear medical physician with the clinical expertise, correlative input and perspective provided by the cardiologist.

Selected References

1. Gottlieb, S., Sheps, D., Myerburg, R.J., and Miale, A., Jr.: Applications of Diagnostic Ultrasound and Radionuclides to Cardiovascular Diagnosis, Part I. Acquired Cardiovascular Disease in Adult. Sem. Nucl. Med., 5:353, 1975.

2. Gottlieb, S., Groch, M., Kallos, N., Ghahramani, A. and Miale, A., Jr.: A Mobile Dual Scintillation Probe System for the Bedside Assessment of Left Ventricular Performance. J. Nucl. Med., 16:531, 1975.

FIGURE I

24 Hours After AMI

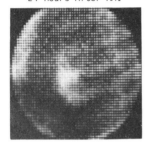

10 Days after AMI

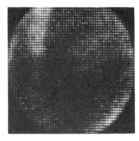

A hot spot scan using Technetium 99 m pyrophosphate in a patient with acute myocardial infarction (AMI). There is an area of increased uptake in the center of the left panel (lighter color) corresponding to the area of injury. A followup scan in the right panel shows the later disappearance of uptake as expected. The lighter area in the upper left of each panel is the sternum, which also takes up the isotope (see text).

FIGURE II

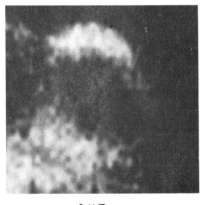
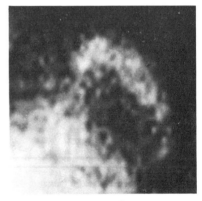

ANT   RAO

A cold spot scan after Thallium 201 injection reveals a large area of abnormally decreased radionuclide concentration involving the anterior heart wall extending to the apex. This pattern is consistent with a large anteroseptal infarction. This patient had clinical and ECG evidence of previous anteroseptal infarction and severe narrowing of the proximal LAD coronary artery, demonstrated by contrast angiography.

FIGURE III

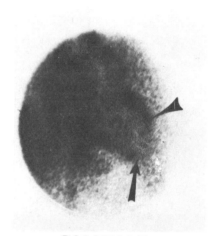
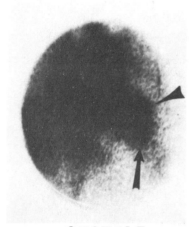

DIASTOLE **SYSTOLE**

ECG-gated scintiphotos that were obtained in diatole and in systole demonstrate poor movement of the anteroapical heart wall (large arrow). The area indicated by the small arrow is akinetic.

SELF-ASSESSMENT QUESTIONS

At the beginning of the Sections on Bedside Diagnosis (p. 209) and Coronary Artery Disease (p. 274), are found teaching cases drawn from our Cardiology Patient Simulator Project. The educational and graphic material presented accompanies two of the diseases currently programmed into the manikin, which can simulate virtually all of the physical findings in any cardiac disease state.

The program on Bedside Diagnosis was developed with Dr. James Ronan of Georgetown University, and that on Coronary Artery Disease with Dr. Andrew Wallace of Duke University. The invaluable assistance of Drs. Stephen Mallon, Stuart Gottlieb and Agis Antonopoulous at the University of Miami is also acknowledged. The National Aeronautics and Space Agency (NASA) contributed all of the graphic work. All involved deserve special thanks.

SELF-ASSESSMENT-BEDSIDE DIAGNOSIS

HISTORY
30 year old female

CHIEF COMPLAINT: Palpitations of 3 year's duration.

PRESENT ILLNESS: The patient has had brief, fleeting "flip-flop" sensations in her chest. At other times she occasionally has sharp chest pains at rest lasting 1 to 3 seconds. There is no past history of rheumatic fever, chest trauma or heart murmur.

FAMILY HISTORY: Her 25 year old sister has a murmur.

Question: Is a specific diagnosis suggested by this history?

Answer: No. Both her palpitations, which suggest premature contractions, and her chest pain, are nonspecific and may be entirely innocent.

PHYSICAL SIGNS

a. GENERAL APPEARANCE - Normal slender young woman with mild scoliosis.
b. VENOUS PULSE - The CVP is estimated to be 3 cm. H_2O.

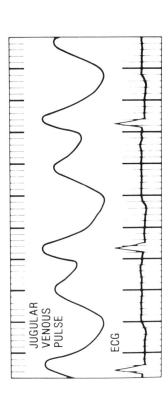

Question: How do you interpret the venous pulse?

Answer: The venous pulse is normal.

c. ARTERIAL PULSE   (BP =120/70)

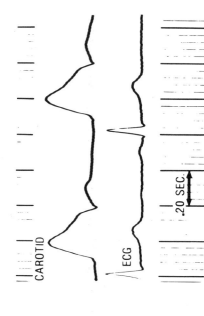

Question: How do you interpret the carotid arterial pulse?

Answer: The arterial pulse is normal.

d. PRECORDIAL MOVEMENT and
e. AUSCULTATION

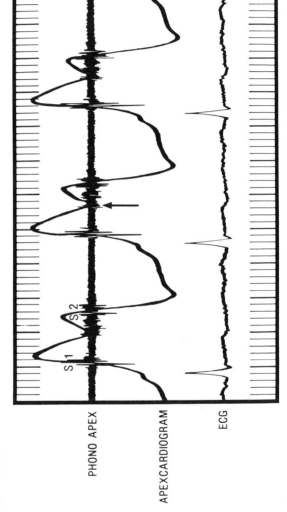

Question: How do you interpret the apical pulsation?

Answer: After the initial normal outward early systolic movement, there is an abrupt inward movement of the ventricular wall (arrow) coinciding approximately with the click on the phonocardiogram. This is followed by a second abnormally prominent systolic outward movement. These findings are consistent with mid and late systolic mitral valve prolapse, in which it is theorized that the prolapsing valve exerts tension on the papillary muscles, which in turn "pull" on the ventricular wall. As late mitral regurgitation occurs, the atrium may acutely expand, thrusting the left ventricle forward again.

Question: In what other disease states may a double apical systolic impulse be palpated?

Answer: Most notably in idiopathic hypertrophic subaortic stenosis, though causes of late systolic mitral regurgitation other than valve prolapse may also cause these movements.

e. AUSCULTATION (continued)

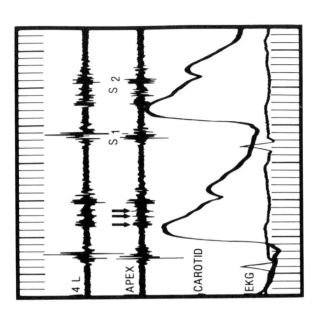

Questions:

1. How do you interpret the acoustic events at the left sternal edge and apex?

2. What additional bedside manipulations will help to assess this murmur?

Answers:

1. There are multiple systolic clicks and a late systolic murmur. These findings indicate mitral valve prolapse. The clicks are likely due to acute tensing of the valve as it everts into the left atrium, or less likely may emanate from the chordae tendineae.

2. Examine the patient standing and squatting as shown below.

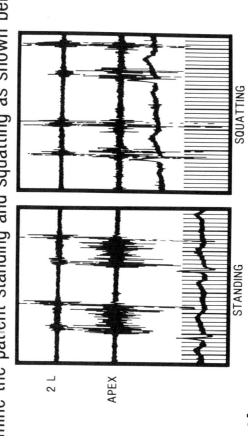

Question: What is your explanation for these postural changes?

Answer: Standing decreases venous return, reducing ventricular size, resulting in earlier and more marked prolapse of the redundant mitral leaflet, and hence earlier and often louder clicks and murmur.

Squatting, by increasing peripheral resistance and hence afterload, increases ventricular size, and the murmur is later and often fainter.

Through similar mechanisms amyl nitrite makes the ventricle smaller (like standing), allows more mitral valve prolapse, and the murmur begins earlier. Vasopressors or isometric handgrip (like squatting) increases ventricular size, allows less prolapse, and makes the murmur begin later in systole.

These changes are in contrast to patients with rheumatic mitral regurgitation. For example, in such patients, a reduction in afterload enhances forward flow, reducing the degree of regurgitation and the murmur.

Proceed

e. AUSCULTATION (continued)

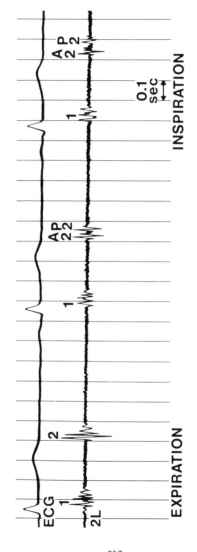

Question: How do you interpret the acoustic events at the upper left sternal edge?

Answer: There is normal splitting of the second heart sound in inspiration.

ELECTROCARDIOGRAM

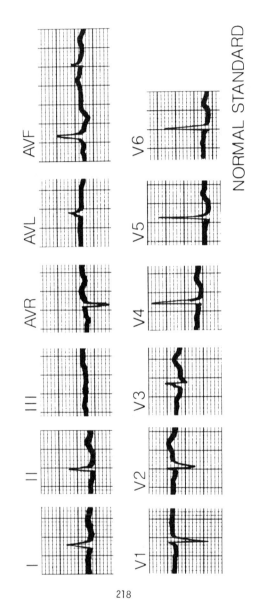

NORMAL STANDARD

Question: How do you interpret this ECG?

Answer: There are minor nonspecific ST-T wave changes and an isolated ventricular premature contraction (VPC) in lead aVF. Such ST-T changes are common in patients with mitral valve prolapse, especially in the inferolateral leads. In many patients, especially those with the isolated clicks and no murmur, the ECG is normal. Premature atrial and ventricular contractions are also common and are the usual cause of "palpitations." Atrial tachycardia and atrial fibrillation are sometimes present. Exercise stress testing results in a high percentage of "false positives."

Proceed

CHEST X RAYS

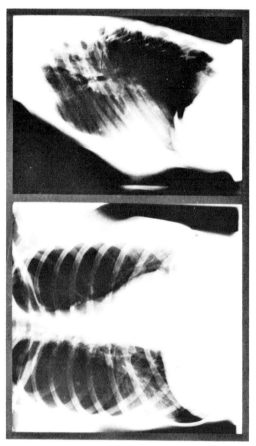

Questions:

1. How do you interpret these X rays?
2. Based on the history, physical examination, ECG and X rays, what is your diagnostic impression and plan to further evaluate this patient?

Answers:

1. The heart and lungs are normal. There is mild scoliosis of the thoracic spine. On the lateral view, the spine is quite "straight," rather than mildly kyphotic as it usually is in normal adults. Thoracic skeletal abnormalities are quite frequent in this syndrome of mitral valve prolapse, particularly "straight back," pectus excavatum, and mild thoracic scoliosis.

2. The history, physical examination, ECG and chest X rays are essentially diagnostic of the systolic click — systolic murmur (Barlow's) syndrome. Echocardiography is a non-invasive procedure likely to show the mitral prolapse and confirm the clinical diagnosis. The patient's study follows.

LABORATORY - Echocardiogram

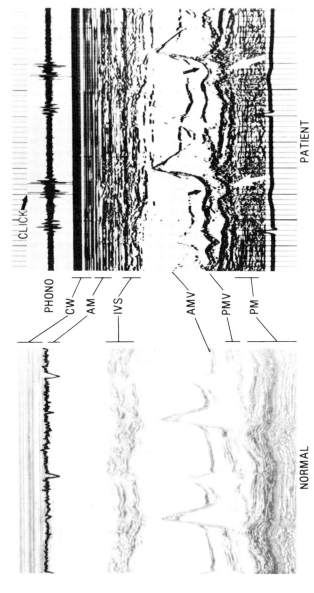

CW = Chest wall, AM = Anterior myocardium, IVS = Interventricular septum, AMV = Anterior mitral valve, PMV = Posterior mitral valve, PM = Posterior myocardium

Question: What are the diagnostic features of this echocardiogram?

Answer: In the normal mitral valve the leaflets migrate together slowly anteriorly during systole. In mitral valve prolapse, there is posterior movement of the leaflets in mid or late systole, usually beginning with the onset of the click or murmur (arrows). This makes the mitral valve echos in systole look like a question mark lying on its side. ⌒ The posterior leaflet is more frequently involved than the anterior leaflet but may be more difficult to visualize on echocardiogram than the anterior leaflet.

Question: Is further study necessary?

Answer: No. The precise diagnosis has been established by non-invasive techniques, the most valuable of which is auscultation. However, if cardiac catheterization were performed, the results would be similar to the following case.

LABORATORY (continued)

LEFT VENTRICULAR ANGIOGRAM
Right Anterior Oblique
- Systolic Frame

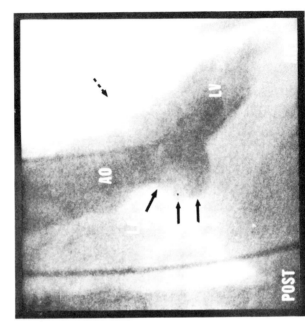

LEFT ATRIUM (LA) = 5 mm. Hg. MEAN
LEFT VENTRICLE (LV) = 120/4 mm. Hg.
AORTA (AO) = 120/70 mm. Hg.
CARDIAC INDEX = 3.5 L./MIN./M.^{2}

Question: How do you interpret the hemodynamics and angiographic data?

Answer: Intracardiac pressures and cardiac output are all normal, as is usually the case since the mitral regurgitation is minimal. The angiogram shows scalloping (arrows) of the prolapsing posterior leaflet as well as some prolapse of the anterior leaflet (broken arrow) as they balloon into the left atrium in late systole.

Question: The patient has received conflicting advice about her cardiac status and about antibiotics. Some have told her to take Penicillin-G, 200,000 units twice daily, while others have said to take Penicillin-V, 500 mg. prior to dental work every six hours on that day and for 2 days after. One doctor advised both. What is your advice?

Answer: Regarding her "cardiac status," the patient should be reassured, as the natural history of the great majority of patients with the systolic click - murmur (Barlow's) syndrome is benign.

She requires prophylaxis against infective endocarditis, not against rheumatic fever. Therefore, she should take antibiotics whenever she is exposed to a bacteremia, e.g., dental work, including cleaning and filling of the teeth, cystoscopies, obstetrical procedures, etc. Rheumatic fever prophylaxis is commonly confused with this but should be reserved for certain patients who have had rheumatic fever previously.

The patient was advised that her younger sister should be checked, as she also has a murmur, and this syndrome may occasionally be familial. Her sister's evaluation follows.

The patient's sister's evaluation was entirely normal, but for auscultation carried out standing. The examination must include listening in multiple positions (and occasionally even at different times), as these vasoactive maneuvers may vary ventricular size and hence vary the murmur.

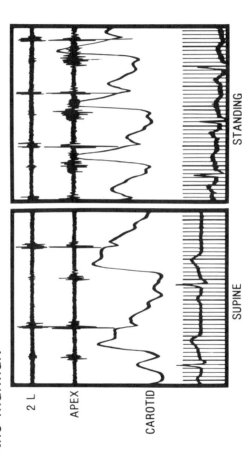

This patient was also instructed to undergo infective endocarditis prophylaxis for any surgical or dental manipulative procedures.

Proceed for Summary

SUMMARY

Mitral valve prolapse is an extremely common disorder, probably occuring in about 1% of the population, and is sometimes familial. Young women are most commonly affected. It is usually a very mild disorder, and in some cases may also involve the tricuspid valve.

In most instances its cause is unknown. However, irregular dilatation of the posterior or both leaflets and myxomatous changes microscopically have been found in the valve in many of the cases studied at autopsy or surgery. These changes are similar to those seen in Marfan's and the "floppy valve" syndrome which, however, are more severe and progressive disorders. The gross pathology of a patient who developed infective endocarditis follows.

While the natural history of the systolic click-murmur syndrome is generally benign, this specimen is from a patient who died of embolic complications of infective endocarditis.

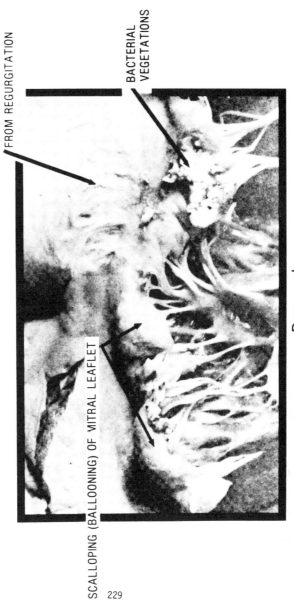

Proceed

SUMMARY (continued)

The systolic click is the hallmark of the prolapsed valve. There is some evidence that the myocardium might contract asynergistically, pushing the papillary muscles upward, allowing the click and murmur to occur. It is rarely caused by rheumatic fever although clicks and systolic murmurs have been found in patients with mitral stenosis who have had mitral commissurotomy.

The late systolic murmur is frequently seen with it but may also be seen with other forms of mitral regurgitation such as papillary muscle dysfunction, rheumatic heart disease or calcified mitral annulus.

To Review This Case of Systolic Click - Murmur (Barlow's) Syndrome:

The **HISTORY** is typical, including palpitations reflecting VPC's and atypical chest pain of the musculoskeletal type. Occasionally there is chest pain which sounds "ischemic" in nature. This may be due to extreme tension on the papillary muscles due to the taut and stretched chordae tendineae. The syndrome may occasionally be familial, as in this case.

PHYSICAL SIGNS:

a. The GENERAL APPEARANCE reveals her slender build with slight scoliosis and a "straight back," common in this syndrome
b. The JUGULAR VENOUS PULSE is normal in mean pressure and wave form.
c. The ARTERIAL PULSE is normal.

d. PRECORDIAL MOVEMENT reveals midsystolic retraction and late systolic outward movement which may be seen in some of these cases, but is not diagnostic.

e. AUSCULTATION reveals normal splitting of the second sound at the upper left sternal edge. Midsystolic clicks and a later systolic murmur are heard best at the apex and are less intense at the left sternal edge. The latter may reflect some degree of tricuspid valve prolapse.

The acoustic events are notoriously variable, and maneuvers which decrease ventricular size augment the findings, with the clicks and murmur appearing earlier in systole. No examination for Barlow's Syndrome is complete unless the patient is examined in the standing position.

On occasion the murmur associated with prolapse of the mitral valve has a quality which has been described as a "honk."

The **ELECTROCARDIOGRAM** shows nonspecific ST-T changes and occasional VPC's. Serious arrhythmias occur rarely.

The **CHEST X RAY** shows no abnormality of the heart or lungs, reflecting the fact that the lesion is hemodynamically insignificant. Associated musculoskeletal abnormalities are seen, including slight scoliosis and a "straight back."

LABORATORY STUDIES include the echocardiogram which shows late systolic posterior movement of the posterior leaflet. While invasive study is unnecessary, a typical angiogram shows the late systolic posterior leaflet prolapse and normal intracardiac pressures and cardiac output.

TREATMENT is mainly reassurance and infective endocarditis prophylaxis for the isolated click or click-murmur syndrome. Arrhythmias are usually untreated because they are brief, infrequent, and of little consequence. Considering the common occurrence of this disorder, the rare instances of serious ventricular arrhythmias which have been reported should not set the standard for therapy. Arrhythmias which are frequent, prolonged, bothersome to the patient or cause him symptoms should probably be treated.

In those cases where chest pain has an "ischemic" quality, beta-adrenergic blocking agents may be effective in reducing the symptoms.

SELF-ASSESSMENT - BEDSIDE DIAGNOSIS

1. Which of the following structures receives a portion of its blood supply from a diagonal branch of the main left coronary artery?

    a. The sinus node
    b. The AV node
    c. The posterior papillary muscle of the left ventricle
    d. The anterior papillary muscle of the left ventricle
    e. The interventricular septum

2. Which of the following pressures is highest?

    a. Left ventricular end-diastolic pressure
    b. Left ventricular systolic pressure
    c. Aortic diastolic pressure
    d. Left atrial "v" wave
    e. Right atrial "a" wave

3. Which of the following is the most common source of blood supply to the AV node?

    a. The left main coronary artery
    b. The left circumflex coronary artery
    c. The right coronary artery
    d. The left anterior descending coronary artery
    e. The diagonal coronary artery

4. Which of the following mechanical events occurs earliest?

    a. Aortic valve closure
    b. Mitral valve closure
    c. Tricuspid valve closure
    d. Aortic valve opening
    e. Pulmonic valve opening

5. Which of the following structures within the conduction system has a dual coronary artery blood supply?

    a. The sinus node
    b. The AV node
    c. The distal right bundle branch
    d. The left anterior fascicle
    e. The left posterior fascicle

235

6. The bedside cardiovascular examination includes evaluation of:

   a. The general appearance
   b. The jugular venous pulse
   c. The arterial pulse
   d. Chest wall movement
   e. Percussion
   f. Auscultation

7. The normal apical impulse occurs at about the time of the second heart sound. True or False.

8. A third heart sound is often heard at the apex in which of the following?

   a. A normal 70 year old man
   b. A normal 7 year old boy
   c. A patient with severe mitral stenosis
   d. A patient with severe mitral regurgitation

9. During the beat following a ventricular premature contraction, the murmur typically becomes louder in which of the following?

   a. Aortic valvular stenosis
   b. Mitral valvular stenosis
   c. Idiopathic hypertrophic subaortic stenosis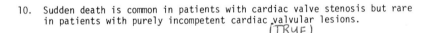
   d. Mitral valvular regurgitation

10. Sudden death is common in patients with cardiac valve stenosis but rare in patients with purely incompetent cardiac valvular lesions. (TRUE)

11. A previously health 45 year old man is seen in the Emergency Room with severe substernal chest pain and shortness of breath. On examination, his blood pressure is 160/100 and his skin warm and dry. He has scattered basilar rales. Chest wall examination reveals a palpable early diastolic movement at the apex in addition to a normal apical impulse at the time of the first heart sound. On auscultation he has a fourth heart sound and a grade 1/6 midsystolic apical murmur. Which of the following are likely true in this case?

    a. He is in cardiogenic shock
    b. A palpable third heart sound and basilar rales indicate left ventricular failure and suggest he has sustained an extensive infarct
    c. The presence of a fourth heart sound in this setting indicates severe failure and an extensive infarct.

    (Question 11 is continued on the next page)

11. (Continued)

    d. The murmur is innocent
    e. The murmur is consistent with mild papillary muscle dysfunction
    f. The murmur is consistent with severe mitral regurgitation and early angiography is indicated as a prelude to surgery
    g. His elevated blood pressure should be treated, as the increased afterload on the heart increases his myocardial oxygen consumption

12. A 22 year old female is seen in the Emergency Room. Earlier that day she had an episode of rapid irregular heart action, after which she noted pain in her left leg which progressed. She has known rheumatic heart disease with mild mitral stenosis. Which of the following are likely true in this case?

    a. She has sustained a peripheral arterial embolic occlusion
    b. Her electrocardiogram shows marked right ventricular hypertrophy (LATE FINDING)
    c. There is an increased first sound at the apex, an opening snap .05 seconds after A_2, and a long diastolic rumbling murmur.
    d. At the apex there is an increased first sound, an opening snap .10 seconds after A_2, and a short diastolic rumbling murmur
    e. She has pathologic C-V waves in the jugular venous pulse

13. A previously healthy 52 year old man is seen in the Emergency Room with severe substernal chest pain and shortness of breath. On examination his blood pressure is 140/80, his heart rate, 95. His carotid vessel is rapid rising. On auscultation you hear a fourth sound at the apex and a grade 3-4/6 systolic decrescendo murmur. Which of the following are likely true in this case?

    a. The patient has ruptured his posterior papillary muscle
    b. The chest X ray shows marked enlargement of the left atrium
    c. The patient has mitral regurgitation from papillary muscle dysfunction
    d. The etiology of the patient's mitral regurgitation is rheumatic
    e. The patient is in sinus rhythm

14. The following phonocardiogram was taken on an asymptomatic 60 year old man with a history of myocardial infarction 2 years ago.

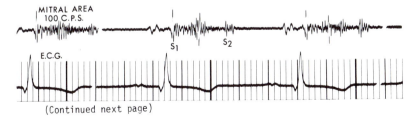

(Continued next page)

14. Continued

    Which of the following are true in this case?
    - a. There is a fourth sound at the apex
    - b. There is a third sound at the apex
    - c. There is a systolic murmur at the apex
    - d. There is a diastolic murmur at the apex
    - e. The etiology of his murmur is likely papillary muscle dysfunction
    - f. The murmur is "innocent," i.e., "functional"
    - g. The murmur is likely due to mild mitral regurgitation
    - h. No therapy is indicated
    - i. He should take antibiotics for dental and surgical procedures to prevent infective endocarditis
    - j. The patient likely has significant aortic stenosis and further study is indicated

15. A 55 year old male is brought to the Emergency Room with severe chest pain. On examination, his cuff blood pressure is 80/60 and he is cold and clammy, cyanotic and confused. A systolic outward movement can be palpated between the left sternal border and apex. He has a third sound at the apex. His ECG shows diffuse non-specific ST-T wave abnormalities and A-V dissociation. Which of the following are true in this case?
    - a. The patient is in cardiogenic shock
    - b. His cuff blood pressure is the most accurate bedside index of his cardiac output and correlates directly with the amount of tissue infarcted
    - c. The absence of a fourth sound suggests a good prognosis
    - d. The third sound is a useful clinical index of the degree of pump failure in this setting, but less important than the patient's general appearance
    - e. The chest wall movement indicates a previous infarction with a ventricular aneurysm
    - f. A presumptive diagnosis of myocardial infarction is appropriate, even though his ECG shows no indicative changes
    - g. Conversion to normal sinus rhythm is the most important first therapeutic goal

16. A 22 year old pregnant female comes to the Emergency Room with recurrent deep vein thrombophlebitis of the right leg. Which of the following are consistent with superimposed multiple pulmonary emboli with moderately severe pulmonary hypertension
    - a. Giant "a" waves in the JVP (atrial contraction)
    - b. Pathologic "c-v" waves in the JVP
    - c. A sustained mid-left sternal border systolic impulse
    - d. A sustained upper-left sternal border systolic impulse
    - e. A fourth heart sound enhanced during inspiration atrial contraction
    - f. A systolic left sternal border murmur enhanced during inspiration (TR)
    - g. A palpable pulmonary second sound with wide persistent splitting of the second sounds on auscultation

17. A 40 year old slender man is seen in your office complaining of dyspnea on exertion and awakening at night short of breath. A murmur was first heard at the age of 18. Some of his bedside findings are shown below.

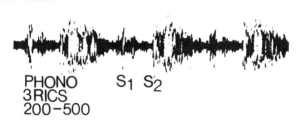

PHONO S1 S2
3 RICS
200-500

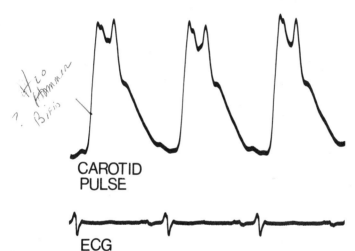

CAROTID
PULSE

ECG

Which of the following are true in this case?
a. There is a systolic murmur consistent with critical aortic stenosis
b. There is a systolic murmur likely due to excess "flow" across the aortic valve
c. There is a diastolic murmur consistent with aortic regurgitation
d. On examination he is likely to have a rumbling murmur at the apex with a soft first heard sound
e. Pulsations are likely visible in the neck
f. The CVP is likely elevated to at least 15 cm. H_2O
g. Rheumatic heart disease is the likeliest etiology
h. Congenital heart disease is the likeliest etiology.

18. A 40 year old man is seen complaining of substernal chest distress with exertion. On examination his blood pressure was 105/80. His cardiac examination is shown below.

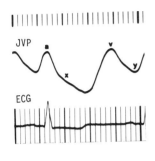
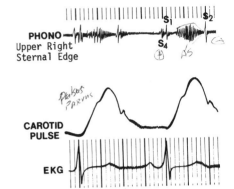

Which statements are true in this patient?

- a. His venous pulse is normal
- b. His carotid pulse is normal
- c. The fourth sound is normal in this setting
- d. His ECG likely shows LVH
- e. He has aortic stenosis and the gradient is likely critical
- f. He has aortic stenosis and the gradient is likely minimal
- g. He has mitral regurgitation due to papillary muscle dysfunction
- h. You should advise the patient that further cardiologic study is indicated

19. A 35 year old male is seen in the Emergency Room with a history of having passed out for several minutes while running to catch a bus. He had no serious injury. On examination, you hear a systolic crescendo-decrescendo murmur at the upper right sternal border, and a diastolic decrescendo murmur at the mid-left sternal broder. Further questioning revealed that the patient had undergone cardiac catheterization one year previously and was told he had a severely narrowed heart valve. Which of the following are consistent with this presentation?

- a. The patient likely has idiopathic hypertrophic subaortic stenosis
- b. The patient likely has a congenital bicuspid valve with dominant aortic stenosis
- c. His carotid vessel is rapid rising
- d. His apical impulse is best felt in the sixth intercostal space at the anterior axillary line
- e. His CVP is 3 cm. H_2O with the "a" wave slightly higher than the "v" wave
- f. The systolic murmur is early peaking and loud
- g. The systolic murmur is late peaking
- h. He has a wide pulse pressure

20. In acute severe aortic regurgitation: (AI)
    a. The first heart sound is loud due to high left atrial pressure
    b. A wide pulse pressure is diagnostic
    c. The murmur is diastolic, decrescendo, long and classically best heard at the mid-left sternal border
    d. The apical impulse is usually in the anterior axillary line as the preloaded ventricle is markedly enlarged (CBl6 LV x RAH @ pmunic)
    e. The left ventricular diastolic pressure is typically elevated

21. In mitral stenosis, the pressure difference between the left atrium and MS left ventricle is determined by:
    a. the cardiac output = LRx SV
    b. the cardiac output and the heart rate
    c. the heart rate and the size of the mitral orifice
    d. the cardiac output, the heart rate, and the mitral orifice size
    e. the cardiac output and the diastolic filling period

22. In mitral regurgitation: (MI)
    a. the predominant hemodynamic abnormality occurs during systole
    b. the left ventricle is protected from overload
    c. diastolic gradients across the mitral valve never occur
    d. the major hemodynamic problem is pressure overload

23. In hypertrophic subaortic stenosis: IHSS
    a. the gradient is at the level of the aortic valve
    b. both the left ventricular septum and the mitral valve participate in the obstruction
    c. pressure gradients are usually identifiable both within the left ventricular outflow tract and at the level of the aortic valve
    d. positive inotropic influences generally do not increase the degree of obstruction FALSE

24. The diastolic filling period across the mitral valve is markedly influenced by the heart rate because:
    a. heart rate increase consistently causes an increase in cardiac output
    b. at fast heart rates, the mitral valve must decrease its excursion because of insufficient time for complete leaflet movement
    c. the decreased cycle length accompanying increased heart rates encroaches more upon diastole than upon systole
    d. the effective valve area is a function of heart rate

25. Digitalis is always contraindicated in the management of patients with obstructive hypertrophic cardiomyopathy. True or False.

26. The distinctive feature of the post PVC response in obstructive hypertrophic cardiomyopathy is the augmentation of the gradient in the post PVC beat. True or False.

27. Each of the following except one will increase the obstruction in hypertrophic cardiomyopathy:
    a. standing (↓VR) ∴ HT contracts further (↓ejection period fraction)
    b. atropine ↑ AV conduction
    c. blood transfusion IHSS)
    d. sodium nitroprusside (vasodil)
    e. isoproterenol ↑ β₁

28. Complete heart block in patients with valvular aortic stenosis usually indicates extension of the calcific process to the most cephalad portion of the muscular ventricular septum where the atrioventricular node is located. (True) or False.

29. The occurrence of left bundle branch block in a patient with valvular aortic stenosis strongly suggests co-existent severe coronary atherosclerosis. True or (False)

30. Sudden death is common in patients with cardiac valve stenosis but rare in patients with purely incompetent cardiac valvular lesions. (True) or False.

31. A 45 year old male patient is seen in the Emergency Room with a history of fever and chills for one week and acute dyspnea of several hours duration. His bedside examination reveals a loud systolic murmur at the apex associated with a thrill. It was not present 10 days previously when he was in the Emergency Room to have a laceration sutured. Which of the following is/are likely true:
    a. there is a fourth heart sound at the apex (ms)
    b. his chest x-ray shows marked enlargement of the left atrium
    c. he is in atrial fibrillation
    d. the murmur has a late systolic crescendo
    e. the anterior papillary muscle is ruptured (post ensp m)anu mI ant ensy " DS.

32. A major advantage of tissue prosthetic valves over synthetic prosthetic valves is that no anticoagulants are needed postoperatively. (True) or False.

33. Match the items in the right hand column with those in the left:
    1. Left atrial myxoma a,b,c,d   a. Attached by a pedicle
    2. Left atrial thrombus c, d   b. Injection of contrast material
                                      c. Mitral stenosis
                                      d. Mitral regurgitation

34. Classic bedside findings in moderate rheumatic mitral regurgitation in a patient with good left ventricular function and in atrial fibrillation include: ↑ SV ↓ CO
    a. an apical holosystolic murmur
    b. a third sound at the apex (tensing chordae tendonae)
    c. a brisk carotid upstroke (m) / ↑S)
    d. a dominant "a" wave in the jugular venous pulse
    e. a non-displaced, sustained left ventricular impulse at the apex following a palpable S4. Imp good LV func

35. Which one of following characteristics does not reduce the likelihood of a good result of operation for valvular heart disease:
    a. A cardiothoracic ratio greater than 0.6
    b. A dilated aortic annulus (95)
    c. Left ventricular end-diastolic pressure at rest greater than 20 mmHg   more 20/10
    —d. A history of syncopal episodes ♦   i.e AS. 6 months
    e. An ejection fraction of less than 40%   80% norm
    f. A "giant" left atrium (dilated)

36. Which one of the following statements regarding isolated mitral stenosis in a young girl is not true:
    a. Heavy calcification is unusual True
    —b. Valve replacement is usually required for correction
    c. The onset of symptoms is usually gradual and insidious True
    d. An opening snap is usually present True
    e. Operation should be considered if the patient is Class II or worse True ?
    f. Operation is often done without need for preoperative catheterization ?
    g. Operation can be performed without cardiopulmonary bypass ??

37. Which one of the following is not an indication that mitral commissurotomy should be performed "open," i.e., on cardiopulmonary bypass:
    —a. A large left atrium
    b. A previous closed commissurotomy
    c. 2+ or greater mitral regurgitation
    d. Left atrial thrombus demonstrated by pulmonary angiography
    e. Associated left ventricular failure with mild aortic regurgitation
    f. Associated coronary arterial disease with mild aortic stenosis

38. Which one of the following statements concerning mitral regurgitation (MR) is not true:
    a. Symptoms usually progress slowly and deceptively True
    b. The "largest left atriums" are usually produced by mitral regurgitation ?
    c. The Carpentier ring can be used to correct this defect
    d. MR is a surgically treatable complication of myocardial infarction True
    e. Afterload reduction plays an important role in the postoperative care of these patients True
    —f. Incidence of emboli following valve replacement for mitral regurgitation is less than the incidence following aortic valve replacement   False

39. A 45 year old man has a typical murmur of aortic stenosis, LVH by chest X ray and electrocardiogram and the recent onset of angina pectoris with two syncopal episodes. The cardiothoracic ratio is 0.53, the ascending aorta is dilated. Which one of the following statements is not true.
    a. Cardiac catheterization is indicated T
    b. Coronary arteriography is indicated T
    —c. Operation should be advised only if the pressure gradient between left ventricle and aorta is 50 mmHg or more
    (Continued next page)

[handwritten top: Little hearts AS / Big hearts AR]

39. Continued
   d. Operative mortality should be less than 5% if the coronary arteries, ejection fraction and LVEDP are normal
   e. An excellent symptomatic improvement and long-term survival can be predicted after aortic valve replacement in this man

40. A 35 year old man with aortic regurgitation after bacterial endocarditis is being followed expectantly. Which one of the following statements is not true:
   a. Operation is indicated when progressive left ventricular enlargement occurs even if the patient remains asymptomatic
   b. Successful surgical correction usually required aortic valve replacement
   c. Such patients usually develop angina pectoris before operation is indicated
   d. Pre-existing mitral stenosis in this patient would lead to much more rapid deterioration and urgency for operation
   e. Aortic valve replacement can be performed in the active acute phase of bacterial endocarditis if hemodynamically indicated

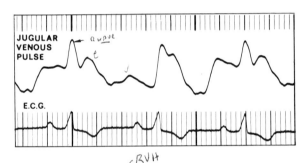

The above tracing was taken from a 15 year old female. On bedside examination there was a sustained left parasternal impulse [RVH] in the 2nd, 3rd and 4th intercostal spaces; a long, late peaking, crescendo-decrescendo grade 4/6 systolic murmur associated with a thrill best heard at the upper left sternal edge and a barely audible pulmonary second sound.

41. The clinical diagnosis is:
    a. Ventricular septal defect
    b. Aortic stenosis
    c. Pulmonary atresia
    d. Pulmonary stenosis
    e. Atrial septal defect

42. The tallest wave (arrow) in the tracing is a:
    a. giant "a" wave
    b. Pathologic C-V wave
    c. Bisferiens pulse wave
    d. Cannon "a" wave

43. The significance of this finding is:
    a. That the patient had severe tricuspid regurgitation
    b. That the atrial contraction is enhanced
    c. That the "C" wave is the "V" wave in this case
    d. That the ECG shows A-V dissociation

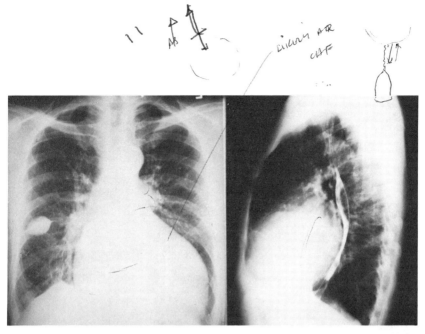

44. The above chest X ray was taken on a 45 year old male whose diagnosis is primary myocardial disease. Which of the following are true:
   a. There is biventricular enlargement
   b. The circular shadow in the right mid lung is likely a tumor
   c. The circular shadow is the right mid lung is due to his heart disease
   d. He likely has a third heart sound
   e. None of the above

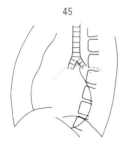

45

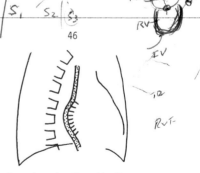

46

Match the statements on the right with the 2 numbered schematic X rays:

45. _____
46. _____

a. Shows left atrial enlargement
b. Best view to assess right atrial enlargement
c. Shows left ventricular enlargement
d. Best view to evaluate mitral and aortic calcification
e. Optimum obliquity 45°
f. Optimum obliquity 60°

245

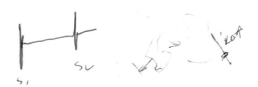

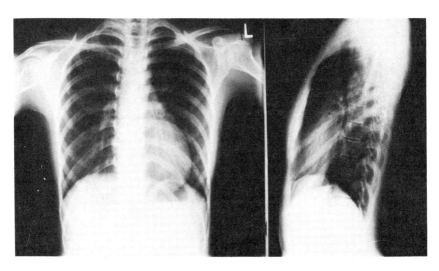

47. A <u>25 year</u> old female is seen by you to evaluate a murmur. Her chest X ray is shown above. Which of the following are likely true in this case:
    a. The murmur is best heard at the upper left sternal edge
    b. The murmur is innocent
    c. There is a fourth sound at the apex
    d. The CVP is 12 cm H_2O
    e. The carotid is bifid
    f. There is a brief impulse palpable at the left sternal edge.

48. This phonocardiogram (at right) taken at the apex, shows:
    a. Mild mitral regurgitation
    b. Mild mitral stenosis
    c. Moderately severe mitral regurgitation
    d. Moderately severe mitral stenosis

    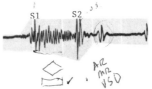

49. Fixed splitting of the second sound is better assessed lying than sitting. True or False.

50. In general, the length of a murmur generated across a stenosed valve is correlated with the severity of obstruction. True or False.

51. Pathologic third and fourth heart sounds may be felt at time when they are inaudible. True or False.

52. An aortic ejection click is common in patients with severe aortic stenosis over the age of 60. True or False.

53. This PA chest X ray is most consistent with:
    a. Severe recent onset mitral regurgitation
    b. Severe chronic mitral regurgitation
    c. Severe recent onset aortic regurgitation
    d. Severe chronic aortic regurgitation
    e. Large ventricular septal defect with left to right shunt
    f. Large ventricular septal defect with right to left shunt (Eisenmenger complex)

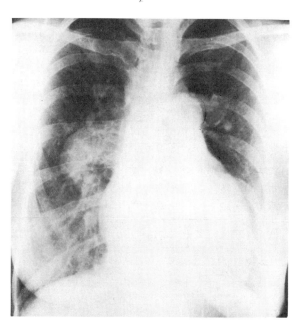

54. This PA chest X ray is most consistent with:
    a. Pulmonary stenosis
    b. Aortic stenosis
    c. Atrial septal defect
    d. Mitral regurgitation
    e. Aortic regurgitation
    f. None of the above

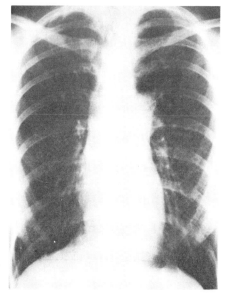

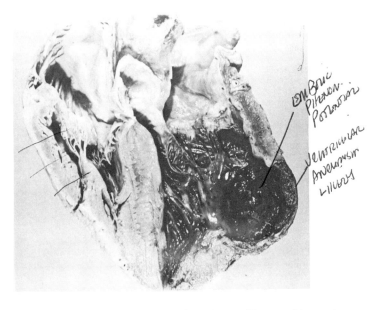

55. The above pathology specimen was obtained from a 60 year old man who died from a stroke. Which of the following are likely true:
    a. The stroke was embolic
    b. He has had a myocardial infarction in the past
    c. He has severe aortic stenosis
    d. He has Tetralogy of Fallot with tricuspid regurgitation
    e. None of the above.

56. The right ventricle may occupy the apex in:
    a. Mitral stenosis
    b. Mitral regurgitation
    c. Atrial septal defect
    d. Aortic stenosis and mitral regurgitation
    e. Aortic regurgitation and mitral stenosis

57.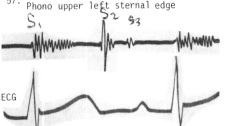

8 year old boy, asymptomatic

Which ones of the following are true regarding the tracing at left:
a. There is a third heart sound present
b. The murmur is innocent
c. The murmur is early systolic
d. The patient has severe aortic stenosis
e. All of the above

58. The "v" wave in the jugular venous pulse is:
    a. A negative wave seen normally   c. Due to tricuspid regurgitation
    b. A positive wave seen normally   d. Due to carotid displacement of
                                             the veins

59. A twice-beating arterial pulse may be felt in:
    a. Aortic valvular regurgitation
    b. Combined aortic valvular stenosis and regurgitation
    c. Idiopathic hypertrophic subaortic stenosis
    d. All of the above

60. In mitral regurgitation, the arterial pulse is hypokinetic even in the
    absence of severe left ventricular failure. True or False

61. A patient is found to have a soft medium frequency early systolic de-
    crescendo murmur at the lower left sternal edge, increasing with inspir-
    ation. Prominent C-V waves are seen in the neck and the pulmonary second
    sound is normal. The likely diagnosis is:
    a. Tricuspid regurgitation with pulmonary hypertension
    b. Chronic tricuspid regurgitation due to biventricular failure
    c. Acute mild tricuspid regurgitation with normal pulmonary arterial
       pressure
    d. Acute severe tricuspid regurgitation with normal pulmonary arterial
       pressure.

62. The presence of a fourth heart sound is of diagnostic significance in:
    (more than one may be correct)
    a. Recent onset mitral regurgitation
    b. Chronic rheumatic mitral stenosis
    d. Aortic stenosis in a 30 year old man
    e. Chronic rheumatic mitral regurgitation

63. Paradoxic splitting of the second heart sound may occur with:
    a. LBBB   c. Angina
    b. Aortic stenosis   d. All of the above

64. In aortic stenosis the degree of obstruction can be determined from
    which of the following parameters. Select two.
    a. Left ventricular end-diastolic pressure
    b. Pressure difference across obstruction
    c. Cardiac output
    d. Dilatation of the aorta
    d. Amount of calcification of the valve

Match the disease states listed in the left hand column with the one best
hemodynamic description on the right:
65. Mitral stenosis   c   a. Systolic pressure gradient
66. Aortic stenosis   a   b. Variable or no gradient
67. IHSS   b   c. Diastolic pressure gradient
68. Myxoma of the left atrium b

MS 69. a,b,d,e,b',i,K,m,u,v,x,b', (g,z,c',d')
MR 70. b,f,h,j,k,g,r,u,x,(c,i,l,n,o,p,y,z)
AS 71. a,b,d,e,h,j,y,K,m,g,p,s,t,u,s,a',b',c' (g,w,x,)
AR 72. g,j,q,l,u,d' (c,f,h,i,k,f,n,z,s T x y)

Match the pathologic features listed below with the valvular lesions listed above them:

69. Mitral stenosis
70. Mitral regurgitation
71. Aortic stenosis
72. Aortic regurgitation

a. Always indicates anatomic abnormality
b. Valvular thickening
c. Valve may be anatomically normal
d. Calcific deposits common
e. Limited etiologies
f. Many etiologies
g. Diffuse pathologic involvement
h. Etiology may be congenital
i. Infective endocarditis
j. Papillary muscle dysfunction
k. May be rheumatic
l. May be traumatic
m. Most frequent fatal valvular lesion
n. Acute onset
o. Most frequent clinically
p. Etiology may be ventricular dilatation
q. Ruptured chordae
r. Marfan's syndrome
s. Dissection

t. Dilated Aortic root
u. Generally takes years to develop
v. Almost always rheumatic
w. Isolated lesion most frequently congenital
x. Left atrium may be enlarged
y. Left ventricular cavity typically dilated with severe longstanding lesion
a'. Risk of sudden death high
b'. Associated involvement of another valve typical
c'. Calcification typical with increasing age
d'. Parachute valve commonest congenital etiology

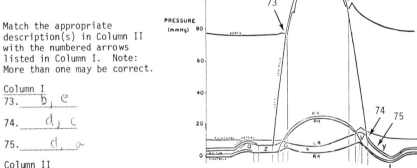

EVENTS OF THE CARDIAC CYCLE

Match the appropriate description(s) in Column II with the numbered arrows listed in Column I. Note: More than one may be correct.

Column I
73. b, e
74. d, c
75. d, a

Column II
a. Rapid ventricular filling
b. Chest wall movement is normally palpable at this point
c. The mitral valve opens at this point
d. The aortic valve is closed at this point
e. The aortic valve opens at this point.

SELF-ASSESSMENT - ECG CORE CURRICULUM

WHAT IS YOUR DIAGNOSIS (Questions 1-40)?

1.
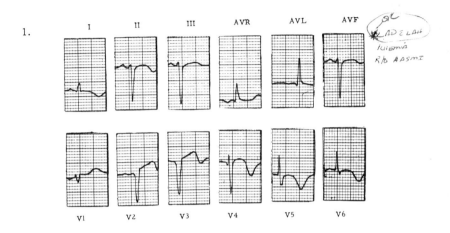

2.
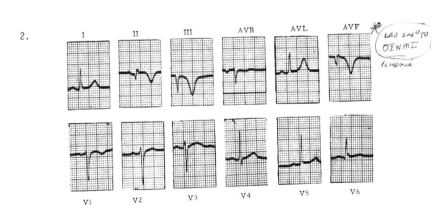

3.

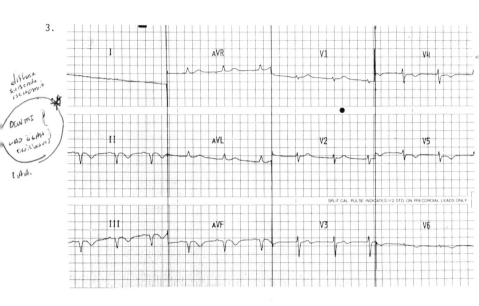

4.

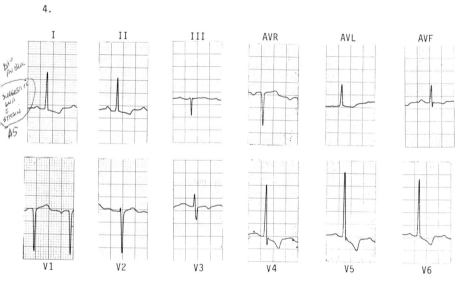

5.

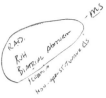

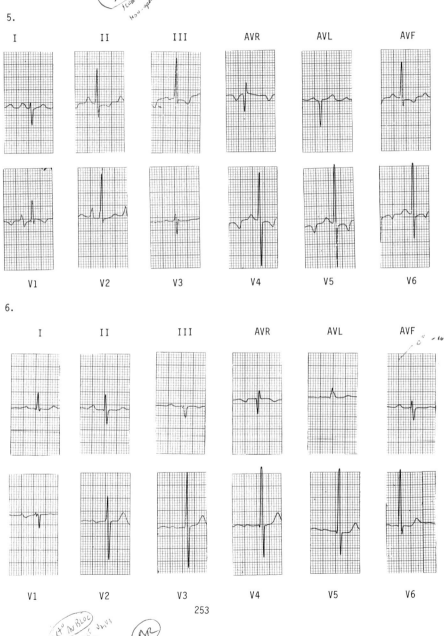

7.

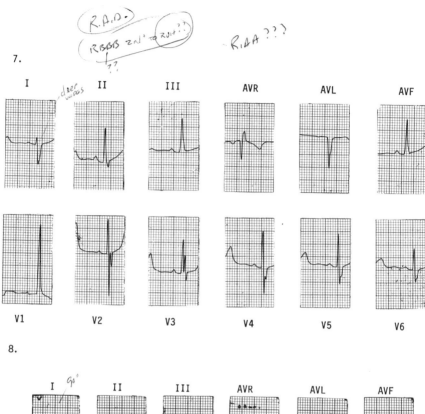

8.

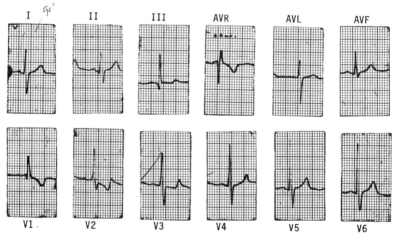

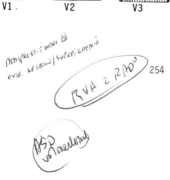

9A. Day of Admission

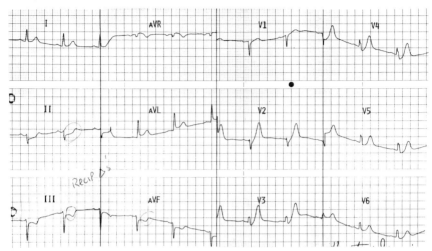

9B. Day after Admission

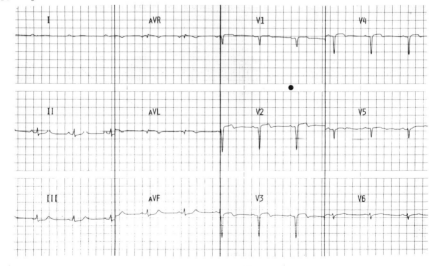

10.

ASMI

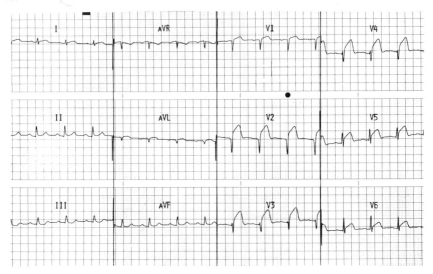

11.

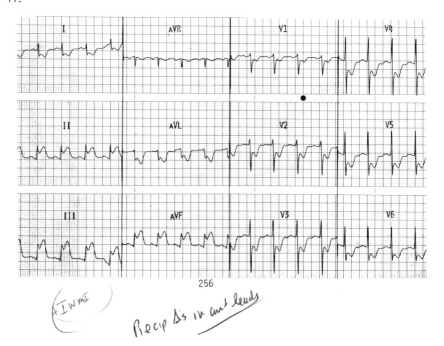

IWMI

Recip ∆'s in ant leads

12.

13.

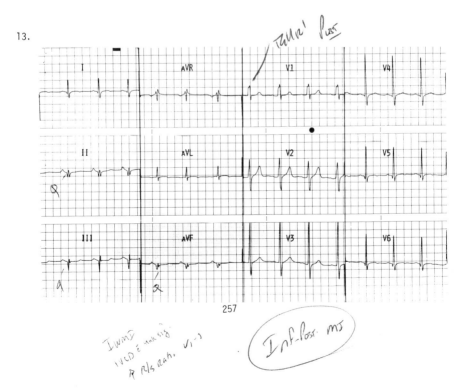

14.

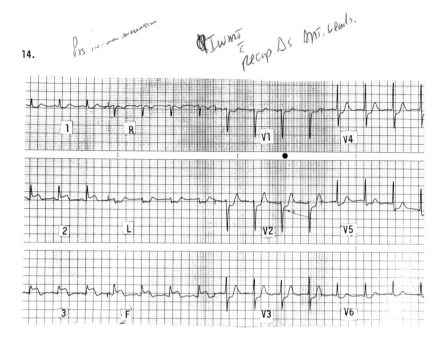

15.

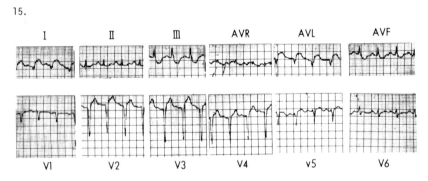

Taken on a 60 year old man with no current cardiovascular complaints.

16.

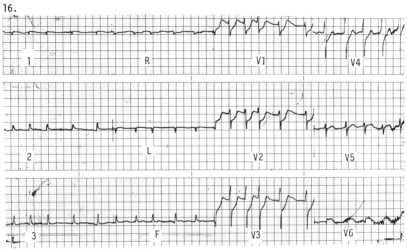

17.

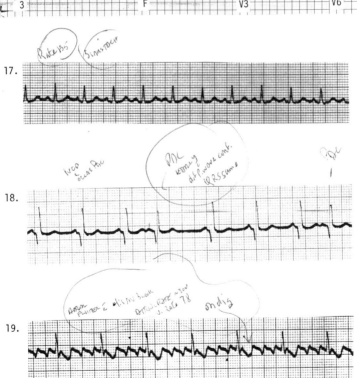

18.

19.

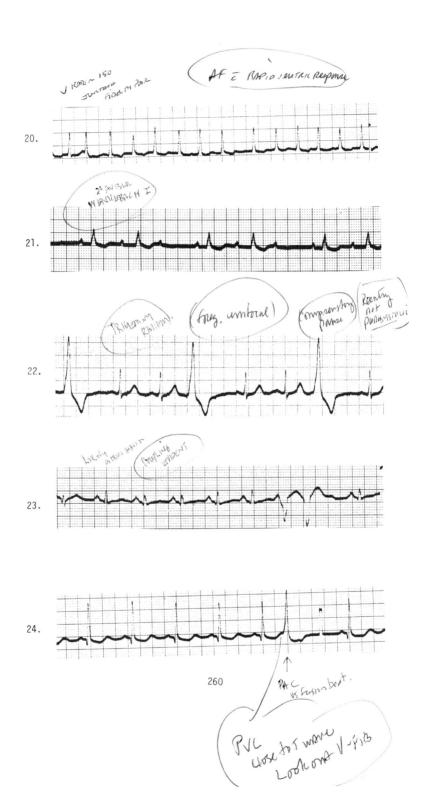

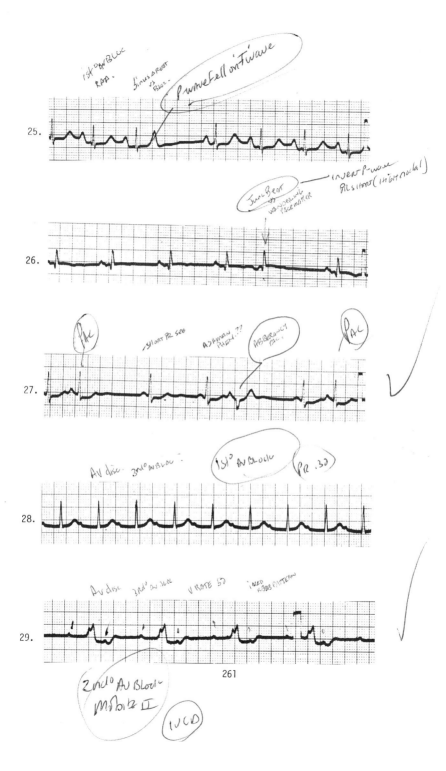

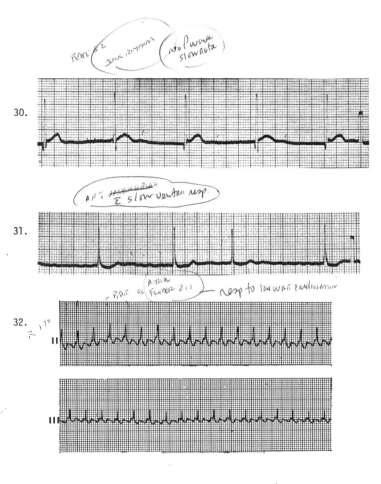

Lead V₁

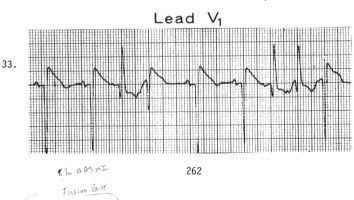

262

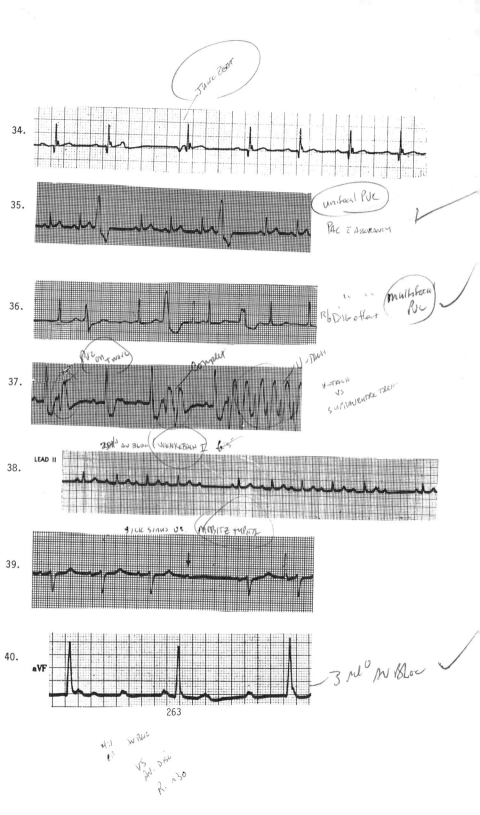

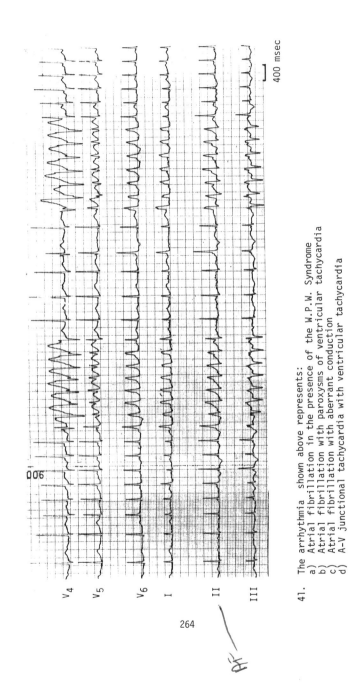

41. The arrhythmia shown above represents:
   a) Atrial fibrillation in the presence of the W.P.W. Syndrome
   b) Atrial fibrillation with paroxysms of ventricular tachycardia
   c) Atrial fibrillation with aberrant conduction
   d) A-V junctional tachycardia with ventricular tachycardia

42. The symmetrically inverted T-waves commonly seen in the presence of ischemic heart disease are a fairly reliable indicator of the ischemic process, since they are not commonly seen in other disease states. True or False.

43. Hyperacute T-waves are characterized by all but which one of the following:
    a. A more acute transition from ST segment to the peak of the T-wave.
    b. Increased peak T-wave voltage
    c. Terminal inversion of the T-wave
    d. Elevation of the ST takeoff

44. A useful generalization to aid in the differentiation of ST-T wave changes due to pericarditis from those due to an acute ischemic event, is that in pericarditis the ST segments usually return to the baseline before the evolution of inverted T-waves, while in acute infarction, the inverted T-waves often co-exist with elevated ST segments. True or False.

45. The downward coving of the ST segment, considered to be a hallmark of digitalis effect is, in fact, quite specific for digitalis effect. True or False.

46. Regarding the ST-T wave changes in Prinzmetal variant angina, which of the following is not true:
    a. The magnitude of the ST segment elevation is the most important differential feature for separating Prinzmetal variant angina from acute myocardial infarction.
    b. After an episode of Prinzmetal variant pain, symmetrical T-wave inversions may persist for many hours.
    c. The duration of ST segment elevation is a useful factor in differentiating Prinzmetal variant angina from acute myocardial infarction.
    d. The ST segment elevations during an episode of Prinzmetal variant angina are often accompanied by reciprocal ST segment depressions in the leads opposite to those demonstrating elevations.

47. Diagnosis of left ventricular hypertrophy on the ECG is best made from which of the following:
    a. Standard limb leads
    b. Unipolar augmented limb leads
    c. Precordial unipolar leads

48. Which of the following is not an ECG sign of LVH?
    a. Increased QRS voltage
    b. Shortened intrinsicoid deflection
    c. ST-T wave changes over the left ventricle
    d. Left axis deviation

49. Which of the following are criteria for the diagnosis of right ventricular hypertrophy?
    a. R/S ratio in V_1 <1.
    b. Deep S-wave in V_6
    c. Q-R pattern in V_1

50. Angina pectoris may occur during rapid tachycardia in a patient with normal coronary arteries. True or False.

51. Choose the three situations in which carotid sinus massage may be dangerous:
    a. Ventricular tachycardia
    b. The elderly patient
    c. Digitalis intoxication
    d. A-V nodal tachycardia
    e. Acute myocardial infarction

52. Which findings during a regular tachycardia are diagnostic for dissociated activity between atrium and ventricle:
    a. Changing loudness of first heart sound
    b. Cannon waves in the jugular venous pulse
    c. Inequality of the arterial pulse
    d. All of the above

53. Which of the following are false about the usual premature ventricular beat:
    a. QRS duration is greater than 80 msec but less than 110 msec.
    b. The coupling interval of the PVC is greater than the normal RR intervals.
    c. The PVC usually propagates retrograde to the atrium.
    d. The PVC usually resets the sinus node.

54. With parasystole, fusion beats are never seen. True or False.

55. Accelerated ventricular rhythm usually occurs with anterior infarction and responds to lidocaine in most patients. True or False.

56. In patients with atrial fibrillation, long RR intervals due to AV block enhance the likelihood of ventricular escape beats which are usually manifest as a widened QRS closely coupled to the first conducted beat after the pause. True or False.

57. Ventricular tachycardia is a common event in coronary heart disease, but rarely if ever complicates aortic or mitral valve disease in the absence of digitalis excess. True or False.

58. Match the lesions on the left with the statement(s) on the right

    I. Right Coronary Occlusions
    II. Left Anterior Descending Coronary Occlusion
    III. Circumflex Coronary Occlusions

    A. Transient Heart Block
    B. Trifascicular Block
    C. Inferior Infarction
    D. Anteroseptal Infarction
    E. Lateral Infarction

59. The endocardium in the most vascular area of the heart. True or False.

60. The earliest electrocardiographic sign of myocardial infarction is:
    a. J point and ST depression with peaked T waves
    b. ST elevation
    c. T wave inversion
    d. Q waves
    e. Loss of R wave amplitude

61. Subendocardial infarction may be diagnosed electrocardiographically when:
    a. ST segment elevation persists for many months
    b. ST segment depression persists for many weeks
    c. T wave inversion persists for many hours
    d. Q waves persist for many years
    e. None of the above.

62. Aberrantly conducted premature atrial beats are more likely to have the QRS configuration seen in:
    a. Right bundle branch block
    b. Left bundle branch block

63. The term "reciprocating" rhythm refers to which one(s) of the following:
    a. Sinus tachycardia
    b. Atrial tachycardia
    c. Atrial flutter
    d. Atrial fibrillation
    e. A-V junctional tachycardia

64. The pause following a premature atrial contraction is not usually a "full compensatory pause" because:
    a. The sinus node is depolarized by the premature beat and the sinus rhythm starts a new cycle beginning with that sinus node depolarization
    b. The sinus node is not depolarized by the premature beat so that it fires at its regularly scheduled time, but is not conducted into the ventricles
    c. The sinus node is not depolarized by the premature beat so that it fires at its regularly scheduled time and is conducted into the ventricles

65. The energy level required for ventricular defibrillation is related to the body weight of the patient. True or False.

66. Which of the following electrolyte disorders is most likely to be associated with complete A-V block?
    a. Hypercalcemia
    b. Hyperkalemia
    c. Hypokalemia
    d. Hyponatremia
    e. Hypocalcemia

67. Which of the following medications is contraindicated in a patient with untreated complete heart block?
    a. Atropine
    b. Prednisone
    c. Quinidine
    d. Isoproterenol
    e. Hydrochlorothiazide

68. Which of the following modes of therapy is the best treatment for sinus bradycardia associated with right bundle branch block, left axis deviation and first degree AV block in a patient with an acute anteroseptal myocardial infarction?
    a. Intravenous isoproterenol
    b. Intravenous steroids
    c. Intravenous atropine
    d. Transvenous ventricular pacemaker catheter
    e. Transvenous atrial pacemaker catheter

69. Which of the following is a major disadvantage of the fixed rate ventricular pacemaker as compared to the demand ventricular pacemaker:
    a. A shorter battery life
    b. A greater incidence of ventricular perforation
    c. An increased incidence of ventricular fibrillation
    d. An increased incidence of bacterial endocarditis
    e. An increased incidence of non-pacing

70. Prolongation of the HV interval represents:
    a. Intranodal conduction
    b. Intraatrial conduction
    c. His Purkinje conduction

SELF-ASSESSMENT - ADVANCES IN ELECTROCARDIOGRAPHY

1. In young adults, the most important prognostic indicator in premature ventricular activity is:
   a. The age of the patient
   b. Presence or absence of co-existent heart disease
   c. The coupling interval of the premature beats
   d. The QRS duration of the premature beats
   e. The frequency of the premature beats

2. Sino-atrial block in adolescents and young adults is:
   a. Not always associated with organic sinus node disease
   b. Always associated with sinus node disease
   c. Usually associated with disease of both the sinus node and the A-V node
   d. Usually a serious conduction disturbance
   e. Associated with propensity for paroxysmal atrial fibrillation

3. In adolescents and young adults, paroxysmal atrial fibrillation:
   a. Is usually best managed by rest and sedation as a first approach
   b. Usually requires cardioversion because of a rapid ventricular response compromising cardiac output
   c. Is associated with organic heart disease in the majority of cases
   d. Is the most uncommon of the supraventricular tachyarrhythmias in young individuals with normal hearts
   e. Often occurs in patients with the Wolff-Parkinson-White syndrome or other bypass tracts

4. The Wenckebach phenomenon in the A-V node in young adults does not always indicate organic heart disease, may occur transiently in the presence of acute febrile illnesses, and in the absence of organic heart disease may disappear when the patient sits up. True or False.

5. Procainamide has no effect on the length of the refractory period of the accessory pathway in patients with the Wolff-Parkinson-White syndrome. True or False.

6. Which accessory connection is most commonly found in patients with pre-excitation:
   a. Kent bundle
   b. Mahaim fiber
   c. James fiber

7. Digitalis shortens the refractory period of the accessory pathway in patients with the Wolff-Parkinson-White syndrome and is a dangerous drug in patients with this syndrome suffering from atrial fibrillation. True or False.

8. The effect of a drug on antegrade and retrograde conduction over the accessory pathway in patients with the Wolff-Parkinson-White syndrome is the same. True or False.

9. To diagnose the W-P-W Syndrome, one should require the constant presence of:
    a. P-delta interval of 0.12 seconds or less
    b. A delta wave
    c. A QRS width of 0.12 seconds or more
    d. All of the above
    e. None of the above

10. In the Wolff-Parkinson-White syndrome, the duration of the QRS complex during the supraventricular tachycardia is usually:
    a. Normal without a delta wave
    b. Normal with a delta wave
    c. Broad without a delta wave
    d. Broad with a delta wave

11. In the supraventricular tachycardia of the Wolff-Parkinson-White syndrome any beneficial effect of digitalis therapy is through its action on:
    a. The sinus node
    b. The A-V junction
    c. The anomalous pathway
    d. The Purkinje fibers

12. In patients with supraventricular tachyarrhythmias either the arrhythmia can be prevented with drugs or the ventricular rate can be controlled with drugs most of the time so that surgical therapy is only rarely considered. True or False.

13. Atrial pacing can be used to prevent bradycardia, but is of little or no value in preventing or terminating supraventricular tachycardias. True or False.

14. Experimental evidence and limited clinical study suggests that surgical sympathectomy of the heart may exert a useful antiarrhythmic influence in carefully selected patients. True or False.

15. Successful interruption of aberrant pathways in the W-P-W syndrome can be accomplished with sufficient probability to warrant surgical consideration in patients with life-threatening arrhythmias. True or False.

16. Surgical creation of AV block is a feasible approach in selected patients with recurrent supraventricular arrhythmias in whom drug therapy fails to produce adequate control of the ventricular rate. True or False.

17. Tachycardia dependent A-V block:
    a. Results in a transient total interruption of A-V conduction
    b. Is a frequent mechanism for the development of AV block in patients with myocardial infarction
    c. May occur on acceleration of the sinus rate in patients with acute myocardial infarction given atropine.
    d. a and c
    e. All of the above

18. Mobitz type II paroxysmal A-V block is commonly seen with:
    a. Acute anterior wall myocardial infarction
    b. Acute inferior wall myocardial infarction
    c. Digitalis toxicity
    d. None of the above
    e. All of the above

19. Physiological tachycardia-dependent aberration of the QRS is commonly:
    a. A right bundle branch block pattern
    b. A left bundle branch block pattern
    c. A left anterior hemiblock pattern
    d. A left posterior hemiblock pattern
    e. None of the above

20. The tachycardia-bradycardia syndrome refers to:
    a. A concomitant tachycardia-dependent and bradycardia-dependent bundle branch block
    b. Alternating periods of atrial tachyarrhythmia and sinus bradycardia or sinoatrial block
    c. The sick sinus syndrome
    d. b and c
    e. None of the above

21. Time-dependent refractoriness can be seen in:
    a. Normal sinus node cells
    b. Normal A-V nodal cells
    c. Depressed His-Purkinje cells
    d. Depressed ventricular cells
    e. All of the above

22. The following treadmill stress test was performed in a 48 year old male. He was taking digoxin .25 mgm. daily. What is your interpretation:

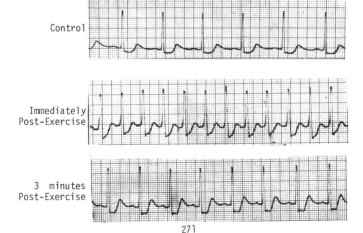

Control

Immediately Post-Exercise

3 minutes Post-Exercise

23. What is your interpretation of the following treadmill stress test?

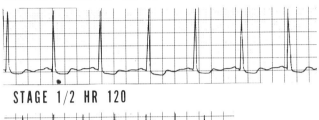

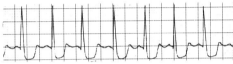

24. What is your interpretation of the following treadmill stress test?

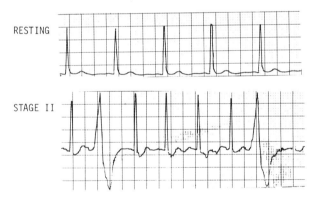

25. In ectopic atrial tachycardia:
    a. The mechanism is reentry
    b. The mechanism is a reciprocating rhythm
    c. Carotid massage often abolishes the arrhythmia
    d. Carotid massage often slows the ventricular response
    e. Digitalis intoxication is a common etiology

26. Match the column on the right with that on the left:
    1. Kent bundle
    2. Mahaim fiber
    3. James fiber

    a. LGL syndrome
    b. WPW syndrome
    c. Delta wave
    d. Short P-R interval
    e. Supraventricular tachycardias
    f. Connects atrium to ventricle
    g. Connects AV node to ventricle
    h. Connects atrium to His bundle
    i. Normal P-R interval

27. Surgical and pacemaker therapy of supraventricular tachyarrhythmias include:
    a. Atrial stimulation to terminate reentrant tachycardias
    b. Rapid atrial pacing to enhance A-V block through concealment
    c. Ablation of localized atrial disease
    d. Division of accessory pathways
    e. All of the above

28. The overall sensitivity in detecting coronary artery disease by treadmill stress testing is approximately
    a. 95%   b. 85%   c. 75%   d. 65%

29. The per cent of false positive responders to treadmill stress tresting is approximately:
    a. 5%   b. 10%   c. 15%   d. 20%

30. Hyperventilation induced "ischemic" ST depression is commonly observed in patients with angiographically proven coronary artery disease. True or False.

31. The Master's test provides the same incidence of positive ECG responses as a maximal treadmill stress test. True or False.

32. ST depression greater than 1 mm., regardless of type, is generally considered positive for ischemic heart disease. True or False.

33. To demonstrate a significant training effect, at least 60% of submaximal heart rate has to be achieved. True or False.

34. Physiologic adaptations to physical training include an increase in work capacity and a decrease in myocardial oxygen demand both at rest and at a given workload. True or False.

35. Which of the following impose limitations on the interpretation of exercise stress tests:
    a. The presence of rheumatic heart disease
    b. The presence of hypertension
    c. Nitroglycerin taken 12 hours before the test
    d. Propranolol taken 2 days before the test
    e. Digoxin taken 3 days before the test
    f. Hydrodiuril taken 1 day before the test

SELF-ASSESSMENT - CORONARY ARTERY DISEASE

HISTORY

48 year old male

CHIEF COMPLAINT: Chest distress of 2 months duration

PRESENT ILLNESS: His substernal chest pressure radiates into the jaw and arms. It occurs with heavy labor, sexual intercourse and emotional upset, and is relieved by rest in 15 minutes. Hypertension has been noted in the past, but not treated. He has smoked a package of cigarettes daily for years.

FAMILY HISTORY: His father had hypertension and died of a myocardial infarction at age 56. Several family members have diabetes.

Question: Given only this history, what is your diagnosis?

Answer:

The history is typical of atherosclerotic heart disease with angina pectoris.

PHYSICAL SIGNS

a. GENERAL APPEARANCE - Slightly obese 48 year old white male
b. VENOUS PULSE - The CVP is estimated to be 4 cm. H_2O

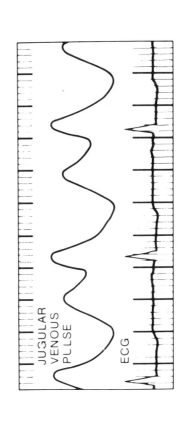

Question: What is your interpretation of the venous pulse?

Answer:

The venous pulse is normal.

c. ARTERIAL PULSE (BP = 150/100)

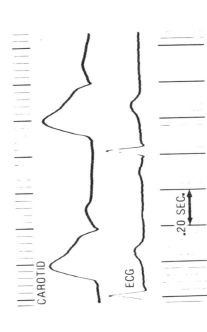

Question:
What is your interpretation of the arterial pulse?

Answer:

The arterial pulse is normal.

d. PRECORDIAL MOVEMENT and
e. AUSCULTATION

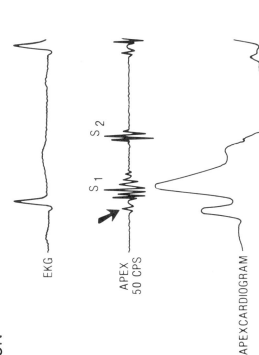

Question: What is the acoustic event shown by the arrow?

Answer: A pathologic fourth sound. Because of its low frequency it is also palpable as the simultaneous "a" wave on the apexcardiogram.

ELECTROCARDIOGRAM

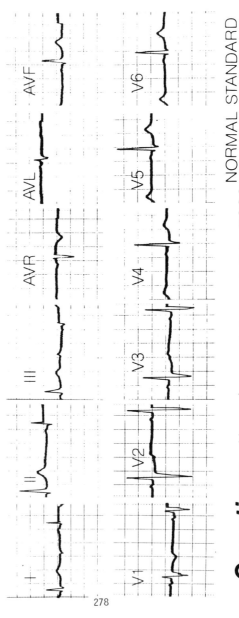

Question: How do you interpret this ECG? Does it change your diagnosis?

Answer: The ECG is normal. It should in no way change your initial diagnostic impression. Patients with angina pectoris commonly have normal resting ECG's.

CHEST X RAYS

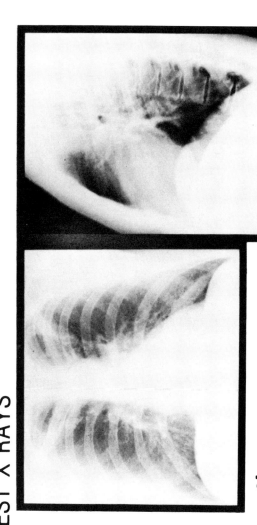

Questions:

1. How do you interpret the chest X rays?
2. Based on the history, physical examination, ECG and chest X rays, what is your diagnosis and plan to further evaluate this patient?

Answers:

1. The chest X rays are normal, a common observation in patients with angina pectoris.

2. Based on the history alone, the best diagnosis is angina pectoris due to atherosclerotic heart disease. Other less common causes of angina, e.g., left ventricular outflow obstruction, are virtually excluded by the physical examination, ECG and chest X rays.

   Evaluation for diabetes and hyperlipidemia will further characterize the patient's coronary risk and will be helpful in his longterm management.

LABORATORY

Blood Tests

Fasting Sugar 140 (Normal 60-110)
Cholesterol   325 (Normal <250)
Triglycerides 258 (Normal <150)

Question: What non-invasive procedure would help to further confirm the diagnosis?

Answer: A graded treadmill exercise stress test.

LABORATORY (continued) TREADMILL EXERCISE STRESS TEST

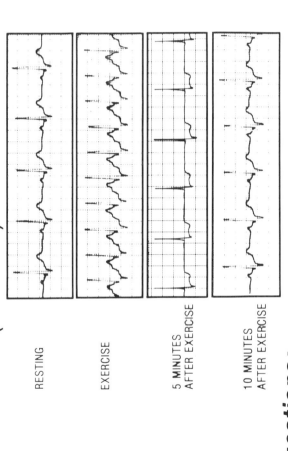

RESTING

EXERCISE

5 MINUTES AFTER EXERCISE

10 MINUTES AFTER EXERCISE

Questions:

1. What is your interpretation of the treadmill stress test?
2. How would you treat this patient?

Answers:

1. The treadmill test is positive with greater than 1 mm. of "ischemic" (horizontal or downsloping) ST segment depression. If it were negative, the diagnosis of angina would still be tenable, as the overall sensitivity of this study is 75%. In addition, up to 10% of male patients may have false positive stress tests.

2. The treatment of angina pectoris is directed at preventing progression of disease and reducing the frequency of attacks.

In an effort to prevent progression of disease, the patient was instructed in methods of eliminating risk factors, including hypertension, hyperlipidemia, diabetes and smoking. Each may increase the risk for coronary artery disease 2 to 3 times.

A diet was provided with restriction of calories, sugar, saturated fats (diary products and animal fats) and salt. If these are unsuccessful, drug therapy may be indicated for hypertension, hyperlipidemia and diabetes.

Proceed

The frequency of attacks may often be reduced by nitrites and/or beta-adrenergic blocking agents. The mechanism by which these agents act is shown below, with the most important of these starred:

Determinants of Oxygen Consumption

	Nitrite	Beta Blocker
Contractility	Reflex increase	★ Direct decrease
Heart Rate	Reflex increase	★ Direct decrease
Preload (Ventricular diameter)	★ Decrease by venous pooling	Increase by decreased rate
Afterload (Systolic pressure)	Decrease by peripheral arterial dilatation	Direct decrease

It is not clear if the direct dilating effect of nitrites on coronary arteries results in greater oxygen delivery to the myocardium.

Proceed

The patient was started on sublingual isosorbide dinitrite 5 mgm. q.2-3h. and propranolol titrated up to a dose of 40 mgm. q.i.d. He also took nitroglycerin 1/150 gr. prn. for angina. There was some initial response, including classic relief of angina by nitroglycerin in less than 5 minutes. However, his symptoms worsened and seriously interfered with the quality of his life even though his medication was pushed to maximum tolerated doses and his risk factors were controlled.

Questions:

1. In addition to intractable angina, what other serious clinical events may occur in the course of coronary artery disease?

2. What other therapy should be considered at this time?

Answers:

1. Myocardial infarction, congestive failure and arrhythmia which may result in sudden death.

2. Coronary artery bypass surgery. Before this can be considered, the exact anatomy of the coronary arteries must be known. The patient's study follows:

LABORATORY (continued)

LEFT CORONARY ARTERY ANGIOGRAM - Right Anterior Oblique

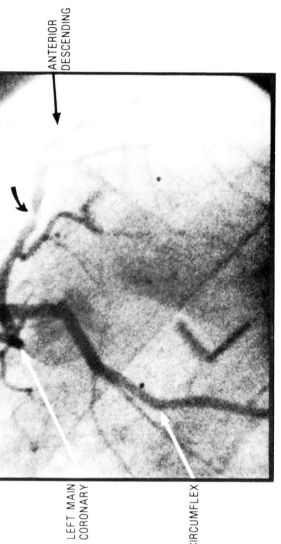

The right coronary and left ventricular angiograms were normal as were the intracardiac pressures and cardiac output.

Question: What is your interpretation of this study and your plan for further therapy?

Answer:

Injection of dye into the left main coronary artery shows 90% obstruction of the left anterior descending branch distal to the first septal perforator (arrow).

The major clinical indication for surgery is refractory angina which is significantly improved in up to 90% of cases by bypass surgery with a mortality which may be < 5%. However, up to 15% of grafts occlude in the first 12 months after surgery.

Because of this patient's youth and excellent ventricular function, which reduce surgical mortality, and because of his high grade focal anterior descending obstruction with good distal runoff, the patient underwent aorto-coronary saphenous vein bypass surgery with complete relief of his symptoms.

Proceed for Summary

SUMMARY

Atherosclerotic heart disease is a disease of obscure etiology in which many risk factors have been identified. These include a positive family history, hypertension, hyperlipidemia, diabetes and cigarette smoking.

The disease afflicts five million individuals in the United States and is the leading cause of death. Angina pectoris is the most common presentation, with 150,000 to 200,000 new cases recorded each year.

The angiographic estimate of the number of diseased vessels has important prognostic significance, as shown in the following figure which expresses annual mortality with medical management. The typical pathology follows.

The basic pathology is the lipid rich atherosclerotic plaque. Shown below is a section through the left anterior descending coronary artery of a man with angina pectoris who died suddenly. An atherosclerotic plaque fills the vessel. The small lumen (arrow) is obstructed by thrombus.

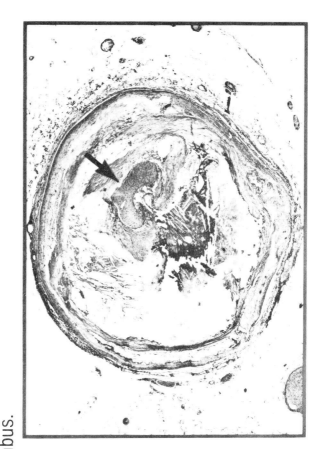

The gross pathology of myocardial infarction follows.

The infarction includes the anterior free wall and part of the septum (shown between arrows). These lesions are in the distribution of the left anterior descending coronary artery.

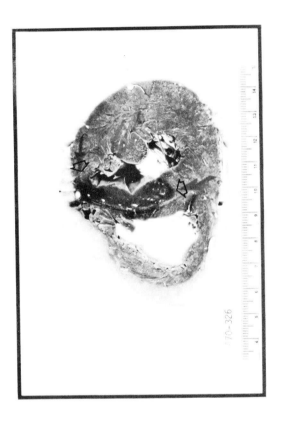

Proceed for Case Review

To Review This Case of Atherosclerotic Heart Disease with Angina Pectoris:

The HISTORY makes the diagnosis of angina pectoris, and in this patient the symptoms were classic. Historical risk factors include a positive family history and heavy smoking.

PHYSICAL SIGNS:

a. The GENERAL APPEARANCE shows moderate obesity.
b. The JUGULAR VENOUS PULSE is normal in mean pressure and wave form.
c. The CAROTID ARTERIAL PULSE is normal and the blood pressure is modestly elevated.
d. PRECORDIAL MOVEMENT reveals a palpable fourth sound followed by a normal left ventricular apical impulse.
e. AUSCULTATION confirms the fourth sound. Note also normal splitting of the second sound at the upper left sternal edge.

The resting ELECTROCARDIOGRAM and CHEST X RAYS are normal.

LABORATORY WORK reveals additional risk factors including diabetes and hyperlipidemia. The treadmill exercise stress test is definitely positive with >1 mm. of "ischemic" ST depression. Coronary angiography reveals a high grade proximal left anterior descending obstruction.

Medical TREATMENT consisted of risk factor elimination and the reduction of oxygen consumption with vasodilators and beta-adrenergic blocking agents. Because of the patient's poor response, coronary arteriography was performed to precisely define anatomical lesions prior to surgery. Such study also provides important prognostic information.

SELF-ASSESSMENT - CORONARY ARTERY DISEASE

ARRHYTHMIAS COMPLICATING AN ACUTE MYOCARDIAL INFARCTION

Louis Lemberg, M.D.

The arrhythmias that may occur as complications of an acute myocardial infarction are presented in a self-assessment format.

A running account of a patient with an acute myocardial infarction is related. Periodically, appropriate clinical information is given in order to help the reader make proper diagnosis and appropriate management decisions in specific clinical settings.

All of the major arrhythmias, their electrocardiograms, diagnosis, and management will have been covered upon completion of this self-teaching program.

Use an overlay to cover the answers in the column on the right. After each response, slide the overlay down to expose the correct answer.

HISTORY

Fifty-five year old white male.

CC: Acute severe substernal chest pressure radiating to the left jaw, shoulders and down the left arm to the little finger.

PI: Essential hypertension - 8 years
Diabetes mellitus managed with
  dietary restriction - 5 years
No previous heart disease

Parents died of atherosclerotic heart disease in their late fifties

The patient was admitted to the Coronary Care Unit two hours after the onset of symptoms. The pain was controlled with I.V. morphine sulfate.

What is the most significant arrhythmia that occurs during an acute myocardial infarction (MI)?

The ventricular premature beat (VPB)
 - Because of its frequency, 80% of acute MI's
 - And its potential for initiating ventricular fibrillation.

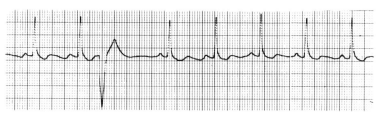

Interpret the trace from the monitoring lead

A VPB falling in the vulnerable period of the preceding beat. The R on T phenomenon.

What VPB patterns are indications for prompt antiarrhythmic therapy in acute MI?

- VPB's occurring 5/min.
- Multifocal VPB's
- VPB's falling during the vulnerable period R on T phenomenon
- Salvas of two or more VPB's

What antiarrhythmic therapy is employed for VPB's during an acute MI?

- Lidocaine 50-75 mg. I.V. as a bolus and may be repeated in three minutes if needed.
- As an alternative, a continuous infusion can be given at a rate of 2 mg/min.
- Pronestyl or quinidine can be used supplementally
- DC countershock is used to convert ventricular tachycardia and to terminate ventricular fibrillation.

The 12 lead ECG revealed characteristic changes of an acute inferior MI.

Bradyarrhythmias complicate the early stages of an acute inferior MI in 30% of patients. They appear more frequently in inferior or diaphragmatic infarctions than in anterior infarctions (3 to 1).

Twelve hours after admission the following rhythm strip was recorded.

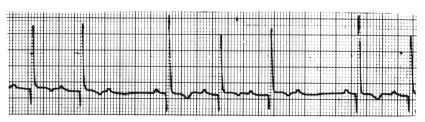

Interpret the trace.

2° AV block
Mobitz I (Wenckebach)
Progressive prolongation of PR intervals ending with a blocked sinus P wave.

The following traces illustrate the types
of bradyarrhythmias that may complicate
acute inferior MI.

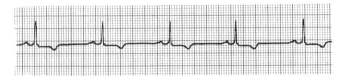

Interpret the trace.　　　　　　　Sinus bradycardia
　　　　　　　　　　　　　　　　Cardiac rate is below 60/min.
　　　　　　　　　　　　　　　　PR interval is normal.

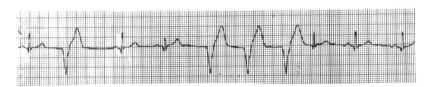

Interpret the trace.　　　　　　　Accelerated idioventricular
　　　　　　　　　　　　　　　　rhythm
　　　　　　　　　　　　　　　　- or nonparoxysmal ventri-
　　　　　　　　　　　　　　　　　cular tachycardia
　　　　　　　　　　　　　　　　- or slow ventricular tachy-
　　　　　　　　　　　　　　　　　cardia.
　　　　　　　　　　　　　　　　This is a ventricular escape
　　　　　　　　　　　　　　　　rhythm associated with
　　　　　　　　　　　　　　　　sinus slowing. Ventricu-
　　　　　　　　　　　　　　　　lar rates are between
　　　　　　　　　　　　　　　　60-100/min.

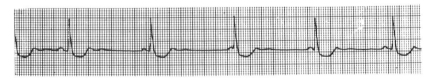

Interpret the trace.　　　　　　　AV dissociation
　　　　　　　　　　　　　　　　Atria and ventricles are dis-
　　　　　　　　　　　　　　　　sociated with the junctional
　　　　　　　　　　　　　　　　rate slightly greater than
　　　　　　　　　　　　　　　　the atrial rate.
　　　　　　　　　　　　　　　　In this arrhythmia, the atrium
　　　　　　　　　　　　　　　　may intermittently "capture"
　　　　　　　　　　　　　　　　the ventricle.

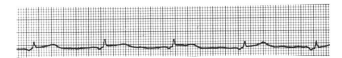

Interpret the trace. Junctional rhythm
A junctional pacemaker controls
the atria and the ventricles.
Retrograde P waves may be
seen before (as in this case),
after, or during the inscrip-
tion of the QRS complex.

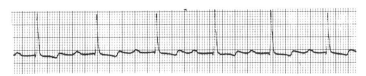

Interpret the trace. 1° AV block
Delay in PR interval.

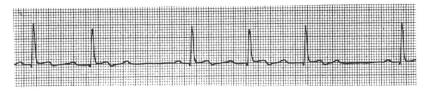

Interpret the trace. 2° Mobitz I (Wenckebach) block
Progressive prolongation of
PR intervals, ending with
a blocked sinus P wave.

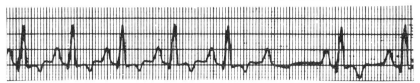

Interpret the trace. 2° Mobitz II block
Blocked sinus P wave preceded
by sinus P waves with fixed
PR intervals. This type of 2°
block is more common in anterior infarction and has a worse
prognosis than Mobitz I block.

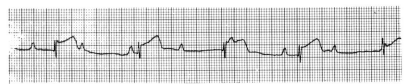

Interpret the trace.

3⁰ complete AV block
- The atrial rate is 96.
- The ventricular rate is 56 and independent of the atria.
- The block is in the AV node.
- The subsidiary pacemaker is in the junctional tissue, has narrow QRS complexes, and rates between 40-60/min.

The following is a strip taken from a different patient admitted to the CCU with severe chest pain, lightheadedness and pulmonary edema on examination.

LEAD V₄

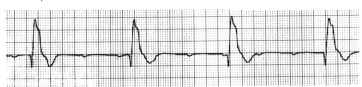

Interpret the trace.

3⁰ AV block
The atrial rate is 98.
The QRS complexes are wide, the ventricular rate is 36 and independent of the atrial rhythm.
An acute anteroseptal infarction is also present, and hence, the block is in the peripheral ramifications of the AV conduction system and referred to as bilateral bundle branch block or tri-fascicular block.
e.g.,
- block of the RB
- block of the anterior division of the LB
- block of the posterior division of the LB

The subsidiary pacemaker is in the Purkinje system of the ventricle.

The following is the sequence of events that
usually occurs in the evolution of trifascicular AV block complicating an acute anterior MI.

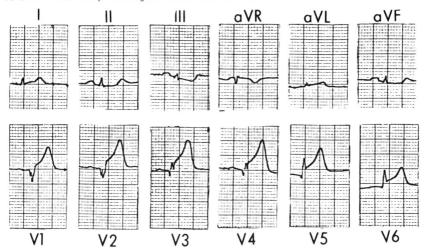

Interpret the trace.   Anteroseptal infarction

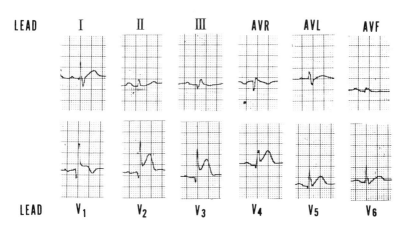

Interpret the trace.   Right bundle branch block
Anteroseptal infarction.

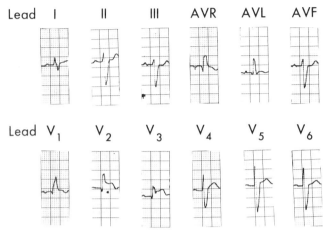

Interpret the trace. Right bundle branch block
Left anterior hemiblock
Anteroseptal infarction.

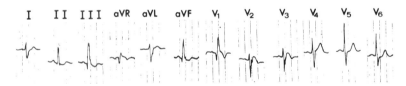

Interpret the trace. Right bundle branch block
Left posterior hemiblock
Anteroseptal infarction

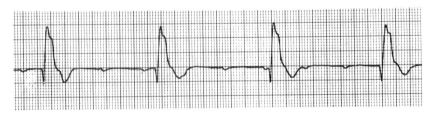

Interpret the trace. Complete AV block
Anteroseptal infarction

The first patient with an acute inferior MI was asymptomatic while in $2°$ AV block Mobitz I. The blood pressure was 115/85 and the lungs were clear to auscultation.

What therapy is indicated for the Mobitz type I AV block in this clinical setting?

None. Peripheral perfusion is adequate and there are no VPB's.

Therapeutic intervention is indicated when bradycardias produce a fall in blood pressure and a decrease in peripheral perfusion because of a reduction in minute volume, and also if VPB's appear because of the bradycardia.

What is the principle of therapy for bradyarrhythmias in the setting of an acute MI?

Cardioacceleration

What modalities of treatment are used?

Pharmacological
  Atropine sulfate
  Isoproterenol
Electrical
  Artificial pacemaker

What modalities of pacing are used?

Modalities of pacing:
  Atrial - if AV transmission is intact.
  Ventricular - QRS inhibited-demand
  Atrial and Ventricular bifocal sequential QRS inhibited - bifocal demand - if the atrial contribution to output is needed.

The treatment and prognosis of acute AV block complicating acute MI is determined by the location of the infarct which determines the anatomic level of the AV block.

What is the treatment of symptomatic AV block resulting from an acute inferior wall infarction?	Atropine sulfate 0.04 to 1 mg. I.V. As an alternative, isoproterenol 1 mg. in 500 ml. 5% D/W is titrated I.V. A temporary QRS inhibited ventricular pacemaker is inserted into the apex of the right ventricle if pharmacological therapy fails.
What is the prognosis?	The prognosis of AV block resulting from inferior MI is relatively good. The AV block is rarely permanent.
What is the treatment of AV block resulting from acute anterior MI?	Prophylactic insertion of a demand pacing catheter when bifascicular block occurs. 50% of patients with bifascicular block following acute anterior wall infarction progress to trifascicular 3° AV block.
What is the prognosis?	The prognosis for this form of complete AV block is poor because of the associated extensive myocardial injury.

On the third day in the CCU, the first patient with an acute inferior MI was dyspneic, the blood pressure was 110/80, moist rales were heard at both bases. The following ECG trace was recorded.

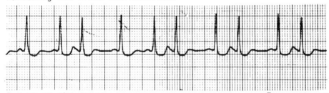

Interpret the trace.   Frequent premature atrial beats

The atrial arrhythmias that occur in the wake of an acute MI are attributed to left ventricular failure and/or atrial infarction. Multifocal premature atrial beats usually precede the appearance of atrial fibrillation. All forms of atrial arrhythmias can be seen, i.e., premature atrial beats, atrial tachycardia, atrial flutter, and atrial fibrillation.

What therapy is indicated?

Digitalis glycosides used primarily for their vagal effect in the event that atrial fibrillation occurs with a rapid ventricular response
<u>and</u>
Diuretic therapy for the associated failure

Digoxin 0.5 mg. was given orally. Lasix 40 mg. was given I.V. One hour later there was a 400 ml. urinary output. The following rhythm trace was recorded.

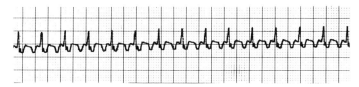

Interpret the trace.

Atrial flutter with ventricular response of 150/min.

What therapy is indicated?

Electrical DC cardioversion is a prompt and effective therapy for paroxysmal atrial tachycardia or paroxysmal atrial flutter.

The paroxysmal atrial flutter was converted to sinus rhythm with a rate of 100/min. using cardioversion with 5 Joules of energy. Low energy outputs are usually effective in the electrical conversion of atrial flutter.

Three hours later the following trace was recorded. The blood pressure was 90/75. The hands and feet were cold.

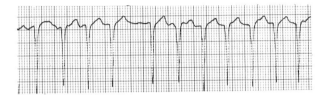

Interpret the trace.

Atrial fibrillation with an average ventricular response of 150/min.

What therapy is indicated?

Propranolol titrated I.V. 0.5 mg. q 2 minute up to an average of 4.5 mg. using electrocardiographic monitoring is usually effective in reducing the ventricular rate and frequently results in conversion of the atrial fibrillation to sinus rhythm. Atropine sulfate or isoproterenol should be available for I.V. use to counter excessive slowing of the heart rate.

DC cardioversion is successful in converting atrial fibrillation to sinus rhythm. However, atrial fibrillation frequently recurs after several minutes in this setting.

The key objective of treatment in this clinical setting is to slow the ventricular rate promptly. The altered hemodynamics that result from atrial fibrillation with a rapid ventricular reponse, produce a reduction in the cardiac output, an increase in O_2 consumption and a decrease in the blood pressure. The net effect is an unfavorable relationship between oxygen supply and demand which further jeopardizes the injured and ischemic zones. This promotes extension of the area of necrosis. Therefore, prompt conversion to sinus rhythm or reduction in ventricular rate will improve cardiac output and raise the blood pressure.

Aggressive management of arrhythmias that complicate an acute myocardial infarction limits the area of necrosis and reduces morbidity and mortality.

SELF-ASSESSMENT - CORONARY ARTERY DISEASE
HOW DO YOU TREAT THIS CASE?

Case I

A 56 year old obese male was admitted to the Coronary Care Unit with pressure-like precordial pain for one hour. This was accompanied by diaphoresis and a faint feeling; blood pressure was 90/60; cardiac rate of 65/min., regular. The admitting 12-lead electrocardiogram is shown.

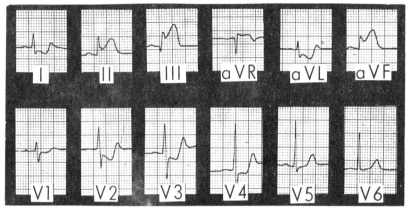

Following intravenous Morphine Sulfate 5 mg., the pain was relieved and the blood pressure rose to 110/70. There were no arrhythmias. The cardiac rate was 60/min. Three hours following admission, another 12-lead electrocardiogram was taken. Through secretarial error, two electrocardiogram requests were sent two hours apart. The second ECG is shown below. Eight hours after admission the patient developed a third heart sound at the apex and crepitant rales in the right base.

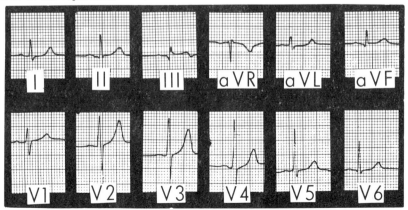

What happened to the ECG?   What is your treatment?

HOW DO YOU TREAT THIS CASE?

Case 2

A 49 year old white male in relatively good health was admitted to the coronary care unit with a three month history of angina. For the past week, his pains have become increasingly frequent, mostly occurring at rest, and usually during the same time of the day; all relieved by nitroglycerin.

In the CCU, there was no improvement in spite of doses of propranolol and isordil given to the point of tolerance. Each episode showed acute changes lasting 10-15 minutes as shown in the figures below. Serum enzymes and electrolytes were within normal limits.

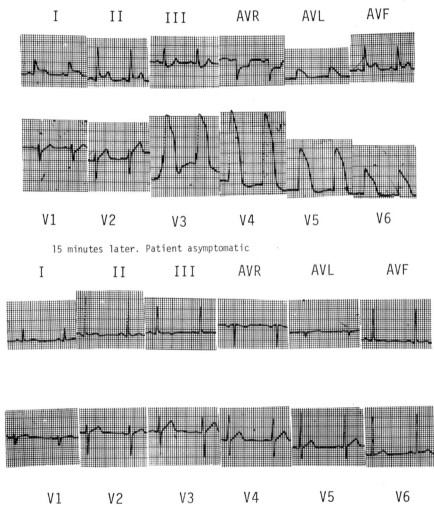

What is your diagnosis and management?

HOW DO YOU TREAT THIS CASE?

Case 3

A 60 year old female enters the emergency room with severe anterior chest pain. An ECG was taken and is shown below. The blood pressure is falling from 120/88 to 80/60. Cardioversion with 100 w/s resulted in transient NSR lasting 30 seconds.

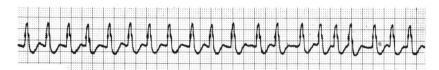

What is your treatment?

Case 4

A 45 year old female is seen in the emergency room complaining of rapid heart action, acute shortness of breath, and nausea. She has known rheumatic mitral regurgitation with a history of failure, but recently compensated on Digoxin and diuretics daily. Her rhythm strip is shown below.

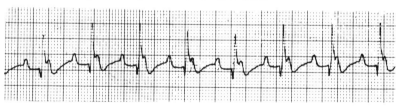

What blood work would you order, and what is your diagnosis and treatment?

Case 5

A 55 year old man is seen in the emergency room with intense substernal pain and an ECG consistent with acute anterior wall infarction. Morphine is given, resulting in relief of pain. He is entirely stable clinically. As the patient is being prepared for transfer to the CCU, you note the ECG rhythm strip from his monitor as shown below.

Is any treatment necessary?

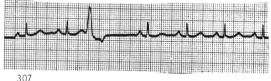

HOW DO YOU TREAT THIS CASE?

Case 6

A 74 year old male with acute inferior wall myocardial infarction is seen in the emergency room. The rhythm strips below were recorded. The patient is in mild left ventricular failure..

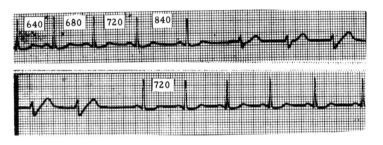

What is your suggestion for management of the arrhythmia?

Case 7

A 53 year old male presents to the emergency room with chest pain, nausea, diaphoresis and and ECG consistent with acute inferior wall infarction. His rhythm strip is shown below.

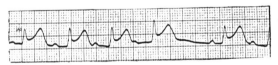

What is your diagnosis and treatment?

HOW DO YOU TREAT THIS CASE?

Case 8

A 55 year old male presents to the emergency room at 7:00 P.M. with severe chest pain radiating into his left arm for the last two hours. His initial ECG is normal and he is clinically stable. After administering medicine for pain, you admit him to the CCU.

At 7:00 A.M. you are called by the CCU nurse to check the patient, since his ECG that morning has changed as shown below, although his clinical state is essentially stable.

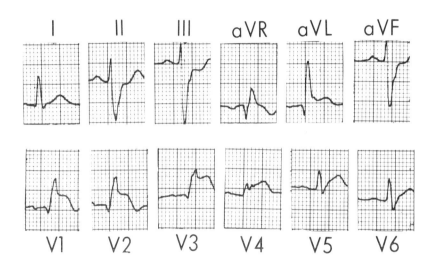

What is your diagnosis and treatment?

SELF-ASSESSMENT - CORONARY ARTERY DISEASE

1. A depressed ST-T segment of the ECG during an ischemic attack or with effort reflects an inadequate blood supply to the:
   a. right ventricle
   b. posterior myocardium
   c. papillary muscle
   d. subendocardium

2. Blood flow in obstructive coronary disease is dependent upon:
   a. aortic pressure
   b. resistance by arteriolar and precapillary sphincter muscles
   c. autoregulatory mechanisms
   d. the diastolic interval
   e. all of the above

3. Trifascicular and right bundle branch block are most commonly due to obstruction of the right coronary artery. True or False

4. The average annual mortality once the diagnosis of angina pectoris is made is ten per cent. True or False

5. The intermediate coronary syndrome is characterized by all of the following except:
   a. prolonged rest angina
   b. incomplete relief of pain with nitrites
   c. diaphoresis
   d. ST-T wave changes on the electrocardiogram
   e. normal serum enzymes

6. Left ventricular dysfunction associated with acute myocardial infarction may be associated with all of the following except:
   a. increased left ventricular end-diastolic pressure (LVEDP)
   b. increased ejection fraction
   c. decreased stroke volume
   d. wide A-V oxygen difference
   e. hypoxemia

7. Systemic vascular resistance in acute myocardial infarction may be:
   a. normal
   b. elevated
   c. either normal or elevated

8. The factors that determine myocardial oxygen consumption are:
   a. preload
   b. heart rate
   c. afterload
   d. inotropic state of the heart
   e. all of the above

9. Sodium nitroprusside, when used in the low cardiac output state of acute myocardial infarction with elevated left ventricular end-diastolic pressure will:
   a. elevate arterial pressure
   b. increase or maintain cardiac output
   c. increase myocardial oxygen consumption
   d. increase venous return
   e. increase systemic vascular resistance

10. Ventricular fibrillation in patients with severe coronary artery atherosclerosis is usually associated with anatomically demonstrable lesions in the atrioventricular node or bundle. True or False.

11. The degrees of coronary arterial luminal narrowing by atherosclerotic plaques are similar in patients with "pure" angina pectoris and in patients with acute myocardial infarction. True or False.

12. Complete heart block during acute myocardial infarction usually indicates necrosis of the atrioventricular node or bundle or both. True or False.

13. In patients dying suddenly from severe coronary atherosclerosis (sudden coronary death) necrotic lesions usually are present in the A-V node or bundle. True or False.

14. In patients with severe coronary atherosclerosis who suddenly arrest but are resuscitated, only about 50% of them will actually develop clinical evidence of acute myocardial infarction (necrosis). True or False.

15. Severe congestive failure commonly coexists with severe angina pectoris. True or False.

16. The occurrence of rupture of a papillary muscle or of perforation of the ventricular septum or left ventricular free wall during acute myocardial infarction usually is indicative of preexisting systemic hypertension. True or False.

17. The major effect of diuretics in heart failure is to:
    a. increase cardiac output
    b. decrease congestion
    c. slow heart rate
    d. increase renal blood flow

18. In acute pulmonary edema, which of the following are employed to decrease venous return and reduce pulmonary congestion:
    a. morphine
    b. diuretics
    c. sitting up
    d. rotating tourniquets
    e. intermittent positive pressure breathing
    f. all of the above

19. Left ventricular failure can be diagnosed if the central venous pressure is:
   a. over 5 mm. Hg.
   b. over 10 mm. Hg.
   c. over 15 mm. Hg.
   d. none of the above apply

20. A 48 year old man enters the CCU with symptoms and ECG findings of an acute myocardial infarction. On the second day, a loud third heart sound is heard. There are no rales.

   A. Would a central venous line be of help in assessing LV function?
      1. yes
      2. no

   B. Assume you decided to put in a central venous line and found the CVP to be 3. Your choice of therapy would be:
      1. volume expansion
      2. diuresis
      3. other

   C. Assume you decided to expand volume with 500 cc. dextran, and the patient went into pulmonary edema. What do you think of central venous pressure monitoring in this situation?
      1. it's just great
      2. expletive deleted

21. A 53 year old man entered the CCU with an acute anterior myocardial infarction. Six hours after admission, his blood pressure was 110/60. He had sinus tachycardia of 110 per minute. Third and fourth heart sounds were present. There were rales in the chest. He was tachypneic and arterial PO_2 was 65. The jugular venous pressure was below the level of the sternal angle. Urinary output was 20 ml/hour. A pulmonary artery catheter was placed. The pulmonary wedge mean pressure was 26 mm. Hg.

   A. Your choice of therapy would be:
      1. Lasix 40 mg. I.V.
      2. Aminophyllin 500 mg. I.V. slowly
      3. nasal O_2 at 6 L/min.
      4. Dextran 100 ml. aliquots until urinary output increases

   B. Assume that diuretics were given and he improved markedly. Twelve hours later he suddenly became very dyspneic. Blood pressure was unobtainable, skin cool, and he was agitated. Rales were loud over both lung fields. Pulmonary wedge pressure was 26 mm. Hg. ECG showed atrial fibrillation with ventricular rate of 160. Your choice of therapy would be:
      1. Lasix 40 mg. I.V.
      2. Digoxin 0.75 mg. I.V.
      3. D.C. synchronized cardioversion
      4. Quinidine gluconate 300 mg. I.M.
      5. carotid sinus pressure

21. Continued
    C. Normal sinus rhythm was restored and he improved, eventually was discharged to home, and all his medications were stopped. One year later, he felt rapid irregular heart rhythm, but was otherwise asymptomatic. He came to the Emergency Room and had atrial fibrillation with a rate of 140 per minute. Cardiac examination was unremarkable except for the arrhythmia. Your choice of therapy would be:
        1. Digoxin
        2. Lasix
        3. D.C. synchronized cardioversion
        4. Quinidine
        5. carotid sinus pressure
        6. Tensilon

22. Disease in a major coronary artery which occludes 50% of the cross sectional area of that vessel is likely to produce a reduction in blood flow at rest. True or False.

23. A myocardial infarction involving 10% of total myocardial mass is usually productive of severe congestive failure. True or False.

24. Digitalis is the drug of choice in congestive failure associated with acute myocardial infarction. True or False.

25. The balloon-flotation (Swan-Ganz) catheter:
    a. may be used to measure pulmonary wedge pressure
    b. requires fluoroscopy
    c. is used primarily to measure the central venous pressure
    d. should be utilized in patients with severe pump failure associated with acute myocardial infarction

26. In a patient with acute myocardial infarction with rales in the lung bases and a third heart sound at the apex, the mean pulmonary artery pressure is likely to be:
    a. between 5-10 mm. Hg.
    b. between 10-15 mm. Hg.
    c. greater than 15 mm. Hg.

27. The primary clinical indication for aortocoronary bypass surgery is:
    a. recent onset of angina pectoris
    b. angina refractory to medical therapy
    c. recent onset of congestive failure
    d. congestive failure refractory to medical therapy

28. The success or failure of aortocoronary bypass surgery is related to:
    a. the degree of pump failure pre-operatively
    b. flow in the graft at the time of surgery
    c. the sex of the patient
    d. the length of time the patient had angina prior to surgery

29. In which of the following is pacemaker therapy indicated in a patient with acute anterior infarction:
    a. preexisting left axis deviation
    b. complete right bundle branch block with abnormal left axis deviation which develops during the evolution of the infarction
    c. complete right bundle branch block with rapid atrial fibrillation
    d. complete left bundle branch block with a sinus rate of 30 not increased with atropine.

30. Which of the following pharmacologic agents is a "cardioselective" beta-adrenergic agonist:
    a. norepinephrine (Levophed)
    b. isoproterenol (Isuprel)
    c. dopamine (Inotropin)
    d. metaraminol (Aramine)
    e. none of the above

31. Nocturnal and spontaneous angina usually indicate triple vessel coronary artery disease. True or False.

32. Abnormal precordial lifts, particularly in the ectopic region, associated with obstructive coronary disease suggest anterior descending artery obstruction. True or False.

33. The right coronary artery transports blood to the right bundle branch. True or False.

34. An acute obstruction of the anterior descending artery just distal to the take-off of the first septal perforator may produce an abnormal left axis deviation. True or False.

35. The clinical setting of a ruptured free wall following a myocardial infarction is an elderly individual with previous history of hypertension and usually no antecedent coronary insufficiency who develops chest pain at 3-7 days after the original infarct. True or False.

36. For a male aged 50 to 60 who has a 6 month history of typical angina which is stable and occurs daily, but only with exertion, which of the following clinical descriptors correlate most strongly with 5 year survival rate: (Select 4)
    a. Blood pressure
    b. Heart size
    c. Presence or absence of PAC's
    d. Glucose intolerance
    e. LVH on resting ECG
    f. Stage achieved on treadmill
    g. Serum uric acid
    h. Body weight

37. The prognosis for men who have survived one myocardial infarction is significantly worse than for men who have a 6 month history of stable angina responsive to nitroglycerin. True or False.

38. Which of the following statements regarding the exercise stress test are true:
    a. The test should not be performed in patients with unstable angina of a severe degree.
    b. False negative tests are so frequent that the test is of little value.
    c. False positive tests are so frequent that angiography is required to make a diagnosis of coronary artery disease.
    d. The stage achieved has prognostic information which is of significant value.
    e. Improved treadmill performance is rare even after successful coronary bypass surgery.

39. Which of the following statements about coronary arteriography are true:
    a. Significant complications occur in less than 1% of studies done in well-equipped labs by experienced arteriographers.
    b. In over 95% of arteriograms there is little or no observer variability regarding the presence and severity of obstructive lesions in the major coronary arteries.
    c. The severity of disease in the coronary arteries by arteriography correlates well with prognosis.
    d. Significant abnormalities of ventricular function are rarely detected by ventriculography if heart size by X ray is normal.

40. The incidence of late arrhythmias (5-21 days) and other significant late complications is so great after acute myocardial infarction that hospitalization and monitoring for 14-21 days is indicated in nearly all such patients. True or False.

41. Left bundle branch block is rarely the consequence of acute anteroseptal infarction. True or False.

42. Complete infranodal (trifascicular) heart block is always preceded by bifascicular block. True or False.

43. In the patient admitted with acute myocardial infarction, the configuration of the QRS complex in lead V1 is of help in differentiating between pre-existent and acquired right bundle branch block. True or False.

44. What percentage of patients develop bundle branch block as a consequence of acute myocardial infarction:
    a. 2%   b. 5%   c. 10%   d. 20%

45. Prophylactic pacemaker insertion should be carried out in:
    a. All patients with acute anteroseptal infarction
    b. All patients with chronic right bundle branch block admitted with acute myocardial infarction
    c. All patients who develop right bundle branch block after acute anteroseptal infarction
    d. Patients who develop right bundle branch block and a frontal QRS axis of less than $-45°$ after acute anteroseptal infarction.

46. A 63 year old woman died suddenly at home 10 minutes after the onset of severe substernal chest pain associated with diaphoresis. The most likely cause of death is:
    a. Cardiogenic shock
    b. Atrial fibrillation
    c. Complete A-V block
    d. Ventricular fibrillation
    e. Pulmonary embolism

47. A 57 year old man was admitted to the CCU with acute myocardial infarction of four hours duration. On physical examination his blood pressure was 140/70, respiratory rate 22, heart rate 106/min., and his jugular veins were distended to 7 cm. He had bilateral rales halfway up the scapula. The left ventricular apex was minimally displaced and an S3 gallop was heard. After treatment with morphine sulfate 6 mg. and Lasix 40 mg., he had a diuresis of 500 ml., and a decrease in pulmonary rales. His blood pressure was 96/60 and he became slightly clammy. Treatment should now include:
    a. Dopamine drip
    b. Levophed
    c. 80 mgs. of Lasix
    d. Sodium bicarbonate, 88 meq. intravenously
    e. Volume expansion with 200 ml. of normal saline.

48. A 61 year old man is seen in the E.R. six hours after the beginning of severe chest pain. The electrocardiogram shows an extensive anterolateral myocardial infarction. Two hours after admission to the CCU he develops complete A-V block. A temporary pacemaker is inserted in the right ventricular apex. The most important factor determining mortality in this patient is:
    a. Pump failure
    b. Primary ventricular fibrillation
    c. Intractable atrial fibrillation
    d. Myocardial rupture
    e. Asystole secondary to complete heart block

49. A 50 year old man was admitted with an inferior wall myocardial infarction. Initial physical examination was unremarkable. On the third day he had severe pain and developed a sinus tachycardia at a rate of 120. On examination he had bilateral pulmonary rales, a palpable S3 and a thrill at the lower left sternal border, along with a III/VI harsh holosystolic murmur louder at the lower left sternal border and radiating toward the apex. After treatment with morphine, digitalis, Lasix and O_2, there was mild improvement, but the clinical and radiologic picture of pulmonary edema persisted. The logical diagnostic procedure to perform is:
    a. Emergency pulmonary angiography
    b. Pulmonary capillary pressure recording by a Swan-Ganz catheter with sampling for oxygen saturation in the right side chambers and pulmonary artery
    c. Coronary angiography to evaluate for coronary artery bypass surgery
    d. Temporary venous pacemaker insertion into the right ventricular apex
    e. Emergency open heart surgery for replacement of the mitral valve

50. After the diagnosis is established in the previous patient, the most acceptable mode of therapy is:
   a. Drug therapy for failure. No consideration for surgery after discharge from the hospital
   b. Immediate corrective open heart surgery
   c. Drug therapy for heart failure, use of afterload reducing agents in the CCU. Not a candidate for cardiac surgery after discharge from the hospital.
   d. Drug therapy for heart failure, treatment with afterload reducing agents. A surgical candidate six weeks after discharge from the hospital
   e. Intra-aortic balloon cardiac assist for 5 days with drug therapy for heart failure. Not a candidate for cardiac surgery after discharge from the hospital.

51. The success of coronary artery bypass surgery is dependent upon:
   a. The severity of clinical symptoms
   b. The size of the coronary artery to be bypassed
   c. The extent of run-off
   d. The quality of the remaining myocardium
   e. All of the above

52. Operative mortality rate in myocardial revascularization procedures is most closely correlated with which one of the following:
   a. A decrease in ejection fraction and a widened A-V O_2 difference
   b. Severity of angina pectoris preoperatively
   c. History of previous myocardial infarction
   d. Elevated left ventricular end-diastolic pressure
   e. None of the above

53. In which of the anatomic lesions described below should coronary artery surgery be considered in the presence of minimal symptoms:
   a. Proximal lesion of the left circumflex coronary artery
   b. Main left coronary artery lesion
   c. Proximal lesions of the anterior descending
   d. Proximal lesion in the posterior descending coronary artery

54. When nitroglycerin precipitates or worsens an attack of angina pectoris, which one of the following diagnoses should be considered:
   a. Single vessel coronary disease
   b. Congestive heart failure co-existing with coronary artery disease
   c. Idiopathic hypertrophic subaortic stenosis
   d. A recent myocardial infarction

55. Previous infarction of the myocardium may be apparent on left ventriculography even when absent by history or ECG criteria. True or False

56. Select the one item in the right column which best matches one item in the left column:
   a. Variant angina   1. Right coronary artery obstruction
   b. Good prognosis   2. Spontaneous angina and ST elevation
   c. Poor prognosis   3. Multiple vessel disease
   d. Transient heart block   4. Ventricular dyskinesis
   e. Palpable ectopic impulse 5. Normal coronary angiogram

57. The mortality in the CCU is correlated with the degree of pump failure. True or False.

58. Choose the three factors which best identify high risk of early death in the post infarction outpatient population:
    a. The quantity and quality of VPC's during continuous ambulatory ECG monitoring
    b. Congestive failure
    c. Level of cholesterol
    d. Angina of effort
    e. Angina of emotion
    f. Angina at rest

59. Physical findings which may accompany an episode of angina pectoris include:
    a. S3
    b. S4, if patient is in atrial fibrillation
    c. Tachycardia and hypertension
    d. Apical systolic murmurs of papillary dysfunction
    e. Fixed splitting of S2

60. The diagnosis of left ventricular failure in acute myocardial infarction is made by three of the following:
    a. S4 gallop
    b. Elevated jugular venous pressure
    c. Moist rales at lung bases
    d. Pathologic S3 (gallop)
    e. Chest X ray evidence

61-70. Match Column I with Column II (Answers in Column II may be used more than once or not at all.)

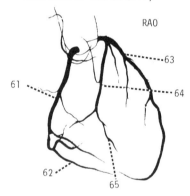
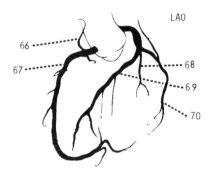

61. _____
62. _____
63. _____
64. _____
65. _____
66. _____
67. _____
68. _____
69. _____
70. _____

a. Right coronary
b. Left coronary
c. Circumflex
d. Posterior descending
e. Sinus node artery
f. Septal perforator
g. Diagonal
h. A-V node artery
i. Anterior descending
j. Obtuse marginal
k. Acute marginal

SELF-ASSESSMENT - PRACTICAL THERAPY, HYPERTENSION, ADVANCES IN DIAGNOSIS

Match the antianginal therapy in Column I with the appropriate answer in Column 2.

___ 1. Sublingual Nitroglycerin

___ 2. Oral long-acting nitrites

___ 3. Oral propranolol

___ 4. Vein bypass graft surgery

___ 5. Digitalis therapy

___ 6. Progressive exercise training

a. Increases coronary blood flow to areas of myocardial ischemia

b. May improve angina in patients with heart failure or atrial fibrillation

c. In the usual dose given, favorable effects on angina are equivalent to that of a placebo

d. Decreases myocardial oxygen demands by decreasing both systolic arterial pressure and left ventricular end-diastolic volume

e. Decreases heart rate, velocity of ventricular contraction and systolic blood pressure during exercise but is contraindicated in the presence of heart failure and bronchospasm

f. Decreases resting heart rate and myocardial oxygen demands at any given workload

7. Patients with rapid paroxysmal atrial fibrillation leading to acute pulmonary edema and shock should be treated with:
   a. Quinidine
   b. Digitalis
   c. Synchronized electrical D.C. cardioversion
   d. Propranalol

8. If drug therapy is the choice in atrial flutter, the first drug used should be:
   a. Quinidine
   b. Digitalis
   c. Procaine amide
   d. Edrophonium

9. In acute myocardial infarction, treatment of VPC's should be started with:

   a. An infusion of Lidocaine at 2 mg./ml.
   b. A rapid injection of 1 mg./Kg. of Lidocaine followed by an infusion of 2 mg./ml. Lidocaine
   c. A rapid injection of 1 mg./Kg. of Lidocaine

10. Usual side effects of Lidocaine are:

    a. Rash
    b. QRS prolongation
    c. Bradycardia
    d. PR prolongation
    e. Confusion or somnolence
    f. Convulsions

11. The treatment of paroxysmal atrial tachycardia is aimed at:

    a. Suppressing the ectopic focus
    b. Accelerating the sinus node
    c. Increasing vagal influence on the sinus node
    d. Blocking the re-entry cycle in the A-V junction

12. Therapy of chronic congestive heart failure should include restriction of activity. True or False

13. The loading dose of digoxin should be about three times the maintenance dose. True or False

14. The drug of choice and first drug to be used in the therapy of pulmonary edema is intravenous digoxin. True or False

15. Intravenous digoxin increases the work of the heart by increasing systemic blood pressure. True or False

16. A 16 year old female is admitted to the Emergency Room with a 24 hour history of sharp substernal chest pain increased with inspiration and by lying down flat. One hour ago she noted the sudden onset of rapid heart action. Her blood pressure was 120/80, her rate 180 and regular. The remainder of her examination was negative. Her ECG is shown below. Her chest X ray was normal. What is your diagnosis and treatment?

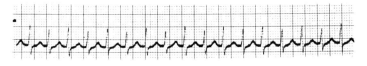

17. A 70 year old man is admitted to the Emergency Room complaining of shortness of breath and orthopnea of 2 weeks duration. He had a brief syncopal spell when he got up to go to the bathroom the night before. His blood pressure was 160/85. Rate 30. He had intermittent cannon "a" waves in his jugular venous pulse and crepitant rales in both bases. His ECG is shown below. His X ray showed congestive failure with small right pleural effusion.

    What is your diagnosis and treatment?

    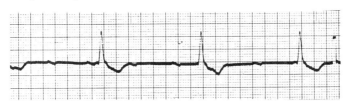

18. A 25 year old anxious female was admitted to the Emergency Room with complaints of palpitations of several days duration. Her examination was entirely normal. While her ECG was being taken, she stated, "That's it," and the tracing showed the arrhythmia demonstrated below:

    What is you diagnosis and treatment?

    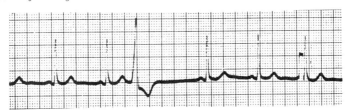

19. A 50 year old man is seen in the Emergency Room with severe chest pain. He was immediately monitored and his ECG showed changes consistent with acute anterolateral infarction. Morphine resulted in relief of pain and his vital signs and examination were normal. His monitor then showed the arrhythmia demonstrated below.

    What is your diagnosis and treatment?

    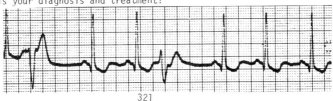

20. The same patient described above did well in the coronary care unit for several hours. The nurse was in his room talking with him at that time and she noted the monitor suddenly showed the following arrhythmia.

What is your diagnosis and treatment?

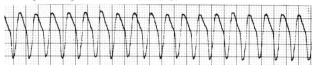

21. A 58 year old man is seen in the Emergency Room with a 2 hour history of shortness of breath. On examination his blood pressure was 150/100, rate 85. He had a third heart sound at the apex and scattered crepitant rales in the bases. His chest X ray showed mild central congestion. His ECG showed an acute anterior infarction. Lead V1 intermittently showed the pattern demonstrated below.

What is your diagnosis and treatment?

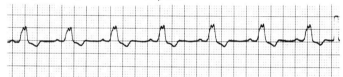

22. A 35 year old female with known rheumatic mitral regurgitation and a history of intermittent atrial fibrillation is admitted to the Emergency Room complaining of nausea of 3 days duration. One week ago she had an episode of rapid irregular heart action which she interpreted as atrial fibrillation. Knowing that her doctors in the past had increased her dose of digoxin when this occured, she took .75 mgm./day instead of the usual .25 mgm./day. Her examination was unremarkable but for a holosystolic grade 2/6 apical murmur. Her ECG rhythm strip (lead II) is shown below.

What is your diagnosis and treatment?

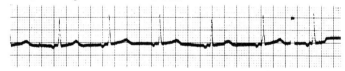

23. Which one of the following is the major determinant of the maintenance dose of digoxin:
    a. Total body weight
    b. Lean body mass
    c. Hepatic function
    d. Renal function
    e. Left ventricular mass

24. Which of the following is the most common precipitating cause of digitalis intoxication?
    a. Magnesium depletion
    b. Calcium administration
    c. Hypothyroidism
    d. Direct current cardioversion
    e. Potassium depletion

25. Which of the following conditions is not associated with an increased incidence of digitalis-induced arrhythmia:
    a. Hypokalemia
    b. Direct current cardioversion
    c. Hypoxemia
    d. Diphenylhydantoin therapy
    e. Hypercalcemia

26. Which of the following statements regarding oral digoxin therapy is incorrect:
    a. The daily excretion of digoxin occurs as a function of the drug present in the body
    b. The size of the loading dose plays little role in determining the tissue concentration during a steady state
    c. Initiation of digitalis therapy by a loading dose is necessary to achieve accumulation of digoxin
    d. Low cardiac concentrations of digoxin produce no effect on myocardial contractility
    e. Digoxin and its metabolic products are excreted completely in the urine

27. Which of the following statements concerning the use of the plasma digoxin radioimmunoassay in patients on digitalis therapy is correct:
    a. There is no overlap in serum digoxin levels between definitely toxic and definitely non-toxic patients on digoxin therapy
    b. The plasma digoxin level is a completely accurate reflection of the myocardial digoxin concentration
    c. Blood must be obtained a minimum of 6-8 hours after the last dose of digoxin for meaningful results
    d. The digoxin blood level rather than the ventricular response should be used for adjusting the dose schedule of digoxin in patients in atrial fibrillation
    e. In patients with electrolyte abnormalities or hypoxemia, the serum digoxin level is more sensitive than the electrocardiogram for diagnosing digitalis toxicity

28. Which of the following conditions is not an indication for the initiation of digitalis therapy?
   a. Paroxysmal atrial tachycardia
   b. Atrial fibrillation
   c. Atrial flutter
   d. Sinus tachycardia
   e. Congestive failure

29. The daily administration of which of the following diuretics is more likely to result in hypokalemic alkalosis, hypovolemia and secondary hyperaldosteronism:
   a. Spironolactone
   b. Triamterene
   c. Chlorothiazide
   d. Meralluride
   e. Furosemide

30. Which of the following diuretic agents inhibits secretion of potassium at the distal renal tubule:
   a. Furosemide
   b. Chlorothiazide
   c. Ethacrynic acid
   d. Meralluride
   e. Triamterene

31. The peak action of intravenous digoxin on myocardial contractility occurs at what period of time after its administration?
   a. 5-10 minutes
   b. 30 minutes
   c. 2-3 hours
   d. 4-6 hours
   e. 8-10 hours

32. The dangers of lidocaine toxicity following a single large intravenous bolus (1-2 mg/kg) would be greatest in which of the following clinical settings:
   a. Hepatic insufficiency
   b. Renal insufficiency
   c. Congestive heart failure
   d. Idiopathic epilepsy
   e. Concomitant propranolol therapy

33. Which of the following pairs of antiarrhythmic agents are most similar in their actions:
   a. Lidocaine - Procainamide
   b. Procainamide - Propranolol
   c. Propranolol - Diphenylhydantoin
   d. Diphenylhydantoin - Quinidine
   e. Quinidine - Procainamide

34. Which of the following modes of therapy would be most dangerous (and should be avoided) in a patient with atrial flutter with 2:1 AV block and a ventricular rate of 150/min.:
    a. Intravenous or oral digitalization
    b. Intravenous or oral procainamide
    c. Edrophonium infusion
    d. Phenylephrine infusion
    e. Propranolol

35. One of the actions of digitalis at the atrioventricular node is to decrease the refractory period. True or False

36. Since digitalis preparations increase the level of cardiac contractility in normal hearts, administration of these agents leads to an increase in cardiac output. True or False.

37. A 45 year old male enters the Emergency Room with a heart rate of 150 per minute. The following clinical clues would be of help in identifying which of these arrhythmias:

    A. Carotid sinus pressure
       1. Will abruptly stop
          a. atrial fibrillation
          b. paroxysmal atrial tachycardia
          c. atrial flutter
          d. ventricular tachycardia

       2. Will slow but not stop
          a. atrial fibrillation
          b. paroxysmal atrial tachycardia
          c. atrial flutter
          d. ventricular tachycardia
          e. sinus tachycardia

       3. Will not affect
          a. atrial fibrillation
          b. paroxysmal atrial tachycardia
          c. atrial flutter
          d. ventricular tachycardia
          e. sinus tachycardia

    B. Cannon waves in jugular venous pulse
       1. atrial fibrillation
       2. paroxysmal atrial tachycardia
       3. A-V junctional tachycardia
       4. atrial flutter
       5. ventricular tachycardia
       6. sinus tachycardia

    C. Heart sounds - varying intensity of first sound, third and fourth heart sounds coming and going
       1. atrial fibrillation
       2. paroxysmal atrial tachycardia
       3. atrial flutter
       4. ventricular tachycardia
       5. sinus tachycardia

38. Match the percentages for the expected frequency of various diagnoses among patients seen with hypertension in a medical center:
    a. essential hypertension   1. 4%
    b. pheochromocytoma   2. 0.5%
    c. renovascular hypertension   3. 90%
    d. chronic renal disease   4. 0.1%
    e. coarctation of the aorta   5. 5%

39. On funduscopic examination, what is the best evidence that hypertension has been present for several years:
    a. papilledema
    b. flame hemorrhages
    c. arteriovenous compression with complete separation of the vein
    d. soft exudates
    e. focal narrowing of arteriolar lumen

40. A 30 year old woman is found to have a blood pressure of 160/100. What medication might be implicated in the genesis of her hypertension?
    a. Dilantin
    b. Prednisone
    c. Valium
    d. Epinephrine-containing bronchodilators
    e. oral contraceptives

41. A 45 year old man is discovered to have a blood pressure of 150/100 in three separate clinic visits. He is asymptomatic and the physical examination is negative. Serum electrolytes, BUN, blood glucose, urinalysis, CBC and ECG are normal. The next step in the management of this patient should be:
    a. determination of plasma renin activity and aldosterone in a 24 hour urine
    b. determination of metanephrines and VMA in a 24 hour urine
    c. intravenous pyelogram
    d. renal arteriogram
    e. none of the above

42. A 31 year old attractive medical secretary is known to have had labile hypertension for the past five years. During the two months prior to her consultation she has been complaining of almost daily frontal headaches and on several occasions her blood pressure has been found to be around 180/120. On three separate clinic visits her blood pressure has been 180 to 200 systolic and 115 to 120 diastolic. On physical examination, she has arteriolar constriction in the eyegrounds, an increase in the aortic component of the second heart sound with an S_4, and a systolic bruit heard in the epigastrium, right flank and right costo-vertebral angle. Positive laboratory findings include a serum K of 3.1 mEq/L, chloride of 92 mEq and CO_2 of 32 mEq/L. An intravenous pyelogram was found to be normal. The next step in the management of this patient should be:

42. Continued
    a. start antihypertensive drug therapy
    b. determinations of plasma renin activity and aldosterone in a 24 hour urine to investigate for primary aldosteronism
    c. determination of a 24 hour urine for metanephrines and VMA
    d. determination of 17 ketosteroids in a 24 hour urine
    e. renal arteriogram

43. Patients with hypertension vary in the extent to which abnormalities of peripheral vascular resistance, cardiac output, intravascular volume, and the activation of the renin-angiotensin - aldosterone and sympathetic nervous system contribute to their elevated blood pressure. On this basis, please match the type of hypertension with the form of drug therapy which seems to be most rational:

    a. renovascular hypertension
    b. primary aldosteronism
    c. fixed hypertension
    d. volume-dependent chronic renal disease hypertension
    e. low-renin essential hypertension

    1. diuretic and salt restricted diet
    2. spironolactone
    3. proproanolol
    4. peripheral vasodilator
    5. loop diuretic

44. Match the drug with its most common and bothersome side effects. Use each answer only once:

    a. reserpine
    b. methyldopa
    c. guanethidine
    d. minoxidil
    e. propranolol

    1. palpitations
    2. congestive heart failure
    3. impotence and diarrhea
    4. drowsiness and fatigue
    5. mental depression

45. After three months of thiazide therapy in doses of 100 mg. daily of chlorthalidone, which is most likely to be found in a young patient with hypertension:
    a. fasting blood sugar of 200 mg%
    b. plasma potassium of 2.3 mEq/L
    c. serum sodium of 120 mEq/L
    d. serum uric acid of 7.5 mgs%
    e. serium calcium of 12 mgs%

46. Regarding adrenolytic agents, which of the following statements is not true:
    a. guanethidine decreases the cardiac output
    b. propranolol favors sodium retention
    c. methyldopa used alone may increase intravascular volume
    d. reserpine in doses of 0.2 mg. daily does not induce a decrease in cardiac output
    e. clonidine has a predominantly central nervous system effect

47. Please indicate whether the following statements are true or false:
    a. Hyperstat used intravenously increases the cardiac output
    b. Nitroprusside intravenously increases the cardiac output

47. Continued
   c. Aldomet used alone may increase blood volume
   d. the use of an oral diuretic for the treatment of chronic hypertension is associated with a decrease in plasma renin activity
   e. Propranolol decreases the level of plasma renin activity
   f. Hydralazine may induce palpitations
   g. lowering the blood pressure with minoxidil alone may induce palpitations and sodium retention
   h. Propranolol is not contraindicated in patients with bronchial asthma
   i. Lasix is far superior to hydrochlorothiazide as an antihypertensive drug in patients without renal failure
   j. Guanethidine is a frequent cause of palpitations

48. Which of the following statements is not true regarding antihypertensive drugs frequently used for the treatment of hypertensive crisis:
   a. Diazoxide (Hyperstat) is a direct vasodilator which increases the cardiac output by an indirect activation of the adrenergic nervous system
   b. Hydralazine given intravenously increases heart rate and cardiac output
   c. Trimethaphan (Arfonad) given intravenously decreases peripheral vascular resistance and cardiac output, but increases heart rate
   d. Sodium Nitroprusside is a direct vasodilator which increases heart rate and cardiac output when given intravenously
   e. Guanethidine should not be given intravenously for treatment of hypertensive crisis because it may initially have a hypertensive effect

49. A middle aged man who is known to have moderately severe hypertension and angina pectoris presents to the Emergency Room complaining of severe headache. On physical examination his blood pressure is found to be 234/146. The neurological examination is essentially within normal limits. In this clinical setting which antihypertensive agent is best to immediately drop the blood pressure without risk of precipitating an episode of angina pectoris:
   a. Diazoxide
   b. Hydralazine
   c. Aldomet (methyldopa)
   d. Nitroprusside
   e. Propranolol

50. Which of the following statements is true regarding the hemodynamic effects of antihypertensive drugs:
   a. Hydralazine intravenously does not increase the cardiac output
   b. Diazoxide given intravenously induces bradycardia
   c. Trimethaphan (Arfonad) is a pure sympatholytic agent
   d. Diazoxide produces increased sodium diuresis
   e. Nitroprusside is a potent direct vasodilator which does not increase cardiac output

51. A 42 year old man presents at the Emergency Room complaining of severe headache, blurred vision, somnolence and vomiting. He has a previous history of hypertension, but has not been taking any medication for the past six months. On physical examination, his blood pressure is 244/146, heart rate 92, and respirations 24. Eyegrounds demonstrate blurred discs and bilateral exudates with flame hemorrhages. Neurological examination showed mental obtundation but no signs of lateralization. Which of the following modalities would you request immediately:

 a. Furosemide (Lasix) intravenously and Guanethidine 75 mg. by mouth
 b. an intramuscular injection of 5 mg. of reserpine
 c. rapid injection of 300 mg. diazoxide (Hyperstat) while arterial pressure is carefully monitored
 d. start an infusion of 500 ml. of Dextrose 5% with 500 mg. of methyldopa (Aldomet) after giving 40 mg. of furosemide intravenously
 e. Propranolol intravenously first to reduce heart rate and then Diazoxide 300 mg. intravenously given rapidly.

52. Match the drugs in Group I with the items in Group II (more than one item in Group II may match with drugs in Group I)

Group I

1. Thiazide diuretics
2. Spironolactone & triamterene
3. Alpha-methyl dopa
4. Guanethidine
5. Propranolol
6. Diazoxide

Group II

 a. Positive Coomb's test
 b. The cornerstone of antihypertensive drug therapy
 c. More effective or specific in low renin hypertension
 d. More effective or specific in high renin hypertension
 e. K+ loser
 f. K+ sparer
 g. Hyperuricemia
 h. Use predominantly limited to acute hypertensive emergencies
 i. Side effects include orthostatic hypotension, diarrhea, and failure of ejaculation

53. An asymptomatic 60 year old white man is found to have a blood pressure of 170/105. The physical examination demonstrated a carotid bruit and a systolic bruit in the epigastrium. The electrocardiogram, chest X ray, urinalysis, biochemical profile and serum electrolytes were normal. The patient was started on a diuretic and reserpine, and the blood pressure was reduced to 130/80 without side effects. Please indicate which of the following statements are true or false regarding this patient.
 a. The reduction of his blood pressure should improve his life expectancy according to present information
 b. An elevation of the BUN from 15 to 25 mg., and of the serum creatinine from 1.2 to 1.6 mgs. is an indication to discontinue antihypertensive medication
(Continued next page)

53. Continued
    c. A triple renal scan and an intravenous pyelogram should have been obtained before instituting drug therapy
    d. The epigastric systolic bruit is compatible with renal artery stenosis
    e. The occurrence of nightmares and insomnia is a strong indication to modify the drug treatment

54. Hypertension is found in at least 50% of patients with which of the following diagnoses:
    a. Sudden death
    b. Angina
    c. Myocardial infarction
    d. Aortic aneurysms
    e. Strokes
    f. Renal failure
    g. Calcific aortic stenosis in the elderly

55. Left ventricular hypertrophy is found at necropsy in at least 50% of patients with which of the following diagnoses:
    a. Sudden death
    b. Angina
    c. Myocardial Infarction
    d. Aortic aneurysms
    e. Strokes
    f. Renal failure
    g. Calcific aortic stenosis in the elderly

56. Morbidity and mortality in hypertension are directly related to the level of systolic and diastolic blood pressures. True or False.

57. In the differential diagnosis of primary versus renovascular hypertension, which of the following would be more compatible with a diagnosis of renovascular hypertension:(more than one many be correct)
    a. Biochemical manifestation of secondary aldosteronism
    b. Black race
    c. Abdominal or flank bruit
    d. Left ventricular hypertrophy
    e. Hypertension of less than five years' duration

58. What is the single most important finding listed above favoring a diagnosis of renovascular hypertension?

59. What is the single most important finding listed above against a diagnosis of renovascular hypertension?

60. Which of the following are characteristic bedside findings in moderate hypertension:
    a. A displaced left ventricular impulse
    b. Midsystolic clicks due to papillary muscle dysfunction
    c. A pathologic fourth sound
    d. A short early systolic murmur at the upper right parasternal area
    e. A loud aortic second sound

61. Match column A with the best single response in column B.

    A - Disease State
    a. Pheochromocytoma
    b. Coarctation of the aorta
    c. Primary aldosteronism
    d. Cushing's disease
    e. Renovascular hypertension
    f. Malignant hypertension
    g. A-V fistula
    h. Polycystic kidneys

    B - Physical Finding
    1. Delayed femoral pulse
    2. Obesity
    3. Black race
    4. Tremor
    5. Muscle weakness
    6. Rapid rising arterial pulses
    7. Abdominal bruit
    8. Palpable irregular abdominal mass

62. The urographic signs of renovascular hypertension include:
    a. Delayed appearance of contrast
    b. Delayed disappearance of contrast
    c. Reduction in renal length
    d. All of the above

63. The simplest screening procedure for renovascular hypertension is:
    a. Conventional intravenous pyelography
    b. Nephrotomography
    c. Renal angiography
    d. Rapid sequence intravenous pyelography
    e. Plain film of the abdomen

64. A 55 year old male has had hypertension for 10 years with diastolic levels of 110 mm. Hg. He sees you as a patient complaining of nocturnal dyspnea. You decide to add a more potent antihypertensive agent to his program. This results in clinical improvement along with a standing diastolic pressure of 80, but his BUN increases from 20 to 60. The changes described are probably due to:
    a. Underlying nephrosclerosis with superimposed diminished renal perfusion due to the lowering of his blood pressure
    b. A toxic reaction to the drug you prescribed
    c. The natural history of his disease
    d. Otherwise undetected gastrointestinal bleeding

65. Which one of the following list of drugs should not be considered "essential" during cardiopulmonary resuscitation:
    a. Lidocaine
    b. Digitalis
    c. Calcium chloride
    d. Sodium bicarbonate
    e. Epinephrine

66. You are walking down the street when an elderly gentleman drops to the sidewalk.

    A. What is your first step in evaluating this man?
       1. Check the carotid for a pulse
       2. Apply precordial thump
       3. Give mouth to mouth resuscitation
       4. Begin external cardiac massage
    (Continued next page)

66. Continued
    B. Assuming you have determined that the patient has arrested, you should:
       1. Check the carotid for a pulse
       2. Apply precordial thump
       3. Give mouth to mouth resuscitation
       4. Begin external cardiac massage

    C. If the patient is not breathing, you should:
       1. Tilt the head to open the airway and give four quick full lung inflations
       2. Turn the head to the left to avoid vomiting and aspiration
       3. Place your fingers on the patient's tongue to avoid his swallowing it.

67. A 52 year old man has just been brought to the Emergency Room by the fire rescue squad with an IV with D5W hanging and O_2 being given at 5L/min. The patient had an episode of chest pain lasting 20 minutes, but now the pain has abated somewhat. You attach him to the monitor. He suddenly develops ventricular fibraillation.

    A. What is your first maneuver, and if no response, your second maneuver:
       1. Single precordial thump
       2. Xylocaine IV 50 mgm stat
       3. Xylocaine IV 75 mgm stat
       4. Intubation to avoid airway obstruction which is imminent in this situation
       5. Countershock

    B. The patient responds immediately by converting to sinus rhythm, but frequent premature ventricular contractions are noted on the monitor. You should:
       1. Institute a xylocaine drip after a bolus of 50 mgm of xylocaine I.V.
       2. Transport immediately to the CCU
       3. Begin Pronestyl p.o. 500 mgm q. 6h
       4. Begin IM Quinidine .3 gm. q. 3h for 4 doses
       5. Give Propranolol IV 5 mgm push

68. A 19 year old male is noted floating unconscious after diving into the shallow end of a pool. When you arrive at his side you note there are no spontaneous respirations. You should institute artificial respiration remembering to:

    a. Leave the head in a neutral position to avoid complicating a neck injury
    b. Leave the head in a tilt position to avoid complicating a neck injury
    c. Leave the head in a neutral position to avoid airway obstruction
    d. Leave the head in a tilt position to avoid airway obstruction

69. You are playing golf with your neighbor when he suddenly collapses to the ground. There is no one within calling distance. You feel for his carotid; there is no pulse. You must perform CPR alone until the group behind you catches up.

   A. In what ratio must artifical ventilation and artifical circulation be instituted:
      1. 15 external cardiac massages to 2 full lung inflations
      2. 5 external cardiac massages to 1 full lung inflation
      3. 2 external cardiac massages to 1 full lung inflation

   B. Help finally arrives. At what ratio should you then institute artifical respiration and artificial circulation?
      1. 15 external cardiac massages to 2 full lung inflations
      2. 5 external cardiac massages to 1 full lung inflation
      3. 2 external cardiac massages to 1 full lung inflation

70. The echocardiogram shows which of the following:
    a. Flail tricuspid leaflet
    b. Asymmetric septal hypertrophy
    c. Pericardial effusion
    d. Reduced a wave
    e. Abnormal posterior leaflet motion
    f. Mitral stenosis
    g. Mitral prolapse in late systole

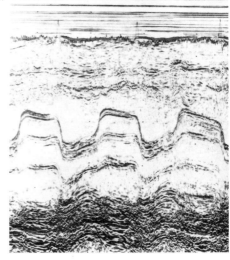

71. The echocardiogram came from a patient whose clinical findings likely include:
    a. BP 180/0
    b. Systolic clicks
    c. Mitral regurgitation
    d. Murmur longer sitting up
    e. S3 and S4
    f. LVH and "strain" on ECG
    g. Bifid carotid

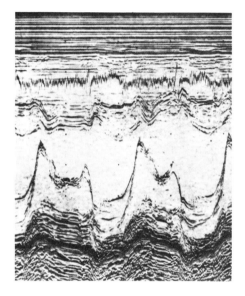

72. The echocardiogram came from a patient whose clinical findings likely include:
    a. Anginal pain
    b. Bifid carotid
    c. S3 and S4
    d. Systolic murmur
    e. Diastolic murmur
    f. Pathologic C-V waves in the JVP
    g. Midsystolic clicks

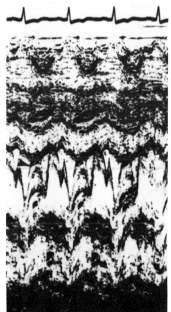

73. The echocardiogram shows which
    of the following:
    a. Pericardial effusion
    b. Asymmetric septal hypertrophy
    c. Mitral prolapse
    d. Mitral stenosis
    e. Flail tricuspid leaflet
    f. Acute aortic regurgitation
    g. None of the above

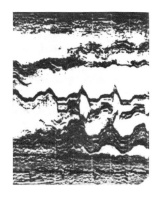

74.

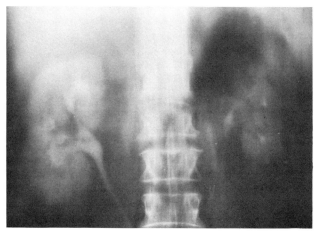

IVP from a patient with moderately severe hypertension. Which of the following is (are) correct:
a. The study is normal
b. The poor function, small size and irregular outline of the left kidney probably indicate that surgical intervention is unlikely to be beneficial.
c. The small size, contracted collecting system and irregular outline probably indicate the need for arteriography and surgery after differential renal vein renin assay.
d. The small size, contracted collecting system and irregular outline bilaterally, suggest arteriography will show parenchymal disease, so one may suggest a left nephrectomy

75.

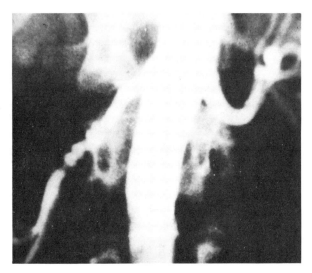

Renal arteriogram from a 40 year old female with moderately severe hypertension. Which of the following is (are) correct:
- a. A left flank bruit is likely
- b. Irregular obstructions and aneurysms of the right renal artery are consistent with atherosclerotic obstruction
- c. Irregular obstructions and aneurysms of the right renal artery are consistent with fibromuscular medial hyperplasia
- d. The arteriogram is normal
- e. The lesion is commonly familial

76. A "hot spot" scan of the myocardium:
- a. Shows concentration of radionuclide in an area of infarction after 2 weeks
- b. Commonly uses Technetium 99 pyrophosphate as the radionuclide
- c. Shows concentration of radionuclide in an area of acute ischemia-injury
- d. Shows false positive results in about 10% of cases
- e. Is commonly positive in the presence of ventricular aneurysm

77. A "cold spot" scan of the myocardium:
- a. Demonstrates a concentration of radionuclide in the area of ischemia-injury or of infarction
- b. Commonly utilizes Thalium 201
- c. Correlates well with angiography when injected into the patient during maximal physical stress
- d. Demonstrates a lack of concentration of radionuclide in the area of ischemia-injury or infarction
- e. Demonstrates a lack of concentration of radionuclide in an area of infarction, but not ischemia-injury

78. Abnormal regional left ventricular wall motion is best assessed by:
    a. A hot spot scan with Technetium 99 pyrophosphate
    b. A cold spot scan with Tahllium 201
    c. ECG gated scintiphotos
    d. None of the above
    e. a and c

79. Using cardiac scintigraphic techniques it is possible to obtain flow curves from which cardiac output and ventricular volumes can be calculated. True or False.

80. Shunt lesions cannot currently be detected by cardiac scintigraphy. True or False.

SELF-ASSESSMENT ANSWERS - BEDSIDE DIAGNOSIS

1. d
2. b
3. c
4. b
5. e
6. a,b,c,d,f
7. False
8. b,d
9. a,c
10. True
11. b,e
12. a,d
13. c,e
14. a,c,e,g,h
15. a,d,f,g
16. a,b,c,d,e,f,g
17. b,c,d,e,h
18. a,d,e,h
19. b,e,g
20. e
21. d
22. a
23. b
24. c
25. False
26. False
27. c
28. True
29. False
30. True
31. a
32. True
33. 1-a,b,c,d; 2-c
34. a,b,c,
35. d
36. b
37. a
38. f
39. c
40. c
41. d
42. a
43. b
44. a,c,d
45. b,c,d,e
46. a,f,
47. a,b,f
48. c
49. False
50. True
51. True
52. False
53. f
54. a
55. a,b
56. a,c
57. a,b,c
58. b
59. d
60. False
61. d
62. a,c
63. d
64. b,c
65. c
66. a
67. b
68. b
69. a,b,d,e,g,h,k,u,v, x,z,b',c',d'
70. c,f,h,i,j,k,l,n,o,p, q,r,x,y,z
71. a,b,d,e,g,h,k,m,t,u,w,x,a',c'
72. c,f,h,i,k,l,n,r,s,t,x,y
73. b,e
74. c,d
75. a,d

SELF-ASSESSMENT ANSWERS - ECG CORE CURRICULUM

1. Left axis deviation due to left anterior hemiblock
2. Left axis deviation due to inferior wall myocardial infarction
3. Left axis deviation due to inferior wall myocardial infarction and left anterior hemiblock
4. Left ventricular hypertrophy with "strain" (systolic or pressure loaded ventricle in a patient with aortic stenosis)
5. Right ventricular hypertrophy with biatrial enlargement and right axis deviation (patient with severe mitral stenosis)
6. Left ventricular hypertrophy with left atrial enlargement, left axis deviation, 1st degree heart block, upright "t" waves (diastolic or volume overloaded ventricle in a patient with aortic regurgitation)
7. Right ventricular hypertrophy with right atrial enlargement and right axis deviation (systolic or pressure overloaded ventricle in a patient with pulmonary stenosis)
8. Right ventricular enlargement and right axis deviation with an rSR' in the right precordial leads (diastolic or volume overloading of the right ventricle in a patient with atrial septal defect)
9. A. Early J point and ST depression and peaked T waves of subendocardial ischemia and injury
   B. Rapid evolution to full blown pattern of extensive acute transmural anterior myocardial infarction with Q waves, ST elevation and T wave inversion in 1, AVL and precordial leads
10. Acute anterior infarction with Q waves and marked ST elevation in precordial leads as well as 1 and AVL.
11. Acute inferior infarction with injury pattern of marked ST elevation in II, III and AVF, and reciprocal changes in the anterior leads.
12. Inferior wall infarction, stable pattern, with Q waves, ST elevation and T inversion in 2, 3 and AVF.
13. Inferoposterior myocardial infarction with Q waves in 2, 3 and AVF, and tall R wave in V1.
14. Acute inferior wall infarction with reciprocal changes in the anterior wall leads.
15. The ECG is consistent with an anterior wall myocardial infarction, possibly acute, but age indeterminate. This 60 year old patient came to the emergency room with a history of "flu" for one week with cough, mild temperature elevation, and ill-defined muscular aching, including chest wall soreness. On examination, he had a sustained anterior chest wall movement between (Continued next page)

15. (Continued)

the left parasternal edge and apex. Because of this, and especially a past history of infarction, the ECG was obtained. The emergency room physician asked for the patient's old ECG from the Heart Station, taken three years previously and shown below. The persistence of ST-T changes in the anterior wall leads, findings on chest wall examination, and negative current cardiac history make the diagnosis: Ventricular aneurysm, asymptomatic (in a patient who now has the "flu.")

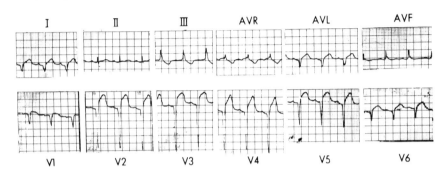

16. Atrial fibrillation. Acute anterior wall subendocardial ischemia-injury or infarction.

17. Sinus tachycardia. The rate is 130, but the P and QRS are otherwise normal.

18. APC's occur on the fourth and last beat. These beats are early and their P waves have a different configuration than the normal beats, while the QRS is the same as the normal beats.

19. Atrial flutter with 4:1 block. Typical "saw tooth" flutter waves are seen at a rate of 320, while the ventricular rate is 80. This patient has received digitalis. (Most untreated flutter has a 2:1 block.)

20. Atrial fibrillation with rapid ventricular response of about 150. There are no clearly identifiable P waves, the QRS is narrow, and the ventricular response is entirely irregular.

21. Wenckebach (Mobitz I) type of second degree heart block. There is progressive lengthening of the P-R interval on the first 2 beats, and the third P wave is not conducted (a beat is "dropped"). The cycle then recurs.

22. Frequent VPC's which are unifocal and occur every third beat (trigeminy). The VPC's are different than the patient's sinus beats and there is a full compensatory pause before the next sinus beat. These are reentry (not parasystolic) VPC's, as they show a fixed coupling interval from the previous sinus beat.

23. Couplet of VPC's.

24. VPC falling on the sinus "t" wave. This is dangerously near the vulnerable period and this pattern can deteriorate into ventricular fibrillation.

25. Blocked atrial premature contraction. The third P wave falls on the preceding "t" wave, changing the "t" wave configuration. The junction is still refractory and hence the P wave is non-conducted.

26. Junctional premature contraction. The P wave of the fifth beat is inverted, and the P-R interval short (so-called high nodal premature).

27. APC's. The second and last beats are early, and their P waves are different in configuration than the sinus beats. The fifth beat is an APC with aberrant conduction. Its P wave is the same as the other APC's, there is no full compensatory pause until the next sinus beat, and the initial forces of the beat are the same as the sinus beats. (Look carefully!)

28. 1st degree heart block. The P-R interval is .30.

29. 2nd degree heart block - Mobitz type II. Every other P wave fails to activate the ventricle. There is also an intraventricular conduction abnormality.

30. Junctional rhythm. No P waves are seen. They are "buried" in the QRS. The inherent junctional rate is 56.

31. Atrial fibrillation with slow ventricular response. Fibrillation waves are present.

32. Atrial flutter with 2:1 block (atrial rate 350, ventricular rate 175). This arrhythmia responds very well to electrical cardioversion at very low watt-seconds.

33. Atrial premature contractions with aberrant conduction.

34. Blocked APC with junctional escape

35. Unifocal VPC's.

36. Multifocal VPC's.

37. Early VPC falling in vulnerable period of patient's "t" wave, then couplet of VPC's and finally, at the end of the strip, ventricular tachycardia.

38. Wenckebach type of second degree heart block (progressive prolongation of P-R interval until a ventricular response is dropped).

39. Mobitz type II second degree heart block (unchanging P-R interval with drop of ventricular response).

40. Third degree or complete heart block (no relationship between P waves and QRS's).

41. Lead 2 clearly shows the basic rhythm is atrial fibrillation. The two episodes showing wide QRS complexes both start and end with QRS complexes intermediate in form between the small and wide QRS complexes present. Apart from these fusion beats two other points make a ventricular origin of the wide QRS complexes likely:
    a. The first episode showing wide QRS complexes starts after a relatively long interval, making aberrant conduction unlikely.
    b. The R-R intervals during the episodes of wide QRS complexes are quite regular.
    An additional but less specific argument for a ventricular origin of the wide QRS complexes is their left bundle branch block configuration.

42. False
43. c
44. True
45. False
46. a
47. c
48. b
49. b,c
50. True
51. b,c,e
52. d
53. a,b,c,d
54. False
55. False
56. False
57. False
58. I. A,C; II. B,D; III. E
59. False
60. a
61. b
62. a
63. b, e
64. a
65. True
66. b
67. c
68. d
69. c
70. c

SELF-ASSESSMENT ANSWERS - ADVANCES IN ELECTROCARDIOGRAPHY

1. b
2. a
3. a
4. True
5. False
6. a
7. True
8. False
9. e
10. a
11. b
12. True
13. False
14. True
15. True
16. True
17. e
18. a
19. a
20. d
21. e
22. Immediately post exercise the tracing demonstrates upsloping ST depression. This is not considered a positive response.
3 minutes post exercise the tracing demonstrates 3 mm. of horizontal ST depression (compared to the control showing 1 mm. ST depression). However, since the patient was taking digoxin, this may be a false positive result. The test should be repeated after the patient is off of digoxin for at least 5 days.
23. Positive. There is marked horizontal ST depression. Even though the baseline control tracing shows some ST depression, there is at least 3 mm. more at stage 1/2 at a heart rate of 120. The significance of this degree of ST depression is highlighted by its occurrence at a relatively low heart rate and light work load.
24. The stress test is negative. The occurrence of VPC's induced by exercise does not necessarily indicate underlying heart disease. It is more common in patients with coronary disease, but occurs in normals with increasing frequency with advancing age.
25. d, e
26. 1. b,c,d,e,f
    2. c,e,g,i
    3. a,d,e,h
27. e
28. c
29. b
30. False
31. False
32. False
33. True
34. True
35. a,b,e,f

SELF-ASSESSMENT ANSWERS - CORONARY ARTERY DISEASE

HOW DO YOU TREAT THIS CASE?

Case 1

The patients first electrocardiogram revealed a recent inferior wall myocardial infarction. Although the tracing recorded a few hours later appeared normal, the patient was treated as an acute myocardial infarction. The second tracing six hours later, and subsequent daily electrocardiograms, showed the typical evolution of a recent inferior wall myocardial infarction. When the patient developed signs of acute left ventricular failure (S3 and rales), 20 mg. of intravenous furosemide (Lasix) was given. Over the next two hours, the patient diuresed 750 cc. of urine, and the S3 and rales disappeared. Rapidly acting diuretics are the treatment of first choice for moderate left ventricular failure in the setting of acute myocardial infarction.

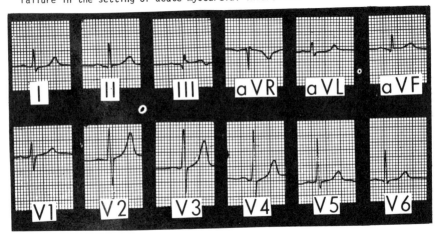

Case 2

The patient's ECG during pain showed striking acute ischemia-injury with resolution between episodes. These observations are consistent with the Prinzmetal variant of angina. Due to his relative youth, good ventricular function clinically and recurrent angina without infarction refractory to medical therapy with beta blocking agents and vasodilators, he underwent coronary angiography. An isolated 90% left anterior descending proximal lesion was found with good "runoff" beyond the obstruction and normal ventricular function. He underwent immediate bypass surgery from the internal mammary to the LAD just beyond the obstruction. His post-operative course was uneventful and he has been pain free and active for the last two years since surgery.

HOW DO YOU TREAT THIS CASE? - ANSWERS

Case 3

The patient is not tolerating the atrial fibrillation and the rapid ventricular rate, as evidenced by progressive clinical deterioration. This, plus the apparent fall in blood pressure and loss of atrial contribution, calls for therapy which will promptly slow the ventricular rate and convert the rhythm to sinus.

The beta-blocking agents given cautiously IV have been found effective in this clinical setting. (Digoxin IV could be given, but is relatively slow-acting in this urgent setting.)

Propranolol was given to this patient at a rate of 0.5 mg. every 2 minutes. The ventricular rate fell to 120/min. and following 4.5 mg. of the drug, sinus rhythm was restored at 98/min. The patient then responded satisfactorily to IV diuretics with subsequent cardiac compensation.

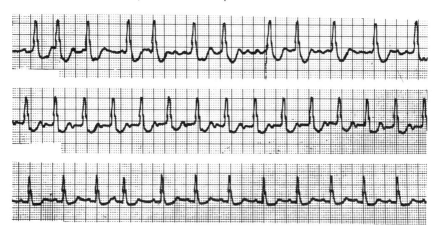

Case 4

The patient's rhythm strip shows PAT with 2:1 block (atrial rate 180, ventricular rate 90), a classic digitalis induced arrhythmia. Her serum potassium was 3.2 (normal 3.5 to 5.0). She was treated with IV KCl and in 45 minutes she converted to normal sinus rhythm as shown below. A serum digoxin level was also drawn and became available the next day. It was 1.8 ng/ml. While this level is not per se "toxic," it was "toxic" for this patient in view of her hypokalemia which potentiated the effect of her digoxin.

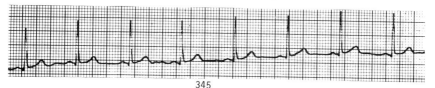

HOW DO YOU TREAT THIS CASE - ANSWERS

Case 5

The ECG shows an early VPC falling dangerously close to the vulnerable period of the patient's "t" wave. This is an indication for IV Xylocaine, as such beats may cause more serious ventricular arrhythmias (V.T. or V.F). Xylocaine 50 mg. was given IV push stat and the patient subsequently remained in sinus rhythm.

Case 6

The patient was given atropine. This increased the sinus rate and the ventricular tachycardia disappeared completely.

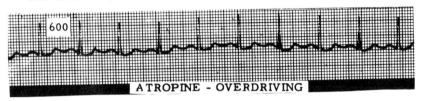

Case 7

The ECG shows Wenckebach type of second degree heart block with progressive P-R prolongation until a ventricular response is "dropped." This is a fairly typical arrhythmia in inferior wall infarction and is often self-limited. However, appropriate treatment was given with atropine, reducing vagal tone and resulting in first degree heart block with ventricular capture related to each P wave as shown below. In the second strip, there is further reduction in the P-R interval to normal sinus rhythm.

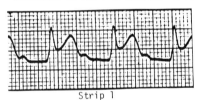 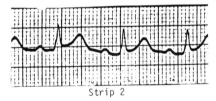

Strip 1   Strip 2

Case 8

The ECG shows an acute anterior wall myocardial infarction. Possibly more important, the patient has developed a right bundle branch block and the axis has shifted to the left. You properly interpret this as acute bifascicular block with involvement of the right bundle, and the anterior-superior division of the left bundle. This implies extensive anterior infarction with diffuse tissue necrosis. You appropriately place a tranvenous pacemaker to have available should the patient progress to complete heart block, which is often preceded by the fascicular blocks described.

SELF-ASSESSMENT ANSWERS - CORONARY ARTERY DISEASE

1. d
2. e
3. False
4. False
5. c
6. b
7. c
8. e
9. b
10. False
11. True
12. False
13. False
14. True
15. False
16. True
17. b
18. f
19. d
20. A-2, B-2, C-2
21. A-1, B-3, C-1
22. False
23. False
24. False
25. a,d
26. c
27. b
28. a,b
29. b,d.
30. e
31. True
32. True
33. False
34. True
35. True
36. a,b,e,f
37. False
38. a,d
39. a,c
40. False
41. True
42. True
43. True
44. c
45. d
46. d
47. e
48. a
49. b
50. d
51. e
52. a
53. b,c
54. c
55. True
56. a-2, b-5, c-3, d-1, e-4
57. True
58. a,b,f
59. a,c,d
60. c,d,e
61. a
62. d
63. i
64. c
65. j
66. e
67. a
68. g
69. i
70. c

SELF-ASSESSMENT ANSWERS - PRACTICAL THERAPY, HYPERTENSION, ADVANCES IN DIAGNOSIS

1. d
2. c
3. e
4. a
5. b
6. f
7. c
8. b
9. b
10. e,f
11. d
12. True
13. True
14. False
15. True

16. The patient's history is typical of pericarditis. Her ECG shows a supraventricular tachyarrhythmia (atrial or junctional). Note also slight electrical alternans as may be seen in pericardial disease. Carotid pressure was applied without change. She was then given Lanoxin .5 mgm. IV, and in 30 minutes carotid pressure resulted in return to sinus mechanism. She was given ASA gr. X q.i.d. and Lanoxin .25 mg.q.d. When seen one week later she was asymptomatic. All medicine was stopped and she did well subsequently.

17. The patient's left ventricular failure and syncope are explained by his ECG which shows complete (3rd degree) heart block. The cannon waves in his jugular venous pulse are due to the atrium intermittently contracting against a closed tricuspid valve. The patient was treated with a temporary transvenous pacemaker and was admitted to the coronary care unit for monitoring. With this treatment alone, he diuresed 5 pounds in two days, felt well and his lungs became clear. A permanent transvenous right ventricular pacemaker was then placed and he did well subsequently.

18. The ECG shows an isolated VPC. The patient was reassured and advised to stop drinking 5 cups of coffee per day as was her usual habit. When seen ten days later, she was asymptomatic and in normal sinus rhythm.

19. The patient's ECG shows multifocal VPC's. In the setting of acute infarction this can deteriorate into more serious ventricular arrhythmias (VT or VF). He was given 50 mgm. of Xylocaine IV push stat, and he remained in sinus rhythm and was transferred to the coronary care unit.

20. The arrhythmia is ventricular tachycardia. A quick chest "thump" resulted in a return to sinus rhythm. Because of his recurrent problems with ventricular arrhythmia, the patient was given a bolus (Continued next page)

20. Continued

of Xylocaine IV 50 mgm. to achieve an immediate therapeutic blood level, and then started on a continuous drip of Xylocaine at 2 mgm./ml/min. He remained in sinus rhythm and was weaned off the drip the next day.

21. The patient has a likely extensive anterior infarction as reflected in his congestive failure with a third heart sound and rales. In addition, the development of right bundle branch block on his ECG is consistent with diffuse anterior wall damage involving the trifascicular system. The fact that pain was not a primary presenting symptom should not change your impression. He was treated with a temporary transvenous right ventricular demand pacemaker, as these patients may go to complete heart block. He was given 40 mgm. of IV furosemide (Lasix) with little improvement. A Swan-Ganz catheter was placed and showed a pulmonary artery mean pressure of 18 mm. Hg. Additional IV Lasix was given. Over the next 6 hours his lungs cleared, the S3 disappeared and he became less short of breath. In several days the pacemaker was discontinued and he slowly improved.

22. The patient has a junctional rhythm with a short P-R interval and negative P waves in lead II, undoubtedly due to digitalis excess. She was instructed to stop digoxin and see her doctor in 48 hours. A digoxin level was drawn and came back elevated at 3.5 ng./ml. The next day when she went to her doctor and her tracing demonstrated sinus bradycardia, he told her to continue withholding digoxin for 48 hours and return. At that time she was in sinus rhythm, her digoxin level was 1.0, and her nausea was gone. She was placed on maintenance digoxin .25 mgm/day and admonished not to manipulate her own medicine in the future.

23. d
24. e
25. d
26. c
27. c
28. d
29. e
30. e
31. d
32. c
33. e
34. b
35. False
36. False
37. A1-b; A2-a,c,e; A3-d; B-3,5; C-4
38. a-3, b-4, c-1, d-5, e-2
39. c
40. b,e
41. e
42. e
43. a-3, b-2, c-4, d-5, e-1
44. a-5, b-4, c-3, d-1, e-2

45. d
46. b
47. a - True
    b - False
    c - True
    d - False
    e - True
    f - True
    g - True
    h - False
    i - False
    j - False
48. d
49. d
50. e
51. c
52. 1 - b,e,g
    2 - c,f
    3 - a, ±i
    4 - i
    5 - d
    6 - h
53. a - True
    b - False
    c - False
    d - True
    e - True

54. All
55. All
56. True
57. a,c,e
58. c
59. b
60. c,d,e
61. a-4, b-1, c-5
    d-2, e-7, f-3
    g-6, h-8
62. d
63. d
64. a
65. b
66. A-1, B-2, C-1
67. A-1,5; B-1
68. a
69. A-1, B-2
70. d,e,f
71. b,c,d
72. a,b,c,d
73. a
74. c
75. c,e
76. b,c,d,e
77. b,c,d
78. c
79. True
80. False